Cancer Is Not a Disease

Also by Andreas Moritz

• • •

The Amazing Liver and Gallbladder Flush

Timeless Secrets of Health & Rejuvenation

Lifting the Veil of Duality

Vaccine-nation

It's Time to Come Alive

Feel Great, Lose Weight

Simple Steps to Total Health

Heart Disease – No More!

Diabetes – No More!

Alzheimer's – No More!

Ending The AIDS Myth

Heal Yourself with Sunlight

Hear The Whispers, Live Your Dream

Art of Self-Healing

Timeless Wisdom from Andreas Moritz

All of the above are available at www.ener-chi.com, www.amazon.com
and other online booksellers, as well as brick-and-mortar bookstores.

Cancer
Is Not
a Disease

It's a Healing Mechanism

Discover Cancer's Hidden Purpose,
Heal Its Root Causes
and Be Healthier Than Ever!

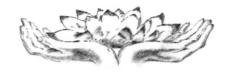

Your Health is in Your Hands

Ener-Chi 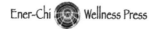 Wellness Press

For Reasons of Legality

The author of this book, Andreas Moritz, does not advocate the use of any particular form of healthcare but believes that the facts, figures and knowledge presented herein should be available to every person concerned with improving his or her state of health. Although the author has attempted to give a profound understanding of the topics discussed and to ensure accuracy and completeness of any information that originates from any other source than his own, he and the publisher assume no responsibility for errors, inaccuracies, omissions, or any inconsistency herein. Any slights of people or organizations are unintentional. This book is not intended to replace the advice and treatment of a physician who specializes in the treatment of diseases. Any use of the information set forth herein is entirely at the reader's discretion. The author and publisher are not responsible for any adverse effects or consequences resulting from the use of any of the preparations or procedures described in this book. The statements made herein are for educational and theoretical purposes only and are mainly based on Andreas Moritz's own opinion and theories. You should always consult with a healthcare practitioner before taking any dietary, nutritional, herbal, or homeopathic supplement, or before beginning or stopping any therapy. The author is not intending to provide any medical advice or offer a substitute thereof, and makes no warranty whatsoever, whether expressed or implied, with respect to any product, device, or therapy. Except as otherwise noted, no statement in this book has been reviewed or approved by the United States Food and Drug Administration or the Federal Trade Commission. Readers should use their own judgment or consult a holistic medical expert or their personal physicians for specific applications to their individual problems.

ISBN-10: 978-0-9892587-4-6
ISBN-13: 978-0-9892587-5-3

Published by Ener-Chi Wellness Press—ener-chi.com, USA
Printed by Ingram/Lightning Source Inc.

First edition, Cancer is Not a Disease, October 2005
Second edition, Cancer is Not a Disease, August 2008
Third edition (minor changes), Cancer is Not a Disease, February 2009
Fourth edition (major changes/additions and new title), Cancer Is Not a Disease – It's a Healing Mechanism, December 2016

Cover Design and Artwork by Andreas Moritz

The picture on the cover is part of *Ener-Chi Art* (See http://www.ener-chi.com), designed to restore balanced Chi flow in all organs and systems of the body. This particular picture is designed to maintain proper Chi presence in the circulatory system/small intestines, an essential prerequisite for healing any cancer in the body.

Editor's Note

At the time of finalizing this updated and greatly-expanded edition, the author had included published academic research as well as information sought from online sources (until 2012) to corroborate his statements, all of which have been carefully presented in the *References, Links and Resources* section. A few links that the author had saved have since expired and are therefore not included. Regarding the Dedication, he specifically wished that this remain unchanged as written in 2009; and so it is.

In Gratitude

Andreas' wisdom and breakthrough insights surrounding natural health and wellness – body, mind and spirit – are a rare gift and blessing to us all. Time-honored, they continue to enrich our lives by expanding our thinking, opening our hearts, and guiding us in new, often unexpected directions. Decades of his dedicated work have impacted the well-being of thousands of lives in countless ways and, gratefully, continue to touch us profoundly.

In essence, Andreas is always with us – through the brilliance of his knowledge, experience and writing, his beautiful healing art, his heart-centered, inspiring messages and all the information that he so generously shared, in order to help us live healthier, happier and more fulfilling lives. His deep spiritual awareness and compassion, combined with a thorough understanding of the human body, have inspired people around the world to lead more vital, uplifting and balanced lives.

May Andreas' deep knowledge and compassionate guidance continue to provide comfort and warmth, wrapped in timeless support and healing from the heart.

The Ener-Chi family and Ener-Chi Wellness Center extend our loving gratitude to you.

Dedication

I dedicate this book to those who trust in
the body's wisdom
and intelligence to heal itself

who wish to work with the body,
not against it

who blame nobody for their illness
or misfortune, including themselves

who perceive everything that happens to them as useful,
regardless of how threatening or painful
it initially may appear to be

who never doubt their body's innate ability to heal.

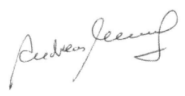

Table of Contents

Introduction

What you are about to read may rock, even dismantle, the very foundation of your beliefs about your body, health and healing. The title, *Cancer Is Not a Disease*, may be unsettling for many, provocative to some, but encouraging for all. This book can help you achieve a profoundly life-changing revelation if you are sufficiently receptive to the possibility that cancer is not an actual disease. If truth be told, you may indeed arrive at the conclusion that cancer must be an elaborate and final attempt by the body to heal itself and stay alive for as long as circumstances permit; circumstances that, as you will discover, are most likely in your control.

It will perhaps astound you to learn that if you are afflicted with any of the root causes of cancer (which constitute the real illness), you would most likely die quickly unless your body actually grew cancer cells. In this work, I provide the logic and understanding that cancer is a healing process that we ought to support, not suppress or fight. I further submit evidence that this rather unorthodox approach to healing cancer is far more effective than the methods that involve destroying it.

I further claim that cancer – one of the body's most sophisticated healing mechanisms – will only kick in after one or both of the following, rarely suspected, preconditions have been met:

1. **The body's main waste removal and detoxification systems have been rendered inefficient**
2. **A major psycho-emotional stress situation has been resolved or is no longer relevant in the person's life**

These two main contributing reasons for developing cancer require an in-depth explanation, and I will elaborate on that through the course of this book. Whereas the first precondition may sound reasonable to those who are familiar with the toxin-cancer connection, the second one will not make sense to you right away, but I promise it will as you read on.

For now I wish to point out that a stress-induced cancer never shows up *during* an actual stress-event, but occurs *after* such a situation has reached some kind of resolution or completion. Stress-events may include being without work for some time, going through a painful divorce, an ongoing severe sickness of a loved one that may lead to their death, being emotionally or physically abused, suffering a traumatic accident, losing one's home or possessions, etc. If cancer truly is a healing mechanism, as I claim it to be, then it makes sense for healing symptoms, such as tumor growth, to occur *after* and not *during* a psycho-emotional crisis or conflict.

There is evidence that this mechanism is not only at work in cancer development, but also in most other health conditions. While the two reasons often coincide (occurring at the same time), they don't have to.

In extreme circumstances, exposure to large amounts of cancer-producing agents (carcinogens) can bring about a collapse of the body's defenses within several weeks or months. This may subsequently require a rapid and aggressive growth of a cancerous tumor to deal with the assault. By and large, though, it takes a lot longer for so-called malignant tumors to form and become diagnostically noticeable.

Unfortunately, basic misconceptions or complete lack of awareness about the true reasons behind malignant tumor growth have turned *abnormal* cells into vicious monsters that discriminately attempt to kill us, perhaps in retaliation for our sins or for abusing the body. However, as you are about to find out, cancer is on our side, not against us. It is also not a senseless, accidental occurrence.

Unless we change our perception of what cancer really is, it will most likely resist treatment, particularly the most *advanced* and commonly used medical methods. If you have cancer, and cancer is indeed part of the body's complex survival responses and not a disease, you must find answers to the following important questions:

- What reasons coerce your body into developing cancer cells?
- Once you have identified these reasons, how will they help you heal your body?
- What determines the type and severity of cancer with which you are afflicted?
- If cancer is indeed a healing mechanism, what will you need to do to avoid having the body employ such extreme measures of self-preservation, now and in the future?

- Since the body's original genetic design always favors the continuance of life and protection against adversities of any kind, how then could the body possibly permit a genetic change to occur that leads to its demise?
- Why do so many cancers disappear by themselves, without any medical intervention?
- Do radiation, chemotherapy and surgery actually cure cancer in some people, or do cancer patients heal themselves, in spite of these radical treatments loaded with side effects?
- What roles do fear, frustration, low self-worth and repressed anger play in the origination and outcome of cancer?
- Why do so many children now develop brain tumors or leukemia?
- What is the spiritual growth implication of cancer, if any?

To heal the root causes of cancer, you ought to find satisfying and practical answers to the above questions. You will uncover them as you continue to read through the pages of this book. Whenever you find an answer, you will get an undeniable feeling of confidence and inner knowing of the truth, coupled with relief and even euphoria.

If you feel the inner urge to make sense of this life-changing event (the cancer), you will greatly benefit from continuing to read on. Cancer can be your greatest opportunity to help restore balance to all aspects of your life, but it can also be the harbinger of severe trauma and suffering if you perceive it as a threat to your life. Either way, you will discover that you are always in control. You may not be able to change a particular situation such as a cancer diagnosis, but you are most certainly in control of your response to it. Your response is the ultimate determinant of whether you become whole again, or remain fragmented in the perception of being a victim of a terrible disease.

To live in a human body, you must have access to a certain amount of life-sustaining energy. You may either use this inherent energy for nourishing and healing the body, or waste it on fighting a battle against a disease that medical theory believes is out to kill you. The choice is ultimately yours.

In case you consciously or unconsciously choose to neglect your body (or go into battle against it) instead of giving it loving attention and self-respect, it will likely end up having to fight for its life. Ultimately, the main issue in question is not whether you have cancer, but how you perceive it and what you are going to do about it.

Cancer is only *one* of the many possible ways the body forces you to alter the way you see and treat yourself, including your physical body. You may either make out cancer to be something dreadful that leaves you victimized and powerless, or see it as an opportunity to stand up for yourself, your values and your self-respect. This inevitably brings up the subject of spiritual health, which I believe plays at least as important a role in cancer as physical and emotional reasons do.

Cancer appears to be a highly confusing and unpredictable disorder. It seems to strike the very happy and the very sad, the rich and the poor, the smokers and the non-smokers, the very healthy and the not-so-healthy. And although cancer occurrence among children used to be extremely rare, it is not rare anymore.

People from all backgrounds and occupations can have cancer. However, if you dare look behind the mask of its physical symptoms, such as the type, appearance and behavior of a cancerous tumor, you will find that cancer is not as coincidental or unpredictable as it seems to be.

What makes 50 percent of the American population so prone to developing cancer, when the other half has no risk at all? Blaming the genes for that is but an excuse to cover up ignorance of the real causes, or lure people afflicted with cancer into costly treatment and prevention programs.

Later in the book, I will discuss the most recent research done on possible genetic inheritance factors in relation to cancers of the breast, lungs and many other parts of the body. You will be astounded to know that genes have little, if anything, to do when members from several generations of the same family develop the same types of cancer. In fact, top genetic researchers now affirm that gene-behavior is ultimately determined by the way we eat, think, emote and live our lives. Genes don't just accidently malfunction in us one day, make us sick, and then cause the same disease in our children and grandchildren. In fact, new research completely contradicts the long-held belief that gene mutation can cause or spread cancer.

Cancer has always been an extremely rare illness, except in industrialized nations during the past 50–60 years. However, human genes have not significantly changed for thousands of years. Why would they change so drastically now, and suddenly decide to attack and destroy the bodies of nearly half of the population? The answer to this question, which I will further elaborate on in this book, is amazingly simple: Although genes may be undergoing mutation for reasons discussed later, even if they became damaged or faulty, they still would not be able to kill anyone.

It is important to know that cancer rarely causes someone to die, although it is undeniable that many people afflicted with cancer also do die. Nonetheless, unless a tumor causes a major mechanical obstruction in a vital organ, or severely impedes the blood flow to it or the lymph drainage from it, a cancer patient is much more likely to die from the reasons that lead to cell mutation and tumor growth than from the cancer itself.

Every cancer therapy should be focused on the root causes of cancer, yet most oncologists typically ignore them. For example, a diet consisting of junk foods, that are usually deprived of any nutritional value and real energy, causes chaotic, traumatic conditions in the body that are identical to those experienced during physical starvation. In this book, I will elaborate on how such a process of self-destruction is bound to require a major healing response on behalf of the body.

It is becoming increasingly evident that almost all cancers are preceded by some kind of traumatic event in the past, such as a divorce, the death of a loved one, an accident, the loss of a job or possessions, an ongoing conflict with a boss or relative, severe national disaster, or exposure to powerful toxins. The body has no other choice than to respond to such profound stress factors with predictable biological survival or coping mechanisms that may involve temporary *abnormal* cell growth. Although most doctors still agree with the theory that the resulting tumor is a disease, and not a healing mechanism, it doesn't mean it is true.

Cancerous tumors are merely symptoms of disease that are caused by something else that may not be obvious at first. It is clear, though, that they don't just pop up for no reason. For one thing, constant emotional conflicts, resentment, anxiety, guilt and shame can easily suppress the body's immune system, digestive functions and basic metabolic processes, and thereby create the conditions for the growth of a cancerous tumor.

Fortunately, the psychological stress/cancer connection no longer lingers in the realm of fiction and uncertainty. Supported by ample scientific evidence, the *Centers for Disease Control and Prevention (CDCP)* make this important statement on their website: "Intensive and prolonged stress can lead to a variety of short- and long-term negative health effects. It can disrupt early brain development and compromise functioning of the nervous and immune system. In addition, childhood stress can lead to health problems later in life including alcoholism, depression, eating disorders, heart disease, cancer, and other chronic diseases."[1]

In spite of the undeniable evidence that backs up the CDCP's claims, most medical doctors rarely acknowledge or attempt to treat these root causes of disease, but instead focus on eradicating its symptoms. Perhaps this crucial and potentially fatal inaccuracy permeating almost the entire medical field is rooted in the lack of acknowledgement of the stress/disease connection; the mind/body relationship is certainly not taught at medical schools.

After having seen thousands of cancer patients over a period of three decades, I began to recognize a certain pattern of thinking, believing and feeling that was common to most of them. To be more specific, I have yet to meet an adult cancer patient who does not feel burdened by some poor self-image, unresolved conflict, persistent worry, or past emotional conflict/trauma that still lingers in his subconscious mind and cellular memory. I believe that cancer, the physical disease, cannot occur unless there is a strong undercurrent of emotional uneasiness and deep-seated frustration.

Adult cancer patients often suffer from lack of self-respect or sense of worthiness, and usually have what I call "unfinished business" in their life. Cancer can actually be a way of revealing the source of such an unresolved, inner conflict. Furthermore, cancer can help them come to terms with such a conflict, and even heal it altogether. The way to take out weeds is to pull them out along with their roots. This is how we ought to treat cancer; otherwise, it may recur eventually.

I often hear the argument that the emotional stress/cancer connection may apply to adults, but certainly cannot apply to young children who have fallen ill with leukemia or brain cancer. I tend to disagree. The CDCP's position in this matter confirms my understanding. Childhood stress **can** lead to cancer, according to the CDCP, and studies have shown that human beings experience stress early, even before they are born.

---

[1] http://www.cdc.gov/violenceprevention/pub/healthy_infants.html

It is a scientific fact that some of the most powerful influences that a child can experience occur while it is still in the mother's womb. It has been clearly demonstrated that what a mother goes through emotionally and physically has a strong impact on the emotional and physical health of her child. For example, research cited in my book, *Timeless Secrets of Health & Rejuvenation,* describes in detail the severe reactions of fetuses to obstetric ultrasounds, which can lead to developmental problems later on.

There is further evidence that not having a normal childbirth, but being born by Cesarean section, can have traumatic effects on babies. In addition, not breastfeeding a baby or keeping it in a separate room from the mother can cause a biological separation trauma which can even cause crib death. Not sensing and feeling the heartbeat of the mother can be severely anxiety-provoking for an infant. Prematurely born babies may become traumatized by separation anxiety.

Furthermore, vaccine shots cause biological shock reactions, similar to mini strokes, besides exposing the baby to the numerous carcinogenic toxins they contain. More and more children have strong allergic reactions to vaccine ingredients, which can traumatize them and even cause them to die. In sensitive children, the pain of the injection and the resulting healing response may also have trauma-evoking consequences.

Absence of breastfeeding is known to cause psychological, emotional and developmental problems in a young child.

Direct exposure to the radiation emanated by cell phones, while in the womb and thereafter, can profoundly affect the health of children. (See Chapter Two, *Deadly Cell Phones and Other Wireless Devices.*)

An inadequate diet that includes sugar, pasteurized cow's milk, animal protein, fried foods and other fast/junk foods greatly affects children, too. And if the mother drinks alcohol, smokes, eats junk food or takes medication during pregnancy, or has been vaccinated herself, this also has detrimental effects on the fetus's health and development.

A very troubling finding shows that x-rays given to young girls increases their breast cancer risk. On the heels of recent reports that revealed too many diagnostic tests are being done on adults, new reports have come out, with warnings that some of these tests not only can cause cancer in children, but can induce new cancers in children who are being treated for cancer. For example, researchers at Memorial Sloan-Kettering Cancer Center in New York City reported that girls who receive radiation to the chest to treat childhood cancer have a high risk of developing breast cancer at a young age. Even those who received lower doses of the common cancer treatment face an increased risk of breast cancer later, the scientists said.

In a different report, the British medical journal *Lancet* reported that CT scans can also give children cancer. The scans can produce life-saving images of head injuries, complicated pneumonia and chest infections. But if a child is exposed to the radiation from just two or three scans, their risk of developing brain cancer is tripled. Five to ten scans can triple the risk of leukemia.

In addition, treating babies for infection with antibiotics is severely damaging to their growing immune systems.

One study by the Environmental Working Group (EWG) has shown that that blood samples from newborns contained an average of 287 toxins, including mercury, fire retardants, pesticides, food additives, chemicals from body care products, air pollutants, toxic plastic compounds, and Teflon chemicals. Many of these toxins are highly carcinogenic.

According to the EWG report, in the month leading up to birth, the umbilical cord transfers the equivalent of at least 300 quarts of blood from the placenta to the developing child. This means that the newborn child has the same chemical load as the mother. Furthermore, mothers who are not in good health and still breastfeed their babies actually continue contaminating them.

Just the plastics chemical bisphenol-A (BPA), an endocrine disrupter that can lead to chromosomal errors in the developing fetus, has been found to trigger spontaneous miscarriages and genetic damage. This toxic chemical was found in 96 percent of the pregnant women tested.

Overall, the study detected a veritable chemical cocktail in 99–100 percent of pregnant women, sufficient to initiate the beginning stages of cancer growth in unborn children.

In addition, a large epidemiological study done in 2006 showed clear evidence found in 151 independent studies that vaccinating children against childhood diseases significantly increases their risk of developing cancers later in life. I will cover this important piece of research in Chapter One in greater detail.

In a series of studies, the poison fluoride, added to the municipal drinking water in the United States and other countries, has been clearly linked to causing cancer of the bone (osteosarcoma), as well as other types of cancer. The good news is that after having endorsed fluoride in drinking water for decades, the CDCP issued an urgent warning in January 2011 that the current levels of fluoride in drinking water can cause serious harm to children. Unfortunately, many uninformed mothers still use fluoridated tap water to prepare baby formula.

Clamping the umbilical cord too early, instead of the required 40–60 minutes after birth, can reduce the oxygenation of the blood in the baby by over 40 percent, and prevent toxins being filtered out of the blood by the placenta. This relatively new practice is found to have severe negative effects on the growth of children.

Whatever affects a child physically, also affects it emotionally and psychologically. In other words, one doesn't need to be a grownup to be gripped by emotional trauma.

Research findings also demonstrate that childhood stress can impact adult health. One of the largest studies of its kind, the Adverse Childhood Experiences (ACE) Study, demonstrates a link between:
1. Specific violence-related stressors, including child abuse, neglect and repeated exposure to intimate partner violence *and*
2. Risky behaviors and health problems in adulthood[2]

The ACE Study, a collaboration between the Centers for Disease Control and Prevention (CDCP) and Kaiser Permanente's Health Appraisal Clinic in San Diego, covered over 17,000 adults participating in their research from 1995 to 1997. It collected and analyzed detailed information on the participants' past history of abuse, neglect, and family dysfunction as well as their current behaviors and health status.

The ACE Study findings have been published in more than 30 scientific articles. They revealed that childhood abuse, neglect and exposure to other adverse experiences are common. Almost two-thirds of the study participants reported at least one adverse childhood experience, and more than 1 in 5 reported three or more. The ACE Study findings suggest that certain experiences are major risk factors for the main causes of illness and death, as well as poor quality of life in the United States. Remember, prolonged emotional stress can compromise the immune system and thereby render the body susceptible to virtually every type of illness, including cancer. I will return to this important subject later.

---

[2] http://www.ncbi.nlm.nih.gov/pmc/articles/PMC3232061/

Lastly, exposing children to ionizing radiation through CT scans after they have received a bump on their head is a very risky and often unnecessary medical practice that can easily and quickly lead to cancer of the brain and other serious health conditions. According to a large study of more than 40,000 children with blunt head trauma revealed that simple observation is the best and most healthy approach. Results appeared in the June 2011 issue of *Pediatrics* (published online May 9, 2011). Of course, children's developing brains have very little or no protection against ionizing radiation.

The first chapter of this book provides profound insights into what cancer really is and stands for, seen from a physical perspective. It is an understanding of cancer you may never have come across before. This new and yet timeless comprehension of cancer allows for new approaches targeted at actually healing the causes of cancer, instead of merely fixing its symptomatic manifestations.

In this chapter, you will also learn about the astonishing discoveries made by leading cancer researchers that prove cancer is not caused by cell mutation alone, but requires the support and participation of the entire organism. Furthermore, check out the new findings that show why so many diagnosed cancerous tumors are actually completely harmless and disappear on their own.

Chapters Two and Three deal with physical and emotional/spiritual causes, respectively. For the sake of clarity, I have tried to separate these categories, although I am very much aware that such a division is arbitrary and non-existent. I have done this for one purpose only: to emphasize that healing the causes of cancer must include restoring one's physical, emotional and spiritual well-being. Leaving out just one of these factors would undermine the chances of full recovery and eventually lead to the recurrence of cancer (a large number of medically treated cancers reoccur). At minimum, such an incomplete approach would seriously affect one's mental and physical health and, foremost of all, one's state of happiness and self-worth.

The following statement, which runs like a red thread through the entire book, is very important in the consideration of cancer: "**Cancer does not cause a person to be sick; it is the sickness of the person that causes the cancer.**" And to this I will add: "**Once a cancer has occurred, its main purpose is to return the sick person to a balanced condition of mind, body and spirit.**"

This is so contradictory to what conventional medicine and the media want you to believe that it may sound outrageous to you. Yet, whether cancer heals you or leads to your demise has actually more to do with what is going on in your personal life than with the cancer itself; that is, how aggressive it is, or how early it is detected.

Take Dave, for example. At age 58, he was diagnosed with lung cancer during a routine health checkup. Although he felt fine before the diagnosis, his health declined rapidly during the following two weeks. He lost his appetite, he couldn't sleep anymore, his breathing became very shallow and he suffered severe panic attacks and chest pain. He died 20 days after the diagnosis. The death certificate said he died from lung cancer, but it is clear that without the cancer diagnosis, none of these overwhelming, stress-induced effects would have occurred.

There is no doubt anymore that emotional stress can shut down your immune system and not only prevent your body from healing, but also actually make you very ill. There is medical evidence to show that during severe stress, people can die from a massive heart attack without any prior heart condition or clogged arteries.

Your ability to recover your health requires you to become and feel whole again on all levels of the body, mind and spirit. Once the root causes of cancer and other impediments to feeling whole have been properly identified, it will become apparent what needs to be done to achieve complete recovery. This is the subject matter of the later chapters of this book.

It is a medical fact that every person has millions of cancer cells in the body at all times in their life. This is not an indication that there is something wrong with us. On the contrary, as we shall see, this forms an essential part of maintaining the body's healthy equilibrium.

These millions of cancer cells remain undetectable through standard tests. However, they show up as tumors once they have multiplied to several billion. When doctors announce to their cancer patients that the treatments they prescribed have successfully eliminated **all** cancer cells, they merely refer to tests that are able to identify the detectable size of cancer tumors.

Standard cancer treatments may lower the number of cancer cells to an undetectable level, but this certainly cannot eradicate **all** cancer cells. As long as the causes of tumor growth remain intact, cancer may redevelop at any time, in any part of the body, and at any speed.

Curing cancer has little to do with getting rid of a group of detectable cancer cells. Treatments like chemotherapy and radiotherapy (radiation) are certainly capable of poisoning or burning many cancer cells, but they also destroy healthy cells in the bone marrow, gastrointestinal tract, liver, kidneys, heart, lungs, etc., which often leads to permanent, irreparable damage of entire organs and systems in the body.

Is it any wonder that the number one side effect of chemotherapy is cancer? In fact, chemotherapy kills far more people by causing new cancers than it *cures* people from cancer. By shrinking tumors, chemotherapy drugs encourage stronger cancer cells to grow, divide and multiply, and become chemo-resistant. This is what makes secondary cancers so risky. In addition, given the high incidence of well-known and devastating side effects of chemotherapy, nearly every recipient of these cytotoxic drugs experiences a surge in the stress protein HSF-1, or heat shock factor-1. HSF-1 allows cancer cells damaged by these drugs to repair themselves and resume their *cancerous* activities.

The same is true for radiotherapy. Radiation exposure at a dose of 100 mSv[3] is the annual dose at which increased lifetime cancer risk is evident. According to research, 10,000 mSv is a fatal dose.[4] Radiation therapy blasts the body with 20,000–80,000 mSv, depending on the kind of cancer involved. Nothing could be more fatal than radiation treatment. In comparison, the radiation leak that resulted from the Japanese earthquake in 2011 would be considered harmless.

The toxic chemicals contained in chemotherapy drugs can cause such severe inflammation in every cell of the body that even the hair follicles can no longer hold on to the strands of hair. A real cure of cancer does not occur at the expense of destroying other vital parts of the body. It is achievable only when the causes of excessive growth of cancer cells have been addressed and the body is being properly supported through its natural healing process. Cancer **is** the healing process that the body may choose in order to reestablish homeostasis. Not recognizing cancer as a healing mechanism can turn out to be fatal, and often is.

This book is dedicated to uncovering the causes of cancer, and proposes to deal with these rather than with its symptoms. Treating

---

[3] One mSv is the basic unit used to measuring the concentration of radiation.
[4] For details, refer to this article by Mike Adams, NaturalNews.com:
http://www.naturalnews.com/032136_radiation_exposure_chart.html

cancer as if it were a disease is a trap that millions of people have fallen into, and have paid a high price for not attending to its root causes.

While I strongly believe that cancer is a final healing phase, not a disease, I am fully aware that most people consider cancer to be a dreaded disease. I make no claims that my understanding of cancer is the only correct one, but I propose it is one of many correct ones.

The old saying, "Knowledge is different in different states of consciousness", reveals *the truth* to be a subjective projection of the mind, conscious or subconscious. In other words, if you insist that cancer is a terrible disease that may take your life, this death-fright belief of yours is likely to fulfill your dreaded expectation. Remember, emotional trauma suppresses the immune system and prevents healing. Likewise, if you perceive cancer to be a healing phase that deals with an underlying imbalance, your truth is also going to help you achieve a positive outcome, one that matches your uplifting expectation. Recent brain research has revealed that the power of positive expectation is the **only** real inducer of healing in the body.[5]

It is unfortunate that the medical profession has, by and large, discouraged patients to participate in, or affect, their own cures. Patients are rarely included in the process of healing. Instead, medical treatments are now propagated to be the sole remedy for today's ills. In truth, whether a person heals or doesn't is largely controlled by the state of the body, mind and spirit of the individual. Accepting this as fact can have enormous self-empowering effects which I consider essential for healing to occur and be effective.

Please note: Wherever in this book you find me making references to cancer being a deadly disease, to people being killed by cancer, or to cancer being an aggressive or terminal illness, etc., please note that I do this only to present the official interpretations of medical research and theories. However, I wish to make it very clear that my understanding and interpretation of the cancer phenomenon are not compatible with this current medical model. I do not agree with the idea that it is the cancer that kills someone, and I will further elaborate on my position throughout this book.

---

[5] For detailed information, see my article on positive expectation on http://www.ener-chi.com/articles/positive-expectation-a-medical-miracle/

Unless a cancerous tumor leads to a life-threatening mechanical obstruction or swelling and subsequent suffocation of an organ, cancer cannot be considered to harm the body or kill it. Rather, cancer is a healing or survival mechanism that takes place when a person's life is threatened by one or several reasons discussed in this book. Cancer is an indication that the body is critically out of balance and may possibly die from whatever is throwing it off balance. When you hear that ionizing radiation or aspirin pills cause some of the most serious or aggressive cancers, please be aware that the resulting cancers constitute the body's survival or healing attempts, not a disease.

This book clearly distinguishes between the causes of cancer and its symptoms. The symptoms, such as a cancerous tumor growth, merely indicate that the body is already attempting to tackle the underlying causes of the cancer. Unless we support the body through this healing process and do not attack it with harmful medical treatments, cancer – the healing process – may remain incomplete and the cancer may continue to grow and therefore be considered *incurable.*

The purpose of this book is to provide you with the knowledge and confidence in the body's infinite wisdom and intelligence, with which the healing can reach its completion and the body can return to its natural state of balance and vitality.

Chapter One

Cancer Is Not a Disease

Power In The Word

Cancer is considered to be the second leading cause of death for Americans. An estimated total of 1,529,560 new cancer cases and 569,490 deaths from cancer occurred in the United States in 2010, according to the American Cancer Society. Among men, the three most common cancer diagnoses are prostate cancer, lung cancer and colorectal cancer. The leading types of cancers among women are breast cancer, lung cancer and colorectal cancer.

The National Cancer Institute (NCI) listed the top 10 killer cancers (deaths between 2003 and 2007) as follows:

1. Lung and bronchial cancer: 792,495 lives
2. Colon and rectal cancer: 268,783 lives
3. Breast cancer: 206,983 lives
4. Pancreatic cancer: 162,878 lives
5. Prostate cancer: 144,926 lives
6. Leukemia: 108,740 lives
7. Non-Hodgkin's lymphoma: 104,407 lives
8. Liver and intrahepatic bile duct cancer: 79,773 lives
9. Ovarian cancer: 73,638 lives
10. Esophageal cancer: 66,659 lives

Whatever your level of medical training, it appears safe to say that cancer seems to be killing us in record numbers. Yet despite millions of lives lost and billions of dollars spent on research, rates of cancer don't seem to be on the decline.

And the problem goes deeper than simply not understanding cancer's root causes or how best to treat it. Dr. Samuel S. Epstein, in his book, *National Cancer Institute and American Cancer Society: Criminal Indifference to Cancer Prevention and Conflicts of Interest*, clearly demonstrates that much of the blame for cancer's growing presence in our society rests on the National Cancer Institute (NCI) and the American Cancer Society (ACS) – some of the very associations that are supported by the U.S. government (and thus by U.S. taxpayer dollars) and charged with fighting America's *war on cancer* – which are also riddled by conflicts of interest and withholding too much valuable information to truly help Americans prevent and treat cancer. Indeed, roughly half of the ACS board is made up of doctors and scientists closely tied to the NCI, many of whom receive funding by double dipping from both bodies.

The result? Federal money and charitable funds spent on cancer research have increased 25-fold, from $220 million in 1971 to $4.6 billion in 2000. Yet, despite NCI president Andrew von Eschenbach's grand promise in 2003 to eliminate suffering and death from cancer by 2015, cancer rates have increased by approximately 18 percent and show no signs of slowing down.

As a result, cancer affects nearly 1 in 2 men and more than 1 in 3 women; however, the billions of tax and charitable dollars dedicated to cancer research are overwhelmingly focusing only on treatment, with almost no studies being done on prevention. "The best defense is a good offense ", as the old adage goes, yet conventional wisdom surrounding cancer tells us just the opposite.

This is due, in part, to tremendous profits available to pharmaceutical and medical companies for maintaining a treatment- rather than prevention-based attitude towards cancer, as well as an unwillingness to address causes of cancer beyond individual lifestyle choices. In other words, while factors such as smoking and poor diet may be acknowledged as issues, those causes that may negatively affect certain industries, such as environmental pollution, contaminants in consumer products and toxic medical treatments, are being ignored.

When pharmaceuticals become regarded as the only suitable options for treating disease, keeping patients sick and overmedicated is an increasingly lucrative business. Considering this, it is not all that surprising that alternative or *unapproved* treatments are systematically vilified by the medical industry and the cancer establishment. More and more often, those doctors who continue to advocate natural treatment methods and point out the important benefits of holistic cancer prevention are harassed and castigated as quacks if they refuse to fall in line with heavily biased NCI and ACS *guidelines.* It is certainly telling that the FDA has approved around 40 pharmaceutical drugs for cancer treatment, but has yet to endorse even one single non-patented alternative treatment.

By looking at the facts, it is clear that the only people truly benefiting from current cancer culture are the medical professionals and lobbyists in positions of power, and not their patients. As former NCI director Dr. Samuel Broder admitted in a 1998 *Washington Post* interview: "The NCI has become what amounts to a government pharmaceutical company." Indeed, it is the American taxpayer who continues to fund expensive clinical trials for drugs that ultimately end up being sold to them at inflated prices. Whether by misguided funding priorities, selective omission of new research or alternative treatments, or outright suppression of the facts, cancer patients are not being protected by those bodies that are supposed to be protecting them.

All in all, the past few decades, more than any other period in history, have instilled in our society such an inflated fear of cancer that it is hardly surprising that most cancer patients simply do as their doctors tell them: throw more pharmaceutical drugs and toxic treatments at their terrifying *disease.* But by failing to focus on inexpensive and minimally toxic prevention in favor of expensive and extremely toxic *treatments,* ostensibly objective agencies like the NCI have exacerbated the very problem they are charged with solving. As a result, the rates of cancer diagnosis are at staggering levels and continue to rise. And in addition to the diagnosed cases of cancer, there are tens of thousands of underprivileged people who have cancer, but may never receive a diagnosis because they cannot afford health insurance or a doctor's appointment.

It goes without saying that words themselves have tremendous power, and *cancer* is no exception. In many cases, cancer is not just a word, but also a statement that refers to abnormal or unusual behavior of the body's cells. The mere mention of the word cancer is enough to immediately call to mind images of suffering and pain. To pin the word on any individual can instantly inspire debilitating fear and stress into their psyche.

Yet in a different context, cancer is referred to as a star sign, just another member of the Zodiac (astrological) family. When someone asks your date of birth and says you are Cancer, are you going to tremble with the fear of imminent death? **Such a reaction is unlikely, because your interpretation of being of the cancer sign does not imply that you *have* cancer, the illness.** But if your doctor called you into his office and told you that you had cancer, you would most likely feel shocked, paralyzed, numb, terrified, hopeless, or all of the above. The word cancer has the potential to play a very disturbing and precarious role in your life, one that is capable of delivering a death sentence and, as you will discover in this book, actually executing it – often simply because of the role that those six little letters have come to play in our terrified society.

Although being a cancer patient seems to start with the diagnosis of cancer, its causes may have been present for many years prior to the patient feeling ill. Yet within a brief moment, the word *cancer* can turn someone's entire world upside down.

Who or what in this world has bestowed this simple word or statement with such great power that it can preside over life and death? Or does it really possess this power? Could our collective, social conviction that cancer is a killer disease, along with the trauma-generating, aggressive treatments that follow diagnosis, actually be mainly responsible for the current dramatic escalation of cancer in the Western hemisphere? Such a thought is too farfetched, you might reply! In this book, however, I will make the convincing point that cancer can have no power or control over you, unless the beliefs, perceptions, attitudes, thoughts and feelings you have about cancer allow it to do so.

Would you be as afraid of cancer if you knew what caused it, or at least understood what its underlying purpose was? Unlikely! If the truth were told, you would probably do everything you could to remove the causes of the cancer and, in so doing, lay the foundation for the body to heal itself.

A little knowledge in the conventional sense – which I might also call ignorance – is, in fact, a dangerous thing. Almost everyone, at least in the industrialized world, knows that drinking water from a muddy pond or a polluted lake can cause life-threatening diarrhea. Yet relatively few people realize that holding on to resentment, anger and fear, or avoiding exposure to the sun and thereby causing vitamin D deficiency, or not getting enough sleep on a regular basis, or holding a cell phone to your head for an hour each day, or being regularly exposed to x-rays, mammograms or CAT scans, or eating junk foods, chemical additives and artificial sweeteners, are all no less dangerous than drinking polluted water. These *habits* of life may just take a little longer to kill a person than any poison or tiny amoebas do, but there is no doubt that they can.

Mistaken Judgment

We all know that if the foundation of a house is strong, the house can easily withstand external stressors, such as a violent storm or even an earthquake. As we shall see, cancer is similarly just an indication that something has been missing in our body and in our life. Cancer reveals that some aspect of our physical, mental and spiritual life stands on shaky ground and is, to say the least, quite fragile.

It would be foolish for a gardener to water the withering leaves of a tree when he knows that the real problem is not where it appears to be – on the surface of those withered leaves. He knows that the dehydration of the leaves is merely a symptom of lacking water in the less apparent part of the plant – its underground root system. By watering the roots of the plant, the gardener naturally attends to the causative level and, consequently, the whole plant becomes revived and resumes its normal growth. To the trained eye of a gardener, the symptom of withering leaves is not a dreadful disease. He recognizes that the dehydrated state of these leaves is merely a direct consequence of withdrawn nourishment – nourishment that is needed to sustain the roots and the rest of the plant.

Although this example from nature may appear to be a simplistic analogy, it nevertheless offers a basic understanding of some very complex disease processes in the human body. It accurately describes one of the most powerful and fundamental principles controlling all life forms on the planet. However skilled we may have become at manipulating the functions of our body through the tools of allopathic medicine, this basic law of nature cannot be suppressed or violated without paying the hefty price of suffering ill-health on physical, emotional and spiritual levels.

I fervently challenge the statement that cancer is a killer disease. Furthermore, I will demonstrate that cancer is not a disease at all. Many people who received a *terminal* cancer sentence actually defied the prognosis and experienced complete remission. George, my first kidney cancer patient, was one of them. His doctors at one of the most prestigious university hospitals in Germany had just *given* him three more weeks to live when he sought me out for help. According to them, his cancer was too advanced and widespread to consider having treatments of chemotherapy or radiation. As it turned out, not receiving further medical treatment turned out to be a great blessing for George.

Healing Cancer versus Fighting It

George had lost one of his kidneys to cancer a year earlier. After emerging from the operating room, his doctors gave him a clean bill of health. They used the famous "We got it all" utterance to instill hope and encouragement. Of course, it made a lot of sense to him; after all, they had removed the tumor, along with the entire kidney. Nevertheless, just several months later his second kidney also started filling up with cancer, and the only *reasonable* advice they had for him was to take care of his personal affairs.

Fortunately for George, he didn't die. In total defiance of the death sentence that his doctors had pronounced, George felt that there should be something else he could do at least to extend his life by a few months. Within a mere three weeks of dealing with the root causes of his illness, the cancer receded to a tiny speck, and during his next major checkup at the German cancer clinic six months later, the *deadly* cancer was nowhere to be found. Fifteen years later, George still enjoys a state of excellent health, with no indication of a malfunctioning other kidney.

I had given George neither a diagnosis nor a prognosis. This is not what I do, anyway. What would have been the point of telling him how bad and hopeless his situation was? Besides, a doctor's objective statement that his patient's cancer is terminal (leading to his death) is actually a purely subjective viewpoint of a highly unpredictable situation. The doctor derives his convincing, final judgment almost exclusively from past observations he has made with previous patients who suffered from similar symptoms. His absolute judgment, though, rules out the chance of recovery resulting from alternative treatments unknown to the treating physician. Just because the relatively young Western system of medicine does not know how to treat cancer successfully without seriously injuring the patient and risking a recurrence of cancer, does not imply that the ancient forms of medicine are equally useless. There is good reason why certain forms of holistic Eastern medicine, however ancient, have not died out: they have proven throughout millennia that they are indeed effective. So why not be open to their potential?

In the arena of orthodox medicine, patients are not encouraged to expect a spontaneous remission of their cancer. Being realists, doctors want to avoid giving their patients *false* hope. However, I question whether there truly can be such a thing as false hope. Either there is hope or there is none; any genuinely felt hope cannot be wrong or false.

Hope can actually act as a powerful placebo[6] that is often far more powerful than cancer medication could ever be. In addition, hope can even turn a dangerous chemotherapy drug into a placebo, which can subsequently reduce the drug's side effects. Furthermore, research clearly demonstrates that doctors who provide hope and encouragement to their patients have higher success rates with cancer and other health conditions than those who don't. Just imagine what hope, encouragement and joyful elation, combined with a completely natural treatment, could accomplish!

Besides, the future is not written in stone, and doctors are not necessarily psychics who know what the future may hold for their patients. No person in this world can predict with absolute certainty what is going to happen in the near or distant future. A physician may come up with a good guess of what the most likely outcome of a disease might be, but such guesswork can hardly be called scientific or carry the stamp of absolute certainty. All in all, hope should be encouraged by every doctor, never discouraged, no matter how seemingly dire the situation.

To make a point, a young man with an extremely rare and inoperable large brain tumor, whose story was documented on prime time live television in the U.S. in 2007, defied the prognosis of a very short life and continues to lead a quite active and vibrant life several years afterward.

---

[6] For an in-depth analysis of the placebo effect as a major healing power in the body, see Chapter One of my book, *Timeless Secrets of Health & Rejuvenation.*

He even got married later. And that is only one of many similar instances in which patients who were told to have no hope have ended up defying all their doctors' *realistic* expectations, regaining their health and living well past even the most generous prognoses. Medical history is full of such unexplained miracles. We would do well to try to explain them, and perhaps even re-create them.

But back to George, my terminal kidney cancer patient. To avoid the complications that may arise from diagnosing diseases, such as making a person believe he is a helpless victim of some sort, I merely encouraged and motivated George to attend to the various reasons responsible for causing and promoting cancer growth in the first place. In fact, I hardly ever mentioned the word cancer in his presence. Being a smart, successful businessman, George quickly realized that remaining fixated on the idea that cancer had somehow gotten hold of him, dragging him to his death, was of no use to him. He was well aware that such victim mentality would only kill him faster. George already knew the value of self-empowerment and positive thinking. My focus was to share with him the most basic, practical methods of making the body more healthy, vital and resilient. In my opinion, George wasn't even a sick man; he just had forgotten how to live his life in a healthy manner. George suddenly came to the realization that he was no longer a victim of unlucky circumstances, but rather in charge of his body and mind. This notion of self-empowerment made him feel ecstatic, and he soon let his family members and friends who previously felt sad and sorry for him partake in his newly discovered zest for life.

Subsequently, his body naturally started to take care of the details, which included removal of the symptom – cancer. It was a fairly minor feat once the causes of the cancer were non-existent.

The total remission of George's cancer was neither the result of curing what appeared to be a horrible, self-perpetuating disease, nor a miracle. It was a simple process of giving back to the body what it needed to return to its most natural and normal state of balance. George merely ended the reasons why his body needed to fight for its life. As simple as it sounds, he healed himself by taking responsibility for all aspects of his life, including his body and lifestyle.

The lesson that can be learned from George's experience is that true healing requires you to stop fighting and, instead, choose to trust and embrace your body's natural and ancient healing mechanisms – for indeed, *fighting* cancer, as we shall see, is what actually prevents a real and lasting cure.

Searching For Answers

Every type of cancer has been survived by someone, regardless of how far advanced it was. Therefore, if even one person has succeeded in healing his cancer, there must be a mechanism for it, just as there is a mechanism for creating cancer. Every person on the planet has the capacity to do both.

If you have been diagnosed with cancer, you may not be able to change the diagnosis, but it is certainly in your power to alter the destructive consequences that this diagnosis may have on you, just as George did. The way you perceive the cancer and the steps you choose to take following the diagnosis are some of the most powerful determinants of your future wellness, or lack thereof. (See Chapter Three, *Demystifying Cancer.*)

The indiscriminate reference to cancer as a killer disease by professionals and laypersons alike has turned cancer into a disorder with tragic consequences for the majority of cancer patients and their families. Cancer has become synonymous with extraordinary fear, suffering and death. This perception continues despite the fact that up to 90–95 percent of all cancers can appear and disappear of their own accord.

Not a day passes without the body making millions of cancer cells. Some people, under severe temporary stress, produce more cancer cells than usual. These cancer cells cluster together as tumors that will disappear again once the stress impact has subsided and after a healing response (as indicated by symptoms of illness) has been completed. In Chapter Three, I will elaborate on the exact, predictable way this occurs.

I wish to mention at this point that according to medical research, secretions of the DNA's powerful anticancer hormone, Interleukin 2, drop under physical and mental duress, and increase again when the person becomes relaxed and joyful. Low secretions of Interleukin 2 increase the incidence of cancer in the body, and normal secretions of this hormone keep cancer at bay.

However, people are generally not under severe stress all the time. Since the incidence of cancer rises and falls with the experience of severe stress, many cancers vanish without any form of medical intervention and without causing any real concern. Accordingly, **right at this moment, millions of people are walking around with cancers in their body without having a clue that they have them. Likewise, millions of people heal their cancers without even knowing it.** Overall, there are many more spontaneous remissions of cancer than there are diagnosed and treated cancers.

The New York Times published an article in its October 2009 issue that certainly raised some eye-opening questions in view of facts that have become highly inconvenient for the cancer establishment and its advocates. The article, written by Gina Kolata, is entitled "Cancers Can Vanish Without Treatment, but How?"

In the article, Kolata points out that the trajectory of cancer was assumed to point in only one direction, like the arrow of time; that is, to grow and worsen. Yet in October 2009, a paper published in the *Journal of the American Medical Association (JAMA)* noted that "data from more than two decades of screening for breast and prostate cancer call that view into question".

More sophisticated screening technologies find many small tumors that would not cause a problem if they were left alone, undiscovered by screening. These tumors are as dormant and harmless as small scars on the skin. As the paper concedes, these tumors were destined to stop growing on their own or shrink, or even, at least in the case of some breast cancers, disappear.

"The old view is that cancer is a linear process," said Dr. Barnett Kramer, associate director of the Division of Cancer Prevention at the National Institutes of Health (NIH). "A cell acquired a mutation, and little by little it acquired more and more mutations. Mutations are not supposed to revert spontaneously."

Until recently, cancer researchers and doctors alike have falsely assumed (and projected their assumption as scientific fact), that cancer results from cell mutation (alteration of the genetic makeup of the cell), which then takes on a life of its own. However, the leading edge of cancer research points toward the discovery that uncontrolled and senseless cancer cell division does not take place at all.

As Dr. Kramer points out, it is becoming increasingly clear that cancers require more than mutations to progress. They need the cooperation of surrounding cells and even, he said, "the whole organism, the person", whose immune system or hormone levels, for example, can squelch or fuel a tumor.

This, Dr. Kramer said, makes cancer "a dynamic process". His statement obviously raises a very important question. If cancer's only function is to be an ultimately fatal succession of cell mutations, then why would the entire body, including the brain, nervous system, immune system and endocrine system, as well as the personality and all the cells surrounding a cancer, support its growth? The answer to this all-important question is both fascinating and encouraging.

As the title of this book asserts, cancer is not a disease at all; instead, it is a healing mechanism. The entire body supports the growth of a cancer so long as it is in its best interest. Once the healing of its root causes is complete, once the body and mind have returned to their proper and balanced state, the cancer no longer serves a purpose and either transitions into a benign and dormant state, or even disappears entirely.

The new view that cancer does not take a predictably one-dimensional path from mutation to disease was difficult for some cancer doctors and researchers to accept. But apparently, more and more of the skeptics are now shifting gear and acknowledging that, contrary though it may seem to everything they had previously thought, cancers can, in fact, disappear on their own.

One of these converts is Dr. Robert M. Kaplan, the chairman of the department of health services at the School of Public Health at the University of California, Los Angeles. "At the end of the day, I'm not sure how certain I am about this, but I do believe it," said Dr. Kaplan. He added, "The weight of the evidence suggests that there is reason to believe."

One more cancer specialist, Dr. Jonathan Epstein at Johns Hopkins University, says that disappearing tumors are well-known in testicular cancer. According to Dr. Epstein, it has been acknowledged to happen that during an operation on a man's testicle, a surgeon may find only scar tissue in place of what was diagnosed to be a large tumor.

The growing evidence that cancers can stop or even reverse direction is now undeniable, and researchers are left with no other choice than to reassess their notions of what cancer really is and how it develops. Still, in my opinion, unless they recognize that cancer is a healing mechanism orchestrated by the entire organism to correct an underlying imbalance, they will continue to search for ways to fight cancer instead of supporting it through the healing process. However, this requires trust in the body's wisdom and natural healing abilities, not in suspicion that the body is inherently faulty or broken.

This discovery that cell mutation alone cannot cause cancer, but must be supported by surrounding cells and the entire organism, speaks for itself. I have always viewed cancer as a friend of the body that assists it during turbulent times. Certainly the body seems to treat cancer as a friend, not an enemy. I believe that we should do the same.

In her article, Kolata writes about a fascinating statement made by Thea Tlsty, a professor of pathology at the University of California, San Francisco, and one of the world's most distinguished cancer researchers. Dr. Tlsty says that cancer cells and pre-cancerous cells are so common that nearly everyone by middle age or old age is riddled with them. That was discovered in autopsy studies of people who died of other unrelated causes, with no idea that they had cancer cells or pre-cancerous cells. They did not have large tumors or symptoms of cancer. "The really interesting question," Dr. Tlsty said, "is not so much why *do* we get cancer as why *don't* we get cancer?"

In the same context, I want to put forward this most intriguing question: Why do some people feel sick when they have cancer while others who also have cancer live completely normal, healthy lives? I will further elucidate this crucial topic throughout the book.

Kolata raises yet another curious point: "The earlier a cell is in its path toward an aggressive cancer, researchers say, the more likely it is to reverse course. So, for example, cells that are early precursors of cervical cancer are likely to revert. One study found that 60 percent of pre-cancerous cervical cells, found with Pap tests, revert to normal within a year; 90 percent revert within three years." Doesn't this show a different trend than the one previous proposed by cancer theorists?

Of course, this prompts the question of whether it is in fact better to leave many cancers untreated, so that they may either go into dormancy and become harmless, or disappear of their own accord. For many decades, doctors and health agencies have been pushing the agenda of early detection on the general population with claims that it is vitally important to catch and treat cancers at an early stage. They argue that this allows for better and more successful treatment. However, once again, their assumptions may have been wrong all along.

Kolata further explains that "the dynamic process of cancer development appears to be the reason that screening for breast cancer or prostate cancer finds huge numbers of early cancers without a corresponding decline in late stage cancers." In other words, discovering so many extra cancers through new and better screening methods has not reduced the incidence of advanced cancers. This clearly contradicts the assumption which asserts that early detection, which normally leads to early treatment, has any overall preventative or long-term cancer incidence-reducing benefits. It also implies that many cancers are better left alone. This supports the hypothesis that many early cancers go nowhere. With regard to breast cancer, there is indirect evidence that some actually disappear. Screening for breast and prostate cancers has clearly failed to reduce occurrence.

For good reason, Johns Hopkins offers men with small prostate tumors an option of *active surveillance*, instead of having their prostates removed or destroyed. In the rare case that the cancer grows bigger, they can still have it removed. However, the frightening diagnosis of having prostate cancer discourages most men from choosing this *wait and see* route. "Most men want it out," said Dr. Epstein of Johns Hopkins. I credit the decades of senseless fear-mongering by medical professionals and the quick-fix obsession among patients for this unfortunate situation.

I might add that the high doses of ionizing radiation emitted by cancer screening devices, such as Computed Tomography (CT) and mammography, etc., have actually contributed to the incidence of various types of cancers. Cancers associated with such radiation exposure include leukemia, multiple myeloma, breast cancer, lung cancer and skin cancer. (See Chapter Five, *Ionizing Radiation*.)

In a Canadian study, researchers looked at the behavior of small kidney cancers (renal-cell carcinomas) which are among the cancers that are reported to regress occasionally, even when far advanced. The double-blind control study, led by Dr. Martin Gleave, Department of Urologic Sciences at Vancouver General Hospital [*New England Journal of Medicine*; 338:1265-1271, April 30, 1998], compared an immunomodulating drug treatment, interferon gamma-1b, with a placebo in people with kidney cancer that had spread throughout their bodies.

Despite the lack of placebo-controlled trials, Interleukin 2 and Interferon have become the central component of most immunotherapeutic strategies for metastatic renal-cell carcinoma. The study was supposed to show that these immunomodulators could control or reverse these kidney cancers, which are very resistant to chemotherapy. Six percent of subjects in both groups had tumors that shrank or remained stable, which led the researchers to conclude that the treatment did not improve outcomes. This six percent of participants who benefitted somewhat showed that whether they received medical treatment, or not, made no difference, except that those in the placebo group lived on average 3.5 months longer than those who received the drug treatment.

Dr. Gleave states that more patients are having ultrasound or CT scans for reasons unrelated to cancer, thereby learning that there is a small lump on one of their kidneys. The accepted response is to surgically remove those tumors. But based on his findings, he wonders if that is truly necessary.

According to the *New York Times* piece, Dr. Gleave's university is participating in a countrywide study of people with small kidney tumors, asking what happens when those tumors are routinely examined, with scans, to see if they grow. Apparently, about 80 percent do not change or actually regress over the next three years.

The conclusion I draw from this important piece of research is that we are barking up the wrong tree if we believe we can outsmart the body. The body regresses or stops the growth of a tumor when it deems it necessary, not otherwise. If we poison, burn or cut out a tumor, the body may need to grow another one in order to complete its healing activity.

The main flaw in the medical cancer theory lies in the assumption that cancer needs to be subdued in order to save a cancer patient's life. Until recently, nearly all scientists shared the opinion that unless a cancer is treated and stopped, it is destined to grow, spread and eventually kill the person. This is obviously not the case. Millions of people live with all kinds of cancers without a problem, and even without being aware of it, according to the work of Dr. Tlsty and many other top scientists.

The truth is, relatively few cancers actually become *terminal*. A vast number of cancers clearly remain undiagnosed and are not found until autopsy. Often these people don't die from the cancer, but from something else. They might not even have the symptoms that could prompt the doctor to prescribe any of the standard cancer-detecting tests. Doesn't it astonish you that 30 to 40 times as many cases of thyroid, pancreatic and prostate cancers are found in autopsy than are detected by doctors? So is cancer really the dangerous disease we have been told it is?

In 1993, the British medical journal *Lancet* published a study that showed early screening often leads to unnecessary treatment. That might be good for pharmaceutical companies, but it certainly does little, if any, real good for cancer patients.

For example, although 33 percent of autopsies in men reveal prostate cancer, only about 1 percent die from it. After age 75, half of males may have prostate cancer, but mortality rates only range from 0.1–2.4 percent. More specifically, the overall 5-year relative prostate cancer survival rate for 1995–2002 was 99 percent. The 5-year relative prostate cancer survival rates by race were 99.9 percent for white men and 97.6 percent for black men, regardless of whether they had few or no signs or symptoms of prostate cancer, were free of disease, or had treatment. Government recommendations (as of August 2008) call for oncologists to no longer treat men with prostate cancer past the age of 75 years because the treatments do more harm than good and offer no advantages over having no treatment at all.

It must be noted that these low mortality rates especially apply to those who have neither been diagnosed with cancer, nor received any treatment for it. Since by the government's own admission, mortality rates increase when cancers are being treated, it certainly suggests what really does the killing.

Once diagnosed and treated, the vast majority of cancers are never given a chance to disappear on their own. They are promptly targeted with an arsenal of deadly weapons such as chemotherapy drugs, radiation and the surgical knife. Dormant tumors, which would never really cause any harm to the body, may instead be aroused into powerful defensive reactions and become aggressive, not unlike relatively harmless bacteria that turn into dangerous superbugs when attacked by antibiotic medication. It makes absolutely no sense that at a time when you need to strengthen the body's most important healing system (the immune system), you would subject yourself to radical treatments that actually weaken or destroy the immune system.

The problem with cancer patients today is that, terrified by the diagnosis, they submit their bodies to these cutting, burning and/or poisoning *treatments*: procedures that more likely than not will only lead them more rapidly to their deaths until they finally find themselves completely out of options.

The most important question a cancer patient may need to ask is not, "How advanced or dangerous is my cancer?" but, "What am I doing or not doing that puts my body into a situation of having to fight for its life?" Why do some people go through cancer as if it were the flu? Are they just lucky, or is there a mechanism at work that heals them and restores their health? On the contrary, what is the hidden element that prevents the body from healing cancer naturally, that makes it seem so dangerous?

The answers to all these questions lie with the person who has the cancer, and does not depend on the degree of a particular cancer's *viciousness* or the advanced stage to which it appears to have progressed. Do you believe that cancer is a disease? You will most likely respond with a "Yes", given the *informed* opinion that the medical industry and media have spoon-fed to the masses for many decades.

Yet the more important but rarely asked question remains: "Why do you think cancer is a disease?" You may answer, "Because I know cancer kills people every day." I would then question you further: "How do you know that it is the cancer that kills people?" You would probably argue that if many people who have cancer die, it must be the cancer that kills them. That's what all the medical experts say.

Let me ask you another question, a rather strange one: How do you know for sure that you are the daughter/son of your father and not of another man? Is it because your mother told you so? What makes you so completely sure that your mother told you the truth? It is likely that you simply believe her because you have no compelling reason not to. But unless you have your father do a paternity DNA test, you will never really know with absolute certainty that the person you believe to be your father is, in fact, your father. Instead, it is your emotional attachments and lack of deeper investigation that have turned your subjective belief into something that you *know* to be an irrefutable truth.

Such a metaphor may seem strange, yet similar assumptions are incredibly pervasive in our attitudes about cancer. Although no scientific proof exists to show that cancer is a disease instead of a healing process, most people will insist that it is a disease because this is what they have been told to believe. Yet this belief is only hearsay based on other people's opinions. Finally, the infallible doctrine that cancer is a disease can be traced to some doctors who expressed their subjective feelings or beliefs about what they had observed, and published them in some review articles or medical reports. Other doctors agreed with their opinion and, before long, it became a *well-established fact* that cancer is a dangerous disease that somehow gets hold of people in order to kill them. However, the truth of the matter may actually be quite different and more rational, and scientific, than that.

The Gene/Cancer Myth

According to a research paper published in the German medical journal *Deutsches Aerzteblatt*, by renowned molecular and cell biologist, Professor Peter Duisberg (University of California, Berkley), the theory that gene mutation is behind malignant tumors is built on shaky ground. Duisberg's disclosure of major flaws in the current mutation-cancer theory was also published recently by the prestigious journal *Cell Cycle* [2011;10 (13); 2100-14].

For many years, cancer scientists have assumed that malignant tumors develop when the mutation of between three and six genes, called oncogenes, cause otherwise normal cells to undergo abnormal, uncontrolled growth. An oncogene is a gene found in the chromosomes of tumor cells whose activation is associated with the initial and continuing conversion of normal cells into cancer cells.

Most healthy cells die and become replaced with new cells within cycles of 10 days to four months. Plasma cells, for example, live for 10 days before they become replaced. Bone cells have a natural lifespan of three months, and blood cells can live for four months before they die. The current cancer-mutation theory proposes that oncogenes prevent the occurrence of timely cell death, and cause cells to survive and proliferate. In fact, it considers gene mutation to be a necessary event responsible for malignant cell transformation.

The problem with this theory is that all malignant tumors that have a chromosomal abnormality (aneuploidy) often don't contain any of these alleged cancer-causing oncogenes. In addition, carcinomas of the same kind that actually contain mutated oncogenes most often do not even share the same type of mutated oncogenes.

It is just as misleading to propose that a chromosomal abnormality is a precondition for abnormal cell growth when carcinogens like asbestos can cause tumor growth without any mutated oncogenes whatsoever.

Another problem with the current mutation theory is that chromosomal abnormalities can exist for decades before a cancerous tumor is formed, or it may never form at all. On the other hand, a person who has no chromosomal abnormality or gene mutation can just as well develop such a tumor. The idea that a chromosomal abnormality must unfailingly and immediately lead to malignant cell growth is an unproven hypothesis that only serves those who make a living from it.

We cannot have it both ways. Either genetic mutation leads to abnormal cell growth, or it doesn't. If mutated oncogenes don't lead to cancer, not even after 40 years, there must be other reasons for causing it.

Of course, the multibillion dollar drug industry is not interested in discovering the real causes of cancer. Rather, it is focused on developing extremely expensive drugs that are designed to prevent genetic mutation, even though genetic mutation clearly isn't what causes cancers in the first place. Once again, we are all taken for a ride, a costly one at that. So far, the success rate of this approach is depressingly dismal.

Extensive scientific research conducted in the field of cellular biology over the past 10 years has already demonstrated that genes do not cause disease, but are influenced and altered by changes in the environment, from the very first moments in the mother's womb to the last moments of a person's life. We already know from leading cancer researchers like Dr. Kramer that genetic mutations alone, without the cooperation of the surrounding organism, cannot cause cancer to occur or progress.

Cellular biologists also recognize that the conditions and occurrences in the external surroundings and internal physiology and, more importantly, perceptions of ourselves and the world around us, directly influence gene behavior. This means that every thought, feeling, emotion, belief and experience we have, every bite of food we ingest, the air we breathe, the way we interact with others and how we treat ourselves can instantly impact our genes. As Dr. Kramer said, cancer is a dynamic, not an isolated phenomenon or a set-in-stone reality; in essence, a process that is constantly altered by its environment – you and your surroundings.

It is important to understand that genes don't mutate because they become *bored* with being normal or because they *want* to be malignant. Rather, the cells are left with no other choice but to mutate in order to survive in a hostile, toxic tumor-milieu that has been created by non-genetic factors. A tumor-milieu – a cell environment that is poorly oxygenated and highly acidic – is the ideal medium for the growth of cancer cells and microorganisms found in cancerous tumors. And as it will become clear in the book, this is the exact condition the body requires to actually heal itself. Later in this chapter I will explain the important role that microorganisms play in the remission of cancer cells.

As difficult as this may be to stomach, research has clearly demonstrated that gene mutations or *defects* cannot be the cause of cancer. While gene mutation may be a factor in the development of cancer, it is also true that millions of people with *defective* genes will never develop the diseases associated with them.

As demonstrated in lab experiments by world-renowned cell biologist Dr. Bruce Lipton, the New York Times best-selling author of the book, *The Biology of Belief*, it is possible to remove the genetic nucleus of a cancer cell. Yet for several weeks or months, the cell will continue to live and behave in exactly the same *abnormal* way as before. So much for the power that is being attributed to the genes.

Biologists use the word 'silencing' to describe a process by which environment and behavior regulate gene expression and environmental *switches* that activate cancer. Genes comprise a complex blueprint that is constantly adapting to external changes and can either evolve with these changes or degrade with them. If the genetic blueprint degrades, you will experience a genetic mutation.

But these genetic blueprints are not capable of causing or perpetuating diseases. If they were, the cell would malfunction or die as soon as you removed its nucleus. A healthy cell continues to live perfectly normally for weeks on end, even if its nucleus has been removed. Likewise, an unhealthy cell will continue to exhibit unhealthy behavior, with or without genes.

Your DNA's main role is to make a copy (RNA) of its genetic blueprint, using it to produce the many different proteins needed for various functions in the body. To understand what cancer really is, we have to understand this important fact: the genetic blueprint of a cell mutates *only* when the information delivered to the cell from its external environment invokes a continuous stress response within the cell.

So what does this mean in practical terms? Each cell in the body is capable of producing adrenaline and other stress hormones, and it activates the fight-or-flight response when you perceive a threat, which can be either external or internal. People who feel scared often describe a jittery feeling throughout the body. They feel all the cells in the body literally vibrating with that fear response.

An external threat can consist of any number of influences coming from outside the body: artificial food additives like aspartame and MSG, an antibiotic or steroid drug, crossing a busy highway, the fear of facing an angry spouse or authority figure, losing a job, or a profound sense of insecurity.

Under the influence of the secreted stress hormones, normal cell functions become subdued. In fact, the genetic blueprint (DNA) receives atypical information that, in turn, alters the cell's gene behavior. Consequently, the DNA's production of natural chemicals, such as the anticancer drug Interleukin 2 and the antiviral drug Interferon, begins to drop instantly and significantly. The cell's health and defensive capabilities are seriously compromised if the threat or stress persists over a period longer than just a few minutes or hours. This kind of stress is a daily reality for millions of people in today's world. Cells cannot fulfill their normal responsibilities when they are under siege for days, months, or even years. Allopathic medicine has a name for this normal response by cells under prolonged stress – chronic disease.

When the body ingests a man-made drug (all pharmaceutical drugs contain toxic chemicals meant to suppress or otherwise manipulate natural processes in the body), it is injurious to its cells. Likewise, prolonged or regular exposure to such stressors as negative thoughts, fear, angry emotions, aggressive behavior, insufficient nourishment, inadequate amounts of sleep, lack of sun exposure, dehydration and toxins, can all alter the behavior of the body's 60–100 trillion cells.

Cancer occurs when cellular balance is threatened and the cell has to take recourse to extreme measures of defending or protecting itself. The weakest cells are often affected first.

The mutation of a normal cell to a cancer cell is merely a temporary, biologically programmed survival response to a threat that prevents the cell from doing its job according to the body's original genetic blueprint.

To deal with the threat appropriately, the body has to alter the genetic blueprint. But to interpret this necessary gene mutation as a disease process is farfetched and misleading.

The possibility that cancer is a healing and survival mechanism has never been considered in the past and is not part of the cancer discussion today. This has had, and still has, fatal consequences.

Not too long ago, *expert* scientists believed that the Earth was flat and stationary. After all, they saw with their own eyes that the sun fell off the horizon every evening and rose again every morning on the other side of the Earth's sphere. This indisputable *truth* was difficult to challenge because it was a phenomenon that the masses witnessed each and every day. They knew well that the entire natural world depended on sunrise and sunset, the cycles of day and night. Little did they realize that what they thought they saw was not all what was actually occurring.

Today, we only smile at such a notion of ignorance. It needed Columbus's voyage to the Americas in 1492 and finally Ferdinand Magellan's successful circumnavigation of the Earth from 1519–21 to provide the final, practical proofs of the Earth's round shape. Likewise, with modern diseases, and cancer especially, we are living by the same old myths handed down to us from generation to generation. Are we not also falling into the trap of blindly believing what other people have accepted as their subjective, personal truth?

But today it is different, you may argue, because we have objective, verifiable scientific research to prove what is real and what is not. I may have to disappoint you here.

First, almost all scientific research studies are actually based on the subjective ideas, feelings, thoughts and expectations of the scientist conducting the experiment – such is the very nature of a hypothesis.

Second, the research is subjected to an almost infinite number of possible and often highly variable influences, as well as simple human error, which can alter the outcome of the experiment in several unpredictable ways.

Third, because it is usually funded or controlled by agencies that have a certain agenda or bias, modern scientific research is often fraught with deceptive practices designed to manipulate its findings. For example, discoveries made by researchers at the University of California, published in the *Annals of Medicine* in October 2010, have shown that 92 percent of about 145 clinical trials conducted between 2008 and 2009 are invalid because they didn't disclose the type of placebo they used. In one case, by choosing a placebo that actually raises cholesterol in the control group, researchers could easily *prove* that a statin drug like Lipitor is more effective than the placebo. Yet the Federal Drug Administration (FDA) has sanctioned this obviously completely unscientific practice of *objective* scientific investigation.

When such biased and faulty research is allowed to stand on its own, that is bad enough. But often these questionable studies are used to support new studies, which in turn are also faulty. What's worse is when this chain of *scientific* falsehood negatively influences patient care. For example, the Mayo Clinic shocked the cancer establishment when it revealed that not only was an important 2009 study entirely fabricated, but that the discovery may also invalidate a decade's worth of other research, and had already influenced the care that doctors had been providing to their cancer patients.

Even if the fraud is uncovered and drug companies are fined for manipulating studies or for not disclosing known serious side effects, business more or less continues as usual. Large, publicly traded pharmaceutical companies like Merck and Pfizer are simply too big to fail, even if they are found guilty of instigating massive medical fraud.

It is unreasonable to expect that any clinical trial conducted by a drug giant would ever publish results unfavorable to their expectations. The conflict of interest seems clear – yet drug companies fund the vast majority of research studies in the world. This profit-based monopoly on what kind of research is suitable to conduct determines our so highly praised *science-based evidence*. It is such a dramatic conflict of interest that it is almost shocking that more people don't speak out about it.

Fourth, although there are still genuinely altruistic researchers who have no financial, career- or prestige-related interests in specific outcomes of their scientific investigations, much of modern science now rarely discovers anything that it did not already expect to find or validate.

Researchers require grants to conduct research. In order to become eligible for receiving these grants, as well as earn their own livelihoods, they have to make numerous concessions to further the financial gains of their sponsors or investors, who naturally expect a significant return on their investments.

For example, when genetic scientists proposed that genes control the body and behavior, they developed the highly profitable *Human Genome*

Project (HGO) to prove exactly that hypothesis. Sponsored by taxpayers' money as well as the drug companies who wanted a piece of the cake, these scientists had just one major objective: to fulfill the expectations of those pharmaceutical conglomerates to patent genes for new (and expensive) *breakthrough* treatments that could then generate vast amounts of wealth.

The mapping of human genes is widely publicized as an important step in the development of new medicines and other aspects of healthcare. The HGO remains one of the largest single investigative projects in modern science. Having nearly unrestricted access to the genetic makeup of the human body, genomics places medical science in the perfect position to predict more accurately those persons who are at high risk for developing genetic disorders.

As expected, most doctors, health-related organizations and patients consider the HGO to be a true breakthrough for everyone. Who in their right frame of mind could possibly object to the discovery of the genetic causes of disease? That's why, besides pharmaceutical companies, most disease-associated advocacy groups, foundations, governmental agencies, researchers, universities, biotechnology firms and pharmaceutical companies, all are on board with, and in support of, the Genome Project.

And while I am certainly not opposed to using genomics as a means of enhancing the scope and effectiveness of regenerative medicine, which is used to treat acute injuries like spinal cord damage and even to re-grow lost limbs and organs, I do see one major problem with it: the mass screening of the general population for genetic diseases will undoubtedly at least double or triple the number of patients who are deemed to *need* medical treatment, which then may make them legitimately sick. For the sake of *disease prevention,* millions of people will subject themselves to investigatory genetic testing so that they can *ensure* that they will not fall ill in the future, long before any signs of disease could possibly develop – only to damage their bodies through overzealous *treatments* of genetic findings that may otherwise have never caused them any trouble.

Unfortunately, many people in industrialized nations are already rolling out the red carpet for genomics as a foolproof way to live long lives free of sickness. Indoctrinated by the medical industry and coerced by their crippling fear of possible genetic illness, they believe they have no control over their body and therefore must submit themselves to a gene checkup. I consider this to be the ultimate form of medical enslavement; it is, however, being praised by seemingly everyone involved.

Yet the process of making up new diseases by discovering *problem genes* in nearly every person tested (most people have some faulty genes), or by renaming existing diseases as genetic diseases, is already well-established. For example, the identification of the breast cancer-susceptibility genes BRCA1 and BRCA2 evoked widespread interest in genetic testing among women at risk for a mutation in these genes. Among the women who have already tested positive for these mutated genes, over half of them voluntarily undergo full *elective mastectomies*. They choose to have their breasts amputated because they want to ensure they will never develop breast cancer.

But, of course, having one's breasts amputated is no guarantee that all one's potential troubles are over. In a Dutch study published in the *New England Journal of Medicine* in July 2001, [345:159-164], researchers caution that "the protective effect of prophylactic mastectomy must be weighed against possible surgical complications and psychological problems". According to the study, up to 30 percent of the women who undergo the procedure will have surgical complications, depending on the type of surgery and the length of follow-up. A long-term study of prophylactic mastectomy reported unanticipated repeated operations in 49 percent of women. That study also found that this procedure reduces the risk of breast cancer by only about 50 percent. Most shockingly, a later 2010 study demonstrated that indeed this increasingly popular practice of preventive mastectomy provides no benefit to 95 percent of women.

Although this is certainly unfortunate for the affected women, it serves as a great financial boost for the medical industry, including plastic surgeons. But performing these drastic, invasive and ineffective procedures, instead of encouraging women to address the real causes of breast cancer, is, in my opinion, playing a game of medical Russian roulette that is far too risky to be justified, no matter its profit potential.

Amputating an arm or a leg to prevent a possible fracture sounds illogical to most of us. Voluntarily amputating healthy breasts to prevent them from possibly becoming afflicted with cancer is really no less illogical. It is true that removing the entire breast may decrease the likelihood of breast cancer developing, but that is only by virtue of the fact that there is hardly any breast tissue left. This can scarcely be counted as proof that the susceptibility genes have anything to do with actually causing breast cancer. Having these genes show up in breasts suggests a possible correlation, but making the assumption that it is a cause-effect relationship is a questionable leap of logic. The gene mutation may just as well be crucial for the body to adjust to or heal the underlying causal condition: the physical environment that caused the susceptibility genes to mutate in the first place.

Since mutated genes alone are not capable of causing cancer, and the involvement of the cells' external environment, the whole organism and the person are necessary to make cancer even possible, it is much more likely that gene mutation is an effect of abnormal changes in the cell environment than it is a direct cause of cancer. Although a mutated gene may be a necessary co-factor for cancer to develop, if cancer does show up in the body, it merely indicates that your (and/or your parents') environment, dietary habits, lifestyles and psychological states and, most especially, exposure to harmful medical radiation, have already compromised your overall health and vitality. This makes genetic mutation an effect of cancer, not its cause.

Stunning research purportedly published by the American Medical Association (AMA) indicates that the so-called genetic basis for disease is completely bogus. Don't believe doctors who say disease is caused solely by your genetic code. It's all quackery!

According to a study by Dr. Ioannidis from the Stanford University School of Medicine, the popular myth that vigilant over-testing is the only way to prevent impending genetic diseases is extremely overstated. He asserts that contemporary medical research is riddled with mistakes as a result of "statistical vagaries coupled with human nature and the competitive nature of scientific publication". Though not intentionally fraudulent, many studies perpetuate medical inaccuracies because they interpret data to suit specific hypotheses or are based on data from other studies that have not been thoroughly verified by the medical community.

Dr. Ioannidis writes, "This is not fraud or poor study design, it's just statistical expectation. Some results will be stronger, some will be weaker. But scientific journals and researchers like to publish big associations." Researchers' analysis of data, even from well-designed studies, is often colored by their own biases or desire to create results that are accepted by the medical industry, thereby enabling them to support themselves and their work.

X-rayed to Death

Ionizing radiation produced by medical x-ray devices, including mammography and computed tomography (CT), causes electrons to be thrown out of their orbits and get detached from atoms or molecules. This ionizes the electrons and makes them highly reactive and damaging. These high frequency electromagnetic fields (EMFs) can severely damage the cells in your body by producing free radicals which can easily injure the body's DNA and compromise its cellular reproductive abilities.

Ionizing radiation may also directly damage DNA by ionizing or breaking DNA molecules (double-strand breaks), thereby contributing to mutations, chromosomal translocations and gene fusions, according to the Center for Radiological Research at Columbia University Medical Center, New York.

By damaging the cells, ionizing radiation can subsequently lead to cancer. And if cancer, the healing mechanism, is unable to correct or repair the damage, death may likely result. Most scientists believe that the resulting death is a direct cause of the cancer rather than the radiation; but as I will explain, the cancer is merely the body's attempt to deal with the damage of radiation and save itself.

According to a study published in November 2007 in the *New England Journal of Medicine*, since the inception of CT in the 1970s, an estimated 62 million CT scans per year were obtained in the United States, including at least 5 million for children. This is up from just 3 million in 1980.The lead researcher of the study, Dr. David Brenner of Columbia University, also estimated that overuse of diagnostic CT scans may cause up to 3 million excess cancers over the next 20 to 30 years.

CT is the largest contributor to medical radiation exposure in the U.S. population. And this ionizing radiation is particularly injurious to children, as even the NCI states:[7] "As a result, the risk for developing a radiation-

---

[7] http://www.cancer.gov/about-cancer/causes-prevention/risk/radiation/pediatric-ct-scans

related cancer can be several times higher for a young child compared with an adult exposed to an identical CT scan."

Children are in fact 10 times more sensitive to radiation than adults, which puts them at a higher risk of developing leukemia and other cancers than adults. For leukemia, the minimum time period between the radiation exposure and the appearance of disease (latency period) is two years. For solid tumors, the latency period is estimated to be more than five years.

This is indeed troubling news for parents and their children, which is further substantiated by major national and international organizations responsible for evaluating radiation risk. They all "agree there probably is no low-dose radiation 'threshold' for inducing cancers, i.e., no amount of radiation should be considered absolutely safe," says the NCI. According to this online report, "recent data from the atomic bomb survivors and other irradiated populations demonstrate small, but significant, increases in cancer risk even at the low levels of radiation that are relevant to pediatric CT scans."

In other words, concerned parents who take their children to the hospital for a CT scan, for whatever reason, may in fact be gambling with their kids' lives. They may need to weigh the risks between some relatively minor complication and an uncertain potential of leukemia and other cancers. At least, they could request ultrasound scans for stomachaches or mild head trauma, which are just as effective as a CT scan for diagnosing many conditions.

This is not to say that ultrasound is 100 percent safe either. Many studies have demonstrated that prenatal ultrasounds may damage a child's biochemistry, immune system and nervous system. Renowned medical researcher Alice Stewart also found in her Oxford Child Cancer Study that children exposed to prenatal ultrasounds had higher rates of juvenile leukemia.

However, the risk is still lower than the powerful x-rays of CT scans, which were proven to cause leukemia even in the 1950s. As David Brenner of Columbia University told USA Today: "About one-third of all CT scans that are done right now are medically unnecessary ... Virtually anyone who presents in the emergency room with pain in the belly or a chronic headache will automatically get a CT scan. Is that justified?"

It is especially important to understand these risks when caring for children, who are more vulnerable than adults to the effects of these diagnostic procedures. One 2011 study found that an infant has an eight times higher risk of suffering from a fatal cancer caused by an abdominal CT scan than a 50 year old receiving the same procedure. The results of this study were published online on January 3, 2011 in the *Archives of Pediatrics and Adolescent Medicine* [DOI: 10.1001/archpediatrics.2010. 270]. In the study, researchers from the University of Michigan examined the use of x-rays, CT scans and other medical radiation in children and found the average child will, on average, receive seven imaging procedures utilizing radiation by age 18. (This study didn't include dental x-rays, which pose an additional risk.)

The study found that not only are children more sensitive to radiation than adults, but they also tend to receive 2 to 6 times the radiation needed to produce clear images, because CT scans given to kids are often calibrated for adults. Even when safety precautions to reduce the radiation doses for children are in place, they are not widely implemented.

CT scans alone will cause nearly 30,000 unnecessary cancer cases a year, which will lead to about 14,500 deaths, according to another study published in the *Archives of Internal Medicine* [Cancer Risks and Radiation Exposure From Computed Tomographic Scans; 2009;169(22):2049-2050].

A list of cancers considered to be radiogenic was published by the U.S. Environmental Protection Agency, Washington DC, September 1999, *Federal Guidance Report No.13*, EPA 402-R-99-001. They include cancers of the esophagus, stomach, colon, liver, lung, bone, skin, breast, ovary, bladder, kidney, thyroid and leukemia. In other words, any and all of these cancers could develop because of unnecessary radiation absorbed through commonplace diagnostic procedures.

Yet another rarely considered risk is that radiation scans often result in misdiagnosis and false positives, increasing the likelihood of follow-up scans, and subsequently more radiation, possibly starting a vicious cycle.

Ionizing radiation not only increases the risk of cancer, but also causes DNA damage in the arteries, leading to cardiovascular disease. Remember, a CT scan of the chest delivers 100 times the radiation of a conventional chest x-ray. This can be enough to cause irreversible DNA and cell damage in already inflamed coronary arteries. It can, in fact, further increase arterial narrowing and decrease vessel elasticity, thereby increasing arterial blockage.

Even if one CT scan may not immediately kill cells, each additional exposure to x-rays or other ionizing radiation can turn out to be fatal. I therefore consider it highly risky to use ionizing radiation on anyone who suffers from an illness, especially cancer, heart disease and diabetes. Ultimately, ionizing radiation is really not safe for anyone.

What about dental x-rays?

For 30 years now I have warned both patients and dentists about the great risk resulting from dental x-rays and to use alternative ways to detect dental problems instead. According to published research, dental x-rays can cause deadly brain tumors.

Medical Diagnosis –
The Single Most Common Cause of Death?

According to the late medical researcher John Gofman, M.D., Ph.D., (1918–2007), Professor Emeritus of Molecular and Cell Biology at the University of California at Berkeley, evidence suggests that at least 50 percent of deaths from cancer and more than 60 percent of deaths from coronary artery disease may be induced by x-rays. This would include a minimum of 281,437 deaths from cancer and 369,640 from heart disease each year, based on 2010 mortality data for these disorders provided by the Centers for Disease Control and Prevention (CDCP). Accordingly, the total annual number of deaths from radiation injury would amount to 651,077 (as of 2010).

In addition to medical technology leading so many people to their death through ionizing radiation, Dr. Gofman claimed to have evidence that shows it also causes 75 percent of new cancers. Since this is an extremely shocking discovery, it deserves further explanation.

Gofman was the author of several books and more than a hundred scientific papers in peer review journals in fields such as nuclear/physical chemistry, coronary heart disease, the relationship of human chromosomes to cancer and the biological effects of radiation, with special reference to causation of cancer and hereditary injury.

In an article entitled "Radiation: Cure or Cause?", published in *Report Newsmagazine* on January 22, 2001, author Marnie Ko describes Dr. Gofman's research and raises the sort of critical questions we should all have asked the medical community a long time ago. Dr. Gofman was the first eminent scientist who had the guts to confront the scientific community with the scientific evidence that ionizing radiation is the leading contributing factor behind cancer and coronary heart disease.

Dr. Gofman's research findings were unwelcome news for those who claimed they were fighting the battle against cancer, when in reality they were the ones who helped create the reasons for the battle.

Others who were profiting greatly from the cancer business were particularly reprehensible. Among them was Dr. John Radomsky, president of the Canadian Association of Radiologists. Although he admitted he had not read Gofman's study, and a substantial amount of research had already been published on the risk of radiation causing cancer, he nevertheless insisted that "radiation safety is not an issue".

Some could not admit they were directly, albeit unintentionally, contributing to the death of many of their patients by exposing them to deadly rays. In 1996, British radiologists tried to prevent a documentary on Dr. Gofman's work from being shown on 20/20 Television. The Royal College of Radiologists called his conclusions "unsound, inaccurate, misleading, and unnecessarily alarmist". They were not, however, able to pass judgment on the soundness of Dr. Gofman's research which, with or without his conclusions, spoke for itself.

Dr. Gofman was certainly no conspiracy theorist, nor was he a celebrity-seeking oddball who needed to make a name for himself. He was a lecturer at the University of California School of Medicine since 1947. He was a co-inventor of the portable VIDA heart monitor, used by patients to detect and signal episodes of cardiac arrhythmias, and the inventor of a cardiographic electrode still used in many hospitals throughout the U.S. In his early years as a nuclear scientist, Dr. Gofman co-discovered uranium-233 and was instrumental in isolating the first milligram of plutonium. Later, in the 1940s, he led a team of researchers in the discovery of the role of lipoproteins, now known as cholesterol.

Dr. Gofman's research on radiation hazards stemmed from his profound concern about the well-being and future health of humankind.

His warning that most new cancers are the result of ionizing forms of medical radiation from seemingly non-invasive diagnostic tools, including x-rays, computed tomography (CT) scans, mammograms and fluoroscopy, was not based on suspicion, but on existing research data and evidence. Basically, all he did was to analyze the full spectrum of existing scientific data available in this area of research – something that had never been done before. This uncovered the enormous scope of the ever-escalating problem.

Gofman's discovery of the deadly connection between heart disease and low-level radiation led him to produce a demographic and statistical analysis to evaluate the effects of medical radiation on an entire population.

In 1999, Dr. Gofman completed his 699-page study which was published by The Committee for Nuclear Responsibility (CNR), based in San Francisco. It concluded that "since its introduction in 1896, medical radiation has become a necessary co-factor in most fatal cases of Cancer and Ischemic Heart Disease (IHD)". It particularly names x-rays, CT scans and the like – combined with other risk factors such as poor diet, smoking, abortions and use of birth control pills – as the major cause of cancer fatalities.

Gofman carefully analyzed all possible causal factors (co-factors) and separated the cancer-causing effects of ionizing radiation from all other risk factors.

The concept of *necessary* co-factors is not new to modern science. In the famous 1964 Surgeon General's Report on cigarette smoking as a cause of lung cancer, the authors wrote: "It is recognized that often the co-existence of several factors is required for the occurrence of a disease, and that one of the factors may play a dominant role; that is, without it, the other factors (such as genetic susceptibility) seldom lead to the occurrence of the disease."

Gofman's assumption, of more than one cause per case of cancer, has subsequently been confirmed by Dr. Kramer and other leading cancer experts.

Although the rate of breast cancer is higher in women who inherit one mutated copy of a breast cancer susceptibility gene (BRCA1 or BRCA2) than in women without that inheritance, "that inheritance certainly does not guarantee the development of breast cancer in every breast-cell – even though every breast-cell contains the mutation," said Dr. Gofman.

Yet as Dr. Kramer stated, mutation alone is not sufficient to cause cancer or make it progress. Gofman made the assertion that one or more additional causes are necessary in order to turn even one of those breast-cells into a cancer. In Chapters Two, Three and Five, I point to a whole list of co-factors, several of which must be in place for cancer to develop and progress. As we can derive from Dr. Gofman's work, ionizing radiation must be one of the causal factors for cancer to develop.

In other words, radiation alone cannot cause cancer. Likewise, a poor diet alone cannot cause cancer. And as stated before, cigarette smoking alone cannot cause cancer either. Emotional stress alone is also not sufficiently able to induce cancer growth. Cancer involves the whole person: diet, lifestyle, relationships, society and environment. This is a very important point to understand.

If just one of the necessary co-factors is absent, then cancer cannot occur. Consequently, a combination of a chronic vitamin D deficiency due to a lack of regular sun exposure, having a bi-annual mammogram, eating junk foods laced with hydrogenated vegetable oils, and going through a lengthy stressful divorce may be enough to induce breast cancer. Such an outcome would not occur, for example, if this woman ate a wholesome diet and didn't get the mammograms. And if she also spent a good amount of time in the sun, the likelihood of developing cancer would be highly remote.

"By definition, absence of a *necessary* co-factor prevents the result," says Dr. Gofman. Knowing this makes it possible for anyone to prevent and even reverse cancer, simply by removing some or all of the existing co-factors.

Obviously, some co-factors are of a greater consequence than others. Dr. Gofman found that medical radiation, in particular, is a highly important co-factor of cancer and IHD mortality. He says that in the *absence* of medical radiation, many or most of the cases would not have occurred when they did. His research led to this poignant, startling conclusion: While medical radiation has not been the *only* factor contributing to such cases, we mean that it has been a *necessary* co-factor in such cases.

In his study, Dr. Gofman compared death rates from cancer and ischemic heart disease between 1940 and 1990 in each of the nine census divisions of the U.S. with the average number of medical doctors per 100,000 population. He made the assumption that because physicians prescribe most tests or treatments involving x-rays, the number of administered x-ray applications should be approximately proportional to the number of doctors serving the population.

His research uncovered this astonishing connection: Death rates from cancer and ischemic heart disease increased in direct proportion to the number of physicians in each of the nine census districts. In comparison, death rates from almost all other causes declined as physician density increased. In other words, wherever more x-rays were prescribed, that's also where more people died from these two leading *killer diseases*.

Before Wilhelm Conrad Roentgen discovered the x-ray in 1895 and x-ray applications became popular, cancer and coronary arterial disease were uncommon. Although x-rays have helped save many lives since then, they have also taken many more lives than that. While x-rays may be useful for specific diagnostic situations, including bone fractures, there are alternative methods such as ultrasound technology – or better yet, thermal imaging technology – that are at least as effective, but without the same side effects.

Thermal imaging technology is a non-invasive, non-destructive test method which I believe is far superior to x-rays and ultrasound. It can detect the development of a tumor, often years before x-rays can, without the harmful side effects associated with radiation from other diagnostic methods. Seeing a thermal imbalance depicting a circulatory disturbance in the breast, for example, can help a person make the necessary changes to prevent a manifestation of the imbalanced condition into a tumor later in life.

Thermology is the medical science that derives diagnostic indications from diagnostic-quality infrared images of the human body through the use of highly-resolute and sensitive infrared (thermographic) cameras. Breast thermography utilizes the principles of thermology as a diagnostic technique in the early detection of breast cancer in a clinical setting or as a monitor of its treatment. Breast thermography is completely non-contact and imparts no form of radiation energy onto or into the body. Its accuracy rate in detecting cancerous tumors in the breast is (as of 2009) 94.8 percent, according to a comparative study published in the *Journal of Medical Systems* [April, 2009;33(2):141-53]. In comparison, mammography boasts an accuracy rate of only 45–50 percent.

The catch? Thermal imaging cameras are relatively inexpensive compared to CT or similar imaging technologies. Hence, they rake in a lot less money for the medical industry. Perhaps this is the reason they are rarely being employed by hospitals and general practitioners.

Pretty much everyone agrees that when it comes to cancer, prevention is the best cure. Nevertheless, despite the fact that less dangerous (and often more effective) methods of diagnosis and prevention are available, the medical industry continues to insist that only CTs and ultrasounds are reliable. Yet this attitude, however financially profitable, is only exacerbating the problem. In most cases, avoiding ionizing radiation and some other co-factors of cancer are sufficient for a person to remain cancer-free.

We are only just beginning to witness the consequences of overly relying on modern technology rather than human diagnostic skills and medical intuition. The latter were pivotal to such ancient forms of medicine as Ayurveda and traditional Chinese medicine. Today, it seems a lot easier to let a machine determine symptoms of disease instead of using human observational and inquisitive skills to figure out what causes these symptoms.

Sophisticated medical tests appear to reduce errors of medical diagnosis, which is supposed to reduce the incidence or likelihood of lawsuits against medical doctors. Medical diagnosis is also supposed to save lives. Medical errors, however, have never been so frequent and serious as they are now, and malpractice lawsuits abound.

In fact, according to an article written by Dr. Barbara Starfield, M.D., M.P.H., of the Johns Hopkins School of Hygiene and Public Health, published medical errors may be the third leading cause of death in the United States. At least 225,000 deaths per year in the U.S. (as of 2000) result from iatrogenic causes (iatrogenic means doctor-caused, either from misdiagnosis or the medical treatment).[8]

Since according to the FDA only between 1 and 10 percent of medical errors are ever reported, the true figure of doctor-caused deaths each year may actually be in the millions, and as a result far outweigh the death rates from cancer and heart disease combined. According to the report, based on the lowest estimate, more people die from medical mistakes than from highway accidents, breast cancer or AIDS.

Of course I personally don't blame the medical doctors for this malaise. Most doctors are genuine healers and are committed to helping their

---

[8]*Journal of the American Medical Association (JAMA)*, Vol. 284, No. 4, July 26, 2000

patients as best as they can, or rather, according to what they were taught to do, or rather, what they were *not* taught. In a study published in the *New England Journal of Medicine* [1993 (January 28); 328 (4): 246-252], researchers pointed out the near-complete lack of knowledge about use of unconventional forms of medicine by their patients. They made these concluding remarks: "We suggest that medical schools include information about unconventional therapies and the clinical social sciences (anthropology and sociology) in their curriculums. The newly established National Institutes of Health Office for the Study of Unconventional Medical Practices should help promote scholarly research and education in this area."

The prevailing attitude in conventional medicine is that modern medicine as taught in medical schools is the only scientific, proven and trustworthy form of medicine around. Homeopathy, Ayurveda, traditional Chinese medicine, chiropractic, herbal medicine, acupuncture, tai chi, yoga, meditation, exercise and even prayer don't *belong* in the field of *real* medicine, even though in some instances they have been proven far more effective than conventional medicine.

For one thing, unlike conventional medicine, unconventional medicine doesn't kill millions of people each year. What's most astonishing is that conventional medicine is still being portrayed as the most advanced system of medicine we have ever had, when there is actually very little science behind it.

An editorial, "Where is the Wisdom? The Poverty of Medical Evidence," by *British Medical Journal*'s editor, Dr. Richard Smith [*BMJ* 1991 (October 5); 303: 798-799], explains the dilemma of our medical system. The article quotes a sobering statement made by renowned health policy consultant, David Eddy, professor of health policy and management at Duke University, North Carolina. "There are perhaps 30,000 biomedical journals in the world, and they have grown steadily by 7% a year since the seventeenth century," writes Dr. Smith, "**yet only about 15% of medical interventions are supported by solid scientific evidence,**" said Dr. Eddy.

"This is partly because only 1% of the articles in medical journals are scientifically sound, and partly because many treatments have never been assessed at all," according to Dr. Smith. Why is that? One of the reasons is because, as discussed earlier in the book, most of those articles quote from other articles which make unsupported and unfounded claims, according to Dr. Smith.

Dr. Eddy adds an even more disturbing perspective to this predicament. For numerous reasons, he began to question the logic and legitimacy of the treatments he was obliged to use in his medical practice. Dr. Eddy began his medical life as a cardiothoracic surgeon at Stanford University in California. Soon he began to investigate standard medical treatments to assess in detail the evidence supporting those treatments.

To find such evidence, he searched published medical reports dating back to 1906 but could not find randomized controlled trials for the majority of standard treatments. Later he traced back the conventional statements in textbooks and medical journals on standard treatments and found that they had simply been handed down from generation to generation, including treatments ranging from basic glaucoma to blockages of the femoral and popliteal arteries, as well ascolorectal cancer. In other words, he found little *real* science; instead, mostly oral tradition and hearsay. Practitioners and advocates of *unconventional* natural healing methods may find such an accusation awfully familiar.

There are countless examples of medical treatments that have been proven to not work, yet they are routinely administered to millions of patients. In the article, Believing in Treatments That Don't Work *(Well, 2009)*, emergency room physician Dr. David H Newman, M.D., explains how medical ideology often replaces evidence-based medicine.

For instance, medical ideology dictates to give beta-blockers to patients who just suffered a heart attack following an abrupt clotting of a coronary artery. In the early moments after a heart attack, the stunned heart often beats quickly and forcefully. For decades, doctors have administered beta-blockers to calm a straining heart. This *logical* approach, however, is not at all supported by scientific evidence. To the contrary, 26 out of 28 studies show that the early administration of beta-blockers to heart attack victims does not save lives but, in fact, takes lives.

For example, in 2005, the largest study on the drugs showed that beta-blockers in the vulnerable, early hours of heart attacks caused a definite increase in heart failure.[9] "Consequently, it might generally be prudent to consider starting beta-blocker therapy in hospital only when

---

[9] *Lancet*, 2005 November 5; 366(9497):1622-32

the hemodynamic condition after MI has stabilized," say the researchers of this study.

Contrary to the large majority of the medical community, I have always held the belief that the forceful reaction of the heart after a heart attack is about the best possible way to save itself and the body. Giving beta-blockers to reduce the heart's consumption of limited oxygen supplies, but suppressing heart function at this crucial moment, is both questionable and risky. To undo the blockage, the heart needs to pump more forcefully, not less. Yet again, the body has its own perfect survival strategies that have an edge over the interventions provided by man-made medicine.

Although the use of these drugs immediately following a heart attack has been scientifically proven to increase the incidence of fatal heart failure, most doctors still believe it is a validated, science-backed medical treatment. I call it legalized quackery.

This is a list of other examples where doctors' ideology contradicts scientific evidence:

- Antidepressants such as Prozac, though riddled with harmful side effects, continue to be distributed to millions of people despite countless studies which have demonstrated that they are no more effective in fighting depression than the placebo.
- The success record of modern cancer therapy is significantly less than even the weakest placebo response. On average, remission occurs in only about 7 percent of cancer patients.
- Evidence suggests that the antibiotics taken for ear infections, bronchitis, sinusitis and sore throats actually harm them more than help them. Yet doctors continue to prescribe these drugs to more than 1 in 7 Americans every year, causing myriad side effects that often require further treatment, costing about $2 billion per year, and contributing to the development of superbugs that resist all known medical treatments.
- Doctors perform approximately 600,000 back surgeries each year, at a cost of over $20 billion. This is in spite of the fact that, in the majority of cases, these surgeries have not been proven to be any more effective than non-surgical treatments.
- Studies have shown that arthroscopic surgery to correct osteoarthritis of the knee is no more effective than *sham* surgeries,

in which surgeons place patients under light anesthesia while they imitate surgery. These surgeries are also no more effective than non-invasive physical therapy. Nevertheless, over 500,000 Americans undergo approximately $3 billion worth of these surgeries every year.

- Although cough syrups have never been proven to have benefits, but actually have been shown to seriously harm and kill children, they are still routinely recommended by doctors. In young children, over-the-counter (OTC) cold and cough medicines can cause serious side effects, including abnormal heart rhythms, seizures, cessation of breathing and death. In fact, complications and overdoses from these so-called safe OTC medications account for two-thirds of children's emergency room visits, as reported by CDCP researchers in the medical journal *Pediatrics* (November 2010). Two-thirds of these cases resulted from leaving the drugs unsupervised where children could get hold of them, and one-third of these ER visits were in cases where dosage was intentional and in the correct amount. All this is in spite of a 2007 FDA ban on administering cough medicines to children under four years of age.

The expense and dismal success rates of each of these treatments, among many others, beg the question as to why we continue to use them. The allure of treatment based on modern medicine's *there's-a-pill-for-everything* mentality is unmistakable. We subject ourselves to tests and treatments because of our faith in them as symbols, in spite of their actual effects. In failing to understand and trust the body as a comprehensive system with its own natural healing mechanisms, we find comfort in the idea of quick fixes.

But that does not address the uncomfortable truth that many of these expensive, invasive, ineffective and/or harmful interventions ultimately only seem to make us sicker. We must instead ask ourselves the tough questions: Will this antibiotic really help heal my minor sinus infection? Do I really need this back surgery? Is chemotherapy really the only way to get rid of my cancer? Am I ready to look at the data instead of the ideology? Am I ready for the evidence? The truth?

And though the medical industry wants you to feel as though time-tested natural prevention and healing methods are all simply quackery, it's not only medical heretics in the wilderness calling for a re-assessment of our modern medical attitude. The ever-increasing evidence speaks for itself: our beliefs about modern medicine are killing us in increasing numbers.

And even on the rare occasions when those agencies charged with monitoring the medical industry make decisions based on actual patient care instead of the bottom line, these decisions often come much delayed and fail to truly address the root causes of this dire situation.

For example, the FDA made headlines in March 2011 when it announced that it would pull from the market roughly 500 unapproved prescription drugs that it had allowed to be sold for decades. Many of these drugs, including Pediahist, Cardec, Rondec, and hundreds of others, have been prescribed since before the FDA even established its approval process. They claim that the new measures are in response to findings made through their adverse event reporting system. But the crackdown also means that hundreds of drugs will now likely be put through the FDA's approval system, thus bringing in millions of dollars of new revenue. Meanwhile, the FDA seems to be doing very little to address the many reports of serious complications stemming from already-approved drugs, such as the HPV (human papilloma virus) vaccine Gardasil, for instance.

What Happened to Personal Freedom?

It is clear that even government watchdog agencies don't always have a patient's best interests at heart. Ultimately, individual knowledge is our own best defense in a medical environment increasingly obsessed with profits over patients, and built on a shaky foundation of tampered scientific evidence and half-truths.

Yet what is perhaps most frightening about today's medical environment is that, because traditional medical diagnosis is regarded as so sacrosanct, patients have increasingly little choice in how to treat and heal their bodies. Despite the dismal effects of medically orthodox treatments, individual freedom to choose alternative healing methods for treating illness is increasingly under attack, especially when it comes to a parent's right to discern what is best for his or her child. In fact, if you take your child to a medical doctor, the diagnosis may end up causing you to be charged with murder.

The medical industrial complex received an unprecedented victory in recent years in the case of Kristen LaBrie. A 38 year old mother of an autistic son diagnosed with cancer was charged, tried and ultimately convicted of attempted murder, reckless endangerment and several other charges, all for simply trying to protect her son from poisonous chemotherapy. She testified, to no avail, that it was her earnest impression that the chemotherapy treatments were killing her son faster than his cancer ever could have. Rather than continuing to put her child through the pain and suffering that the chemotherapy inflicted, she stopped administering the drugs. But her heartfelt concern for her son was ultimately awarded with 40 years in prison!

It is a deeply disturbing example of the extent to which the government and the medical industry will go to do what it has decided is *best* for children – even if mounting data and evidence suggest that conventional treatments are ineffective or even counter-productive.

Faced with more and more of such costly, ineffective and often downright harmful conventional medical *wisdom*, it is little wonder that people are increasingly turning to alternative medicine. In response, the medical industry is amping up its rhetoric against these often commonsense treatments. Yet the increasing popularity and success of alternative medicine in improving the lives of millions of people in the past 30 to 40 years has led to an increased aggressiveness and arrogance – on behalf of the representatives of conventional medicine who claim theirs is the only science-based medicine and that alternative approaches to medical healthcare are therefore not supported. Most of them actually believe in this fallacy. They still claim that established medical practices are backed by scientific evidence, although no such evidence exists for more than but a small fraction of them.

The 2003 article, Death by Medicine, written by Gary Null, Ph.D.; Carolyn Dean M.D., N.D.; Martin Feldman, M.D.; Debora Rasio, M.D.; and Dorothy Smith, Ph.D. paint a very different picture. Their fully referenced report proves that:

- 2.2 million people experience in-hospital, adverse reactions to prescribed drugs per year

- 20 million unnecessary antibiotics are prescribed annually for viral infections
- 7.5 million unnecessary medical and surgical procedures are performed annually
- 8.9 million people are exposed to unnecessary hospitalization every year
- 783,936 people per year die as a result of medical error and side effects of medical treatment

It is truly ironic that we seem to give more credence to a young and mostly unproven system of medicine than to the ancient systems of medicine that have kept entire civilizations healthy for thousands of years. Today's highly *advanced* diagnostic applications and treatments used by conventional medicine have the power to create a massive cancer pandemic and suppress people's immune systems for generations to come. Meanwhile, natural methods of disease diagnosis and treatment are being ignored, even purposefully suppressed.

When I studied Ayurvedic medicine two decades ago, we were taught the 6,000 year old method of "pulse reading" which allowed us to detect any kind of imbalance in any part of the body within less than one minute. Moreover, any good Ayurvedic physician can trace any symptom of disease back to its root cause without the use of costly blood tests, EKGs or x-rays. Our fascination and focus ought to be with the causes of illness rather than its symptoms.

We have all been taught that modern medicine is the savior of life. Billions of dollars are spent each year on studying everything that could cause us to become ill, including bacteria, viruses, toxins and even sunshine! The work of Dr. Gofman and others shows that the atrociously destructive effects of medical radiation by far exceeds all other causes of illness and death taken together, including drug side effects, medical errors and accidents. Diagnosis of disease is meant to prevent disease or help us find our way back to health, not make us more ill and possibly die.

The Hippocratic Oath, historically taken by medical doctors swearing to practice medicine ethically, states: "I will prescribe regimens for the good of my patients according to my ability and my judgment and never do harm to anyone." It also says, "I will not give a lethal drug to anyone if I am asked."

According to the General Medical Council (GMC), the duties of a doctor must include the following rules:

- Make the care of your patient your first concern
- Protect and promote the health of patients and the public
- Keep your professional knowledge and skills up to date

The Greeks were the first to introduce a complete separation between killing and curing. Until then, in much of the primitive world, the doctor and the sorcerer were one and the same person. He had the power to kill and he had power to cure. In a way, in spite of all the technological advancement in the medical field, we have ironically regressed to a primitive world where those who had the power to cure would also be permitted to kill. Now, once again, doctors have a license to kill. They can ignore such evidence that ionizing radiation kills scores of patients, that vaccines can cause the outbreaks of deadly diseases they are supposed to prevent,[10] or that prescription drugs do nothing to actually cure diseases, they just suppress symptoms and create new diseases because of the side effects they produce.

The United States medical boards punish doctors (as well as bereaved parents like Kristen LaBrie) who wish to do no harm to their patients and do not want to prescribe dangerous medication or diagnostic tests to them. These morally ethical doctors will have their licenses revoked and may also be sued for medical negligence.

I personally experienced the deadly connection between diagnosis and severe illness when I was just 17 years of age. My father was wrongly diagnosed with a rare kidney condition. The administered drug treatment generated horrendous side effects that caused his slim body to swell up four times its normal size within one week. I could not even recognize him. Eventually, the error in the medical diagnosis was acknowledged, but the harsh treatment had already taken its toll, damaging my father's heart. Further treatment perforated his stomach, and he died at the age of 54, after one year of a gruesome, bedridden existence.

Why were these medical technologies never tested for side effects when they were first introduced to hospitals, doctors and their patients? I will come back to this important question later in the book.

---

[10] See my book, *Vaccine-nation: Poisoning the Population, One Shot at a Time.*

Everyday Radiation

Indeed, harmful radiation can come from more than just medical technology. It has invaded our everyday lives in many forms, particularly through technological gadgets and new appliances. For example, according to research which I will discuss in detail in Chapter Two, by getting into close proximity to a cell (mobile) phone, even the emitted non-ionizing radiation causes the single- and/or double-DNA strand to break in regions and produce so-called heat shock proteins (HSP).

Our cells produce these proteins in order to counteract harmful stimuli. Regular exposure to these unnatural forms of radiation can lead to serious stress damage and numerous gene mutations. In other words, repeated or regular exposure to both ionizing and non-ionizing radiation can lead to an entire range of *diseases* that medical science subsequently groups into the category of gene-caused disorders.

The discoveries by genetic researchers of an ever-increasing number of mutated genes in people afflicted with cancers and other alleged diseases have diverted our attention away from the real causes of what is damaging our body. Herein lies the true danger of the Human Genome Project. With all the vast amounts of resources spent on researching the human DNA, in not a single case has the knowledge of the DNA sequence of any particular gene contributed to the cure of cancer. Like all the previous promises made by medical science that "we are about to create a cure for cancer", genomic medicine has already failed to make any significant difference.

Both academicians and laypeople alike believe genetic research is going to shape the future of medicine, but nobody can clearly define exactly what that means. Gene research is not as clear-cut as some want us and genome investors to believe.

An article entitled "State of the Art" in the February 13, 2011 issue of the prestigious German paper *Die Süddeutsche Zeitung* provided a realistic overview of the state of gene research. Although the sequences of most of the 3.2 billion DNA base pairs have been decoded, this only covers the genes' building materials, according to the article. Virtually nothing is known about their interplay and relationship of DNA, RNA, proteins, life circumstances and environmental conditions. The paper states that we know just as little about how many genes the human body has, although it is estimated there are 20–22 thousand.

If the estimates are correct, we have over 60 billion DNA base pairs that we know very little about! What makes genome interpretation so unreliable and potentially misleading is the fact that the DNA sequence in one person will always differ from that of another person. No two people have the same DNA – that much is obvious. But this unpredictability factor makes it impossible to determine what is normal in the genome and what isn't. After all, we are not identical machines, but unique in many more ways than we are the same.

It is widely assumed that the human body uses only 1.5 percent of its genome for the production of proteins. Nothing is known about the role of the other 98.5 percent of the DNA – it has even been arrogantly nicknamed *junk DNA*. It is foolhardy to believe that the body does not make use of it. Yet again, it seems we are playing with something incredibly complex and profound, without being aware that we do not have even the basic knowledge of how it works. To base an entirely new technology on something we are almost completely ignorant about is highly irresponsible.

We have already begun to see, for example, the devastating consequences of producing genetically modified foods: millions of acres of GM crops are now failing because of the manipulation of some of the most powerful laws of nature – thanks to irresponsible shortsightedness and corporate greed. Many of us are already familiar with the serious consequences that arise from tampering with genes in our foods.

Without being aware of it, every day, hundreds of millions of people already consume *Frankenstein* foods that may cause permanent alterations to the DNA. These mutations in the DNA allow us to process these foods that have never existed on the planet before, but this 'adjustment' ultimately results in little-understood, yet permanent, abnormalities. GM foods have never scientifically been shown to be safe for anyone. In fact, no peer-reviewed publications of clinical studies on the human health effects of GM food even exist. We are asked instead simply to trust those who manufacture (and profit from) these genetically altered foods. However, dozens of studies and reviews show that GM foods fed to animals cause cancers, stomach and intestinal damage, and numerous other symptoms of severely disrupted homeostasis – even death.

Which of course begs the question, why in the world would we want to eat these foods? Thankfully, the global conversation has resulted in a few positive steps. Most European countries have banned the importation of GM foods. However, this greatly annoys the U.S. government, which is the world's biggest promoter and producer of GM foods. And since GM food producers in the U.S. are not legally obligated to label GM foods (as of 2012), the GM food-to-cancer link in humans is virtually impossible to establish.

It would seem logical that, if we are not yet capable of safely engineering the genes of even the most basic foods, we are certainly nowhere near being able to genetically *cure* diseases. Yet despite our superficial understanding of all its workings and implications, genomic medicine is widely vetted to become the *new medicine* of this century. In fact, genomics is already playing an increasingly important role in the diagnosis, monitoring and treatment of diseases, creating new and expensive diagnostic technology and costly pharmaceutical drugs.

Not surprisingly, biotechnology companies are already heavily involved in designing diagnostic tests used to confirm a medical opinion when a particular condition is suspected based on genetic mutations and symptoms. And since all diseases have a genetic component – whether inherited or resulting from the body's response to environmental stresses like radiation, viruses or toxins – the implications for increasing the scope and influence (and, therefore, the financial profits) of genomic medicine are simply unlimited.

Drug design is shifting toward creating new classes of medicines related to information on gene sequence and protein structure function, rather than the traditional trial-and-error method. The new drugs target just specific sites in the body, thereby promising to have fewer side effects than many of today's medicines, which in turn makes doctors and patients more open to using them. This new branch of pharmacology is known as pharmacogenomics, and is already being used for all critical illnesses like cancer, cardiovascular disorders, HIV, tuberculosis, asthma and diabetes.

Gene therapy, which uses normal genes to replace or supplement defective genes, is considered to be the most exciting application of DNA science. Although I don't dispute that this approach could be helpful in repairing gene defects in people who have certain specific inherited diseases, such as hemophilia, I have strong reservations about, for example, bolstering immunity by adding a gene that suppresses tumor growth. This is because I believe in the holistic interconnectedness of individual health. To illustrate, would it make sense to replace the floor of a house whose entire foundation has already rotted and started to sink? Certainly not. Instead, it is much wiser and more fruitful to address the foundation first: to repair the decay, prevent further damage and restore its ability to hold up the rest of the building. Similarly, implanting a shiny new gene into a body that is already racked with toxins, malnourished and under stress is hardly a smart way to go about treating disease.

To truly heal a whole person, we must restore homeostasis throughout the body, not just fix a flaw in one or several of its many parts. Boosting the immune system unnaturally can be just as risky as suppressing it. We really don't have a clue about the long-term effects that tampering with our genes can entail, for us and for our offspring. It just hasn't been done before.

It is one thing to be born with an inherited genetic defect that manifests itself as a rare disorder such as thalassemia, hemophilia, Down syndrome, muscular dystrophy, hemochromatosis or neurofibromatosis. But it is an entirely different story when a person acquires gene mutations over a number of years because of lifestyle changes or detrimental influences in the environment.

The majority of disorders are multifactorial or polygenic, which means they involve the effects of multiple genes in combination with lifestyle and environmental changes. Such disorders include cancer, heart disease, diabetes, multiple sclerosis (MS), asthma, hypertension, obesity and infertility. Although these disorders tend to run in families, the inheritance does not fit into simple patterns as with true genetic diseases. Yet the Genome Project attempts to make that connection even in places where it doesn't exist.

More and more diseases are being included into the Genome program through the discovery of mutated genes that show up during or before disease manifestation. However, this only further alienates people from their own body. After all, we are taught to believe that we have no control over our genes. Genes control us, or do they?

Russian researchers have repeatedly demonstrated that genes can be repaired and organs can be regrown without having to take recourse to stem cell therapy or other expensive treatments. And when we talk, or even just think a thought, our DNA listens and responds.

Nowhere does the scientific literature on the Genome Project mention the proven biomedical fact that, ultimately, genes alone do not control anything. The genes' main function and purpose is to reproduce cells which, in turn, are responsible for the health and performance of the organs and systems in the body. How effectively genes do that largely depends on you and what you expose yourself to.

In a taped video recording, Dr. Bruce Lipton explains that through a process known as *epigenetic mechanisms,* we can start with a single gene blueprint and create over 30,000 different versions of products, such as proteins and enzymes. We do this all the time. Our mind (both the conscious and subconscious mind), which triggers a vast number of biochemical reactions in the brain and throughout the rest of the body, is primarily responsible for turning genes off or on.

Although genes cannot really be turned *on* or *off,* it is a term genetic medicine likes to use. In reality, genes either exist, or they don't. Genetic blueprints don't just disappear or turn off. What makes them active or inactive is whether they are being read or not. What allows them to be read or ignored is our thoughts, feelings, behavior, diet, environment and lifestyle. Accordingly, a conflict with another human being or the loss of a job or money (which constitutes a separation conflict) can quickly cause the same separation conflict inside the cells, thereby preventing genes from being read. Genes that are not being read properly cause changes in cell behavior, which is called genetic mutation. And just as we can cause a gene to become defective (not readable), we can also rewrite gene expression and modify it back to readable – meaning to a state of balance and health.

Even in the case of gene defects like Down syndrome,[11] something must be causing the rare, spontaneous DNA damage. For every effect there must be an underlying cause, even if it remains hidden from scientific investigation.

There can be many environmental influences that a growing fetus can be exposed to, any of which can cause, for example, the flaw of building an extra chromosome, as found in the case of Down syndrome. In today's world there are multiple sources that can mutate the DNA and its genes.

We can clearly see that even if we inherit abnormal genes from our parents, it doesn't mean we will also inherit their disease. There is something else at play that affects our health other than just genes.

In fact, all genes in the body are controlled by the cells' environment and its influences, including our personal perceptions and beliefs. If, in fact, a faulty gene is present in the body, just as Dr. Kramer and other leading

---

[11] Down syndrome is a congenital disorder caused by having an extra 21st chromosome, usually in each cell in the body. See http://www.cdc.gov/ncbddd/birthdefects/downsyndrome.html

cancer researchers have discovered and proven, it is not capable of causing or producing cancer growth. It is very likely that every person who suffers from a major illness will **also** have altered genes in their body. This is due to changes in the cell environment, not to accidental occurrence. And regardless of whether genes have mutated, the bottom line is they cannot cause cancer or other presumed diseases. There must be other factors at work that cause the human body's balanced and self-healing system to suddenly experience imbalance and illness.

It is easy to assume that defective genes are responsible, for example, for the occurrence of congenital cataracts among children. Cataracts are clouding of the eyes, and when they occur in children or newborns, can lead to blindness early in life. The suspicion that early cataracts are gene-related is especially convincing when all children in a family share the same problem.

On the other hand, it is equally compelling to believe that a chronic nutritional or hormonal deficiency in the mother can cause cataracts in her children. A paper published in 1996 in the *Lancet* [Edward B. Blau, Congenital Cataracts and Maternal Vitamin D Deficiency, *Lancet* 34 7(9001):626 (March 2, 1996)] showed that a vitamin D deficiency in the mother can cause rapid onset cataracts in her vitamin D-deficient child. Since a vast majority of people are indeed vitamin D-deficient, it follows that this would contribute to many health issues.

Infants inherit a vitamin D deficiency not because of a genetic flaw, but because of a detrimental lifestyle habit. As shown in this finding, the deficiency occurs when the mother neglects exposing her skin to the sun on a regular basis. If she passes on this unfortunate habit to her child who never received enough vitamin D while in the womb, the child will continue to suffer vitamin D deficiency even if it is breastfed. This is hardly surprising since there is almost no vitamin D found in human breast milk, especially when the mother is herself deficient in vitamin D.

A study published in *Pediatrics* (January 2011) showed just how important vitamin D is for the proper development of a fetus and newborn. In the study, researchers measured umbilical cord blood levels of vitamin D for roughly 1,000 healthy newborn babies. They then monitored the children over a 5-year period for respiratory problems and allergies, comparing these findings with their vitamin D levels at birth. They discovered that 20 percent of the newborns had a vitamin D deficiency, and that these deficiencies at birth were associated with a more frequent occurrence of later respiratory problems and allergies.

Vitamin D is essential for healthy immune system function, and mothers who wish to help start their babies off on the right foot can make a big difference simply by ensuring that they themselves are not deficient in vitamin D.

Among other functions, vitamin D (which is actually a steroid hormone) is responsible for calcium homeostasis. A lack of calcium (hypocalcaemia) has been clearly linked with cataracts. A vitamin D-deficient child can therefore experience a rapid onset of cataracts at birth or even before.

In adults, vitamin D deficiency has long been shown to cause the bone disorder rickets,[12] which is still very prevalent in sun-deprived countries like England and Ireland. However, it is becoming increasingly evident that vitamin D deficiency can be held responsible for many other disorders, including cancer.

Indeed, new science suggests that the *Sunshine Vitamin* is intimately involved in regulating genes associated with many diseases ranging from cancer to multiple sclerosis (MS). An Australian study recently discovered, for example, that MS rates are higher in latitudes further away from the equator because of differences in sun exposure.

In addition to being proactive about MS, the average adult can also help prevent type I diabetes, osteoporosis and, of course, cancer, by supplementing 4,000–8,000 IUs daily of vitamin D, according to research conducted at the University of California, San Diego School of Medicine and Creighton University School of Medicine in Omaha, Nebraska.

It is interesting, to say the least, that something as simple and inexpensive as vitamin D can go so far in treating and preventing many of today's diseases and helping the body maintain its natural balance. Perhaps this is part of the reason why the U.S. government continues to insist that only 400–800 IUs daily (a mere 10 percent of what is really required) of vitamin D is necessary, and instead throws its weight behind more financially profitable treatments. Meanwhile, around 90 percent of the U.S. population is chronically vitamin D-deficient, and seemingly getting sicker by the minute. Vitamin D is a particular threat to the current medical

---

[12] Rickets is a condition that affects the bones of infants and children, making them soft and deformed. It is caused by a deficiency of calcium, vitamin D and phosphate ions. Due to lack of sun exposure, the body fails to produce vitamin D, which is needed to add minerals to the bones.

industry because not only is it totally free, thanks to sun exposure, but it is also completely safe and able to prevent some of our society's most profitable illnesses.

What else does mainstream medicine not want us to know about vitamin D? If it regulates so many aspects of health, and is chronically deficient in the majority of people, isn't it logical to conclude that we can expect numerous diseases to result from this widespread issue?

In addition to this and other vitamin therapies that boost health and combat many diseases, it is crucial that people are aware of the many forms of toxicity in today's environment, which is more poisonous than ever before. Food, cosmetics and many other aspects of daily life are riddled with harmful chemicals. Yet many of these known toxins are nevertheless vigorously defended by the many companies that produce, market and use them.

It is important to note that there are other significant risks that can result from taking vitamin D supplements. Not only can it increase your absorption of calcium, but will also increase your assimilation of lead, arsenic and cadmium if your levels of calcium, magnesium and phosphorus are inadequate. So, if you are going to take a vitamin D supplement, be sure that your intake of these nutrients (from either diet or supplementation) is also sufficient. The problem is we can never be quite sure how much of these minerals we have in the blood and in our body's tissues.

The obvious question is why is sun exposure not promoted as a zero-cost method of reducing cancer incidence and mortality? Even vitamin D-generating UV lamps are very inexpensive compared with medical treatments that don't even come close to what vitamin D can do to benefit cancer patients.

I recommend using a UV lamp every three days to keep vitamin D levels optimal throughout the wintertime. During the warmer times of the year, I recommend natural sun exposure. (For more details, see my book, *Heal Yourself with Sunlight*.)

All in all, it is safe to say that taking charge of one's own health by being knowledgeable about supplemental vitamin and nutritional therapies, and avoiding the many toxins that exist in today's environment, is the best time-tested way of preventing and even treating cancer. At the very least, it is a much smarter choice than conventional modern cancer treatments, which are much younger than holistic, natural medicine and have a bleak success rate.

Dismal Success of Anticancer Treatments

Just take the placebo effect[13] as an example. A placebo (which literally means 'I shall please') is included as an indispensable element of every scientific study conducted today. The placebo effect is purely based on the subjective feelings of a person. Each person who is tested for the effectiveness of a medical drug believes in the drug in a unique and unpredictable way. A certain number of people may have a hopeful, trusting disposition, thereby experiencing a stronger placebo response than others. Others, however, may be suffering from depression, which is known to affect a person's ability to respond positively to any kind of treatment.

As a result, one study may *prove* a particular drug to be effective for, let's say, a certain kind of cancer. However, if a repeat experiment is conducted with different subjects, this drug may turn out to be ineffective when compared to the placebo response. For this reason, pharmaceutical companies instruct their paid researchers to publish *only* the most favorable findings from these various experiments. Those parts of the study where the drug has had no advantage (or only an insignificant one) over the placebo effect are simply omitted from the study's final report.

The drug companies reporting their findings to the Food and Drug Administration (FDA) only need to prove that the tested drug has shown some benefit in some people. If the researchers manage to recruit enough candidates with a positive disposition that are likely to produce a good placebo response to the drug treatment, they may hit the jackpot and produce a *convincing* study, and therefore a marketable drug.

This is a no-brainer for drug makers since FDA approval is granted to anticancer drugs based on response rates that are, at best, in the 10–20 percent range (as happened, for example, with the popular drugs, Avastin,

---

[13] A placebo is a term that describes the administration of a sugar pill or dummy procedure in order to test whether a drug or procedure is more effective than the power of belief. In an article in *The Guardian* (June 20, 2002), Jerome Burne reported that "new research suggests that placebos work surprisingly well, in fact, rather better than some conventional drugs."

Erbitux and Iressa). In addition, the *success* of most clinical cancer studies is measured by tumor shrinkage instead of mortality rate. In other words, even if most of the subjects died but had their tumors shrunk through aggressive treatments, the study would be hailed as a great success and a medical breakthrough.

Yet the big problem with popular cancer drugs is that the drugs are so dangerous that they can kill the patients before the cancer could. One such drug, Avastin, apparently raises patients' risk of death by up to 350 percent once combined with chemotherapy. It's been linked with a higher instance of fatal adverse events (FAEs) due to blood clots, GI puncture, brain bleeding, blindness, neurological disorders and even death. This is, of course, is on top of the already disastrous effects of radiation and chemotherapy.

Also, invasive surgeries are usually ineffective for they merely cut out cancerous growth without addressing the root causes that allowed the cancer to flourish. And still some doctors tout the potential of experimental drugs; but these drugs are untested and, because of their chemical nature, often totally unsafe.

Ultimately, any attempt to treat the human body as if it were a machine that simply responds to mechanical or chemical manipulation is bound to have serious setbacks. Such an approach is not only unscientific, but also unethical and potentially harmful. For many cancer patients whose immune systems are already compromised, just one dose of chemotherapy or radiation, just one surgery or an experimental pill, can turn out to be fatal.

Senior cancer physician, Dr. Charles Moertel of the famous Mayo Clinic in Rochester, Minnesota, once aptly summarized the modern cancer treatment dilemma in the following words: **"Our most effective regimens are fraught with risks and side effects and practical problems, and after this price is paid by all the patients we have treated, only a small fraction are rewarded with a transient period of usually incomplete tumor regression."**

The success record of modern cancer therapy is dismal, significantly less than even the weakest placebo response. On average, remission occurs in only about 7 percent of cancer patients. Moreover, there is no evidence that this discouragingly low 7 percent *success rate* results from the treatments offered; it could just as well be in spite of the treatments. This is more likely, since not treating cancer at all has a much higher success rate than treating it. A drug treatment that promises temporary tumor shrinkage in 10 percent of patients is not a promising therapy; rather, it is a dangerous gamble with their life.

In fact, treating any disease, including cancer, first with a placebo may work even better than the most optimistic *therapies*. Most people think of placebos as something that only works if the patient doesn't know it's a placebo – the classic *power of positive thinking* trick.

Yet stunning research from Harvard Medical School and the Beth Israel Deaconess Medical Center suggests that placebos may work even without the deception. Unlike traditional studies, where patients don't know whether they are taking a placebo or an actual drug, the placebo recipients in this study were fully informed that they were only taking sugar pills. Yet they actually reported symptom improvement at twice the rate of the participants taking *real* pills.

My lifelong assertion that much of medical science is literally wishful thinking has now been confirmed by groundbreaking scientific research involving the, so far, underestimated healing power behind patient expectation. The study, entitled "The Effect of Treatment Expectation on Drug Efficacy: the Analgesic Benefit of the Opioid Remifentanil"[14] may completely crush the principles upon which medical science has built its case, to date. Yet, this finding may also open the door to an entirely new way of treating disease.

Prominent researchers from the University of Oxford, University Medical Center Hamburg-Eppendorf, Cambridge University, and Technical University, Munich, found that the ultimate and most influential determining factor of whether a drug treatment is or isn't effective is nothing less than the patient's own mind. Their research, published in February 16, 2011 in the medical journal *Science Translational Medicine* [Vol. 3, Issue 70, p. 70ra14, *DOI:* 10.1126/scitranslmed.3001244], removes any doubt that the placebo effect is responsible for healing – not a drug treatment or even a surgical procedure.

In the study's abstract, the researchers state: "Evidence from behavioral and self-reported data suggests that the patients' beliefs and expectations can shape both therapeutic and adverse effects of any given drug." They discovered how divergent expectancies in patients alter the analgesic

---

[14] http://www.ncbi.nlm.nih.gov/pubmed/21325618

efficacy of a potent opioid (painkilling drug) in healthy volunteers by using brain imaging.

In this study, when test subjects were told that they were not receiving painkiller medications – even though they were – the medication proved to be completely ineffective. In fact, the research showed the benefits of painkillers could be boosted or completely wiped out by manipulating the subjects' expectations, which basically means it's entirely up to the patient whether he gets relief or not.

This particular research also identified the regions of the brain that are affected by patient expectation. "On the basis of subjective and objective evidence, we contend that an individual's expectation of a drug's effect critically influences its therapeutic efficacy and that regulatory brain mechanisms differ as a function of expectancy," according to the study's findings. Now try telling *that* to your doctor the next time you are given prescription medication!

Obviously, this should have important consequences for patient care and for testing new drugs, but I doubt that it ever will. There is no money to be made from telling patients they can heal themselves. Still, alternative and complementary forms of medicine may greatly benefit from incorporating these principles into their approaches.

Now let us look at some of the specifics of this fascinating research. A group of healthy test patients who experienced the same intensity of continuous pain caused by heat application to their feet were asked to rate their pain levels on a scale of 1 to 100. All patients were attached to an intravenous drip so drugs could be administered to them without their knowledge. The patients experienced pain at an average level of 66.

The first phase of the experiment involved giving the patients one of the most effective and potent medications, Remifentanil, without their knowledge. Their rate of pain dropped to 55.

In the second phase, the patients were told that they were receiving an intravenously administered painkiller. With no doubt in the patients' mind that this was true, the pain score dropped to 39.

Then, without actually altering the dose of the drug, the patients were told the painkiller had been discontinued altogether and to therefore expect pain to return; consequently, the pain score went up to 66. Even though the patients still received Remifentanil, they now experienced the same level of pain as they did at the beginning of the experiment, when no drug was given to them.

Professor Irene Tracey, from Oxford University, told the BBC: "It's phenomenal, it's really cool. It's one of the best analgesics we have and the brain's influence can either vastly increase its effect, or completely remove it." She further pointed out that the study was conducted on healthy people who were subjected to pain for just a short period of time.

People with chronic conditions who have unsuccessfully tried many drugs would not be as responsive because their expectations were likely dampened too many times before. Consequently, they may readily turn their own doubts (negative expectations) into a self-fulfilling prophesy of non-recovery. In other words, recovery or cure does not depend on the treatment, but rather on what the patient *believes* it will, or will not, do for him.

"Doctors need more time for consultation and to investigate the cognitive side of illness; the focus is on physiology, not the mind, which can be a real roadblock to treatment," claimed Professor Tracey.

George Lewith, a Professor of Health Research at the University of Southampton, poignantly stated that these findings call into question the scientific validity of many randomized clinical trials: "It completely blows cold randomized clinical trials, which don't take into account expectation."

George Lewith is a person to take very seriously, given his impressive and impeccable record of achievements and contributions to the world of medical science. The University of Southampton awarded a personal chair to Dr. Lewith as Professor of Health Research. He has published over 200 peer review papers and 17 books. The *Times*, in an article on September 6, 2008, included George Lewith in The Lifestyle 50, the newspaper's listing of the "top 50 people who influence the way we eat, exercise and think about ourselves."

What made this study so fascinating and important is that objective brain scans taken during the experiment also showed which regions of the brain were affected by the patients' subjective expectations.

The researchers found significant changes in neural activity in those brain regions involved with the coding of pain intensity. Positive expectancy effects of pain relief were associated with activity in the endogenous pain modulatory system, whereas negative expectancy effects linked with activity in the hippocampus and the medial frontal cortex. Having either a positive or a negative expectation of outcome from a particular treatment, therefore, alters brain chemistry and determines your body's ability to heal.

This is a paragraph taken from the first edition of my book, *Timeless Secrets of Health & Rejuvenation* (1995), which now makes more sense than ever: "The mechanism of placebo healing is centered in the belief of the patient that a drug, an operation, or a different kind of treatment is going to relieve his pain or cure his illness. Deep trust or a sure feeling of recovery is all that the patient has at his disposal to initiate a healing response. Utilizing the previously described powerful mind/body connection, the patient may release natural opioids (morphine-type painkillers) from areas of the brain that are activated by certain thought processes. The corresponding neurotransmitters for pain relief are known as endorphins. Endorphins are about forty thousand times more powerful than the strongest heroin."

Aligning with this, Professor Anthony Jones, Salford Royal NHS Foundation Trust, has stated: "Work from our own lab and those of others indicates that expectations are a key driver to pain perception and to placebo analgesic effects. So this provides further confirmation of that idea in relation to drug effects. This has been demonstrated previously in relation to nitrous oxide analgesic effects, but the current study provides good evidence that this phenomenon is not due to the subject saying what they think the investigator wants to hear."

Most Drug Studies Are Fraudulent

The implications of this study are profound and science-shattering. It seriously undermines the validity of all drug studies ever conducted because they did not include this crucial factor – the subjective expectation of the patient or the test subject who takes the actual drug. To reiterate Dr. Lewith's words, "It blows them cold."

Simply having a placebo group for comparison can neither make a drug trial trustworthy and scientific, nor can it ascertain the true effectiveness of the drug. Those subjects who receive the actual drug have similar subjective, unpredictable expectations as members of the placebo group. Drug companies like to give the impression that the placebo effect can only occur in the placebo group, not in the test subject group. But since members of neither group initially know whether they are getting the real drug or a *dummy* drug, the study results are ultimately determined by each person's expectation of beneficial outcome, regardless of the group to which he is assigned.

Even if a tested drug shows greater benefit than the placebo, this still doesn't prove that the drug is effective. To the contrary, it may merely show that the placebo effect is stronger in the drug group than in the placebo group – which is a big finding, in and of itself.

Principal Flaws in Drug Trials

Why would the placebo be stronger than the dummy drug in those participants that receive the actual drug? Well, since all trial participants hope they will receive the real medicine, not just a placebo pill, they will experience a significantly increased positive expectation the moment they notice the side effects they were told the drug might produce, such as constipation, diarrhea, headaches, dizziness, nausea, dryness of the mouth, etc. Realizing they are among the actual drug recipients because of this self-observation, their expectation of possible recovery boosts the drug's success score. Researchers claim that this is proof of effectiveness of the tested drug, and gives zero credit to the now-elevated expectancy on the part of the participants.

While some of the tested subjects may be very hopeful and enthusiastic about receiving a new medicine, others who have tried many similar medications before, without reaping much, if any, benefit, may have a more reserved or even negative expectation about its benefits. Since patient expectancy is highly relevant, according to this research, all previously conducted scientific studies that didn't account for patient expectancy are misleading and must be thrown out as invalid. This practically applies to all double-blind control studies ever done.

Another reason why clinical drug trials are so unscientific and fraudulent is that they are not conducted in a truly double-blind setting. All participants, regardless of whether they receive the real drug or the placebo pill, are told that the study is for a specific condition. For example, a clinical trial may test a new drug to combat hypertension, lower blood sugar or decrease cholesterol. This simple information, which is advertised during the trial recruitment campaign, already generates an expectation in the participants that, perhaps, the new experimental drug might help them improve their health. This hopeful expectation may, in fact, be the primary reason they enroll in the trial.

There has never been a clinical trial where participants were not told what drug treatment they could expect to receive. On the one hand, the researchers claim their study is foolproof because participants won't know whether they receive the drug or a placebo. On the other hand, they tell all the participants upfront that at least half of them can expect to receive a pharmaceutical drug to improve the specific condition they are suffering from.

In other words, at least 1 in every 2 participants may already experience a placebo effect *before* the trial has even started.

Every clinical scientist knows that the mind's belief in a drug or treatment can produce a healing response. This is the very reason there is a placebo group in every clinical trial. Why, then, do scientists and doctors insist that only drugs can cure conditions?

There is a clear double standard in medical research. If they are correct in that only drugs can cure and treat diseases, then why do they need to include a placebo group in their research?

Telling the participants that one-half of them will receive the experimental drug and the other half will just get a placebo creates a major uncertainty factor of varied, unpredictable expectations in the subjects, one that the research doesn't account for. This is pseudo-science at best, and outright fraud at worst.

The only other way to do an objective study would be to tell every participant that he or she will receive the real drug, but nobody actually will. Instead, all participants will get a placebo. Then start a second phase with the same subjects at a different time, and now give them the real drug while telling them so. If findings from the above pain study are correct, then the subjects are most likely going to get the same results at both phases. If the findings are incorrect, then it will show that the researched medication has true benefits. This would be honest, scientific research.

Dishonest Practices

To prevent getting a poor success score for the tested drug, pharmaceutical companies typically instruct researchers to choose the youngest and healthiest subjects to test it against a targeted disease. However, this practice is both unrealistic and deceptive. In real life, most drugs are being prescribed to the sicker, weaker and older patients who are already less likely to muster positive expectations than younger, stronger and healthier patients. When you are really sick, you are also much more likely to feel disheartened or depressed.

Drug companies know about this dirty little secret and, therefore, refuse really sick or depressed people from participating in drug trials. Think of a time in your life when you suffered from influenza or another type of illness. In all likelihood, you felt weak and lost interest in almost everything that normally excited you. As we now know, you will need to be excited about a treatment (positive expectation) to reap genuine benefits from it or, rather, from the placebo response it can trigger in you.

Even with the drug companies succeeding in manipulating the outcome of the so-called *research* in favor of a new drug, there always are a relatively large number of trials that show outright ineffectiveness of the same drug.

If a drug were truly effective, it would work for every person tested. But since patient expectancy is a highly variable and unpredictable factor, some of these trials show that there are drug benefits, whereas others show there aren't any. Drug companies are legally permitted by the Federal Drug Administration (FDA) to cherry-pick the *good* trials and throw out the *bad* ones.

When the research is finally presented to the FDA and the medical journals for peer review and publication, it will look like a valid scientific study. The research paper carries the stamp of *proof* of drug efficacy.

In truth though, all of the studies conducted in this way are fabricated, worthless and potentially risky for the patient population, leading to the often serious consequences of side effects, including death. No wonder the FDA is compelled to pull numerous drugs off the market each year because they are just too toxic and dangerous. Hundreds of thousands of Americans die each year, poisoned by these Frankenstein pharmaceuticals.

Bottom line, it is impossible to directly prove whether a patient improves his condition because he is taking a medical drug, or because he believes the treatment will make him better. However, this new pain research clearly indicates the latter to be the case.

The 'Miracle' of Spontaneous Remission

The mind/body/spirit triad connection is clearly demonstrated in the now thousands of cancer patients who experience spontaneous remissions of their cancers. Research has shown that the size of a tumor can be reduced dramatically within a few hours of holistic health treatment, when the patient is highly motivated by personal development. Perceiving a spiritual purpose in the disease that affects them can also be enough to achieve remission.

This usually happens when the disease is no longer perceived as a threat, but as a blessing in disguise. In other words, instead of being helpless victims of a senseless disease, they become active participants in the process of becoming whole again. The expectation of being blessed by something they might have previously seen as a dreadful curse evokes some of the most powerful healing responses the body has at its disposal.

The mechanism of expecting, and subsequently experiencing, pain relief from a saline solution placebo is no different than the mechanism that transforms a big tumor, disintegrating it in less than a minute.

I once saw a live ultrasound image where a cancerous bladder tumor, the size of a grapefruit, completely disintegrated and vanished during a 15-second sound-energy healing session by a group of Chinese Qigong masters. Of course, without the patient's hopeful and receptive expectation that healing would occur, nothing can happen. Nobody can enter your home as long as you keep the door closed.

Instead of instilling death fright in a patient, a doctor ought to help the patient to develop hope-filled expectations that can then translate into the necessary biochemical responses in the brain and heart that are required for the patient's body to actually and fully heal itself. On the other hand, telling the patient that he (or she) is suffering from a terminal illness introduces a factor of expectancy that is undeniably capable of executing the doctor's unintended death sentence.

If the doctor or, even worse, a diagnostic machine like a CT scanner (and *machines don't lie*) passes a death sentence on a patient, it is the natural expectation of the patient that the sentence will be carried out that actually kills him, not the disease.

When feeling this vulnerable, patients often see their doctor as their savior, their God. If God tells me I am dying, then it must be true.

Relinquishing one's power to someone who plays God makes one a slave, where the expectation is one of worthlessness and dependency. Letting a diagnosis, or rather the negative interpretation of it, rule one's life, lies at the core of today's health crisis.

Just the title of the first edition of my book, *Cancer is Not a Disease – It's a Survival Mechanism,*[15] has helped thousands of people restore their confidence in themselves and their bodies. Transforming a negative expectation into a positive one is what practicing medicine ought to be about. The aforementioned research should be studied by every doctor and applied to every field of modern medicine, but this would most certainly make most of modern medicine obsolete.

Still, thanks to these brilliant researchers, we now have the model to scientifically explain that healing is largely up to the expectation, state of mind and attitude of the patient, and not necessarily to the doctor and his pharmaceutical treatments.

So far, most medical dogma has turned everything upside down. I sincerely hope, for the sake of the survival of humankind, that modern medicine undergoes a revolution that will set it right again. I am encouraged to see there is some light at the end of the tunnel.

Expectations Shape Reality

Both negative and positive expectations can lead to very unusual events. Many people have heard about the studies that showed heart attacks occurring more often on Mondays, usually at 9 a.m., to be more exact. It is presumed this is due to the expected difficulties and stress that may occur during the work week. Also, fewer people die during the days before Christmas, whereas more people die right after Christmas.

Another phenomenon, discovered by the Yale School of Public Health and the National Institute of Aging, is that young people who have positive expectations about aging are less likely to have a heart attack or stroke when they grow older.

In a study on aging conducted at Yale and also Miami University, middle aged and elderly people lived seven years longer when they had a positive attitude about aging.

---

[15] This new, updated edition is titled *Cancer Is Not a Disease – It's a Healing Mechanism.*

In a classical study, 100 individuals over 80 years of age were placed in an environment that put them back 30 years in time – from old time music playing on the radio, to era-appropriate clothing. Within a few weeks all their physiological and biochemical markers of aging had dropped by an average of 15 years. When they returned to their current homes and living environments, however, they *aged forward* by 15 years in just one day.

In a piece posted on CNN.com, Elizabeth Cohen, CNN Senior Medical Correspondent, wrote about the self-induced, spontaneous remission of cancer in David Seidler, who won an Oscar for the best original screenplay for the movie The King's Speech. Mr. Seidler, age 73, suffered from bladder cancer and used a simple method of visualization to completely disintegrate his large tumor in less than two weeks, just in time before his scheduled operation, much to his physician's astonishment.

There are literally thousands of examples where imagination, expectation, visualization, perception, attitude, etc., have shown to manifest whatever is being seriously entertained by the mind. Mind/body medicine is not some kind of woo-woo or wishful thinking; it is true science, as the following research further confirms.

Would you believe that just looking at the photograph of a romantic partner is enough to significantly dull pain, in the same way that paracetamol or narcotics, such as cocaine, can? Well, a research study by Stanford University discovered just that.

In the study, which was published in the journal *PLoS ONE* on October 13, 2010, [doi:10.1371], researchers took MRI scans of the brains of love-struck students who were asked to focus on photographs of partners while varying levels of heat pain were applied to their skin. On average, the pain levels were reduced between 36 and 44 percent, according to neuroscientist Jarred Younger. Pain drugs don't perform much better than that.

According to a report in the September 2006 issue of the *Hospitalist,* "many patients will only experience a 30%–50% reduction in pain relief." Besides, pharmaceutical painkillers can have side effects, including nausea, dizziness, somnolence, constipation, dry mouth, increased sweating, liver failure and death. In other words, you don't have to rely on drugs to get good pain relief.

In yet another study, published in the journal *Psychological Science* in November 2009, psychologists from the University of California, Los

Angeles, studied 25 women and their boyfriends for a period of six months, subjecting them to different levels of pain.

While experiencing the pain, the women were told to either hold their boyfriend's hand or the hand of a male stranger, both of whom were hidden behind a curtain. The women experienced significantly less pain while holding their partner's or a stranger's hand.

When asked to view a photograph of their boyfriend, or a picture of a male stranger while being subjected to discomfort, the women experienced at least the same pain reduction. In fact, the relief was even greater when a stranger was involved. This means that pain relief doesn't necessarily involve love-induced analgesia. The feeling of closeness or security that the women expected to receive from looking at their lover's picture, or touching someone's hand, is all that is needed for the brain to send out the necessary opiates that bring on relief.

These studies are invaluable in that they show how healing is closely connected to how we feel. We are not robots. To heal from a cancer, we require the support, encouragement and assurance from the world around us, so that we can generate the kind of (positive) expectations necessary for the healing to occur. A negative diagnosis or prognosis, threatening a person by saying, "If you don't take this medicine, you will die," or making him feel that he is a helpless victim of a terrible disease, won't help but may actually be responsible for his declining health or ultimate demise.

Many pharmaceuticals only work because people expect them to work, not because they have any significant biochemical effect on the body. Without the belief of receiving a substantive benefit, the brain will simply block the medication from doing its job.

As we have seen in the first study, giving a person a painkiller while telling him it's not a painkiller, proved to be completely worthless. Mind power either overrides the potential benefit of the drug, or it triggers the same biochemical responses that the drug is designed to produce. In other words, the mind tells the brain whether or not to initiate the biochemical responses necessary for healing to take place.

We know from brain research that all healing in the body is regulated by the brain. This has repeatedly been confirmed by many studies, including those on antidepressant drugs, which have consistently failed to outperform the placebo. What's so encouraging about all this is that we are in charge of our brain. The brain carries out our instructions in the form of beliefs and expectations, positive and negative, conscious and subconscious. In one expression, we are what we believe. So, perhaps, it is now time to change the way we think about the power we have over our own healing ability.

Statistical Fraud

The cancer industry tries to use statistical *evidence* to convince you that you need to entrust your life into its hands. However, many chemotherapy success stories are limited to relatively obscure types of cancer, such as Burkitt's lymphoma and choriocarcinoma, so rare that many clinicians have never seen a single case. Childhood leukemia constitutes less than 2 percent of all cancers, and therefore hardly influences the overall success rate. Chemo's supposedly strong track record with Hodgkin's disease (lymphoma) is a blunt lie. Children who are successfully treated for Hodgkin's disease are 18 times more likely to develop secondary malignant tumors later in life (*New England Journal of Medicine*, March 21, 1996).

According to the National Cancer Institute [*NCI Journal* 87:10], patients who underwent chemotherapy were 14 times more likely to develop leukemia and 6 times more likely to develop cancers of the bones, joints and soft tissues than those patients who did not undergo chemotherapy. Yet if you have a child with lymphoma and refuse treatment for the above well-documented reasons, you face prosecution by the law, and your child may be taken away from you. The bottom line is this: although only 2–4 percent of cancers respond to chemotherapy, it has become standard procedure to prescribe chemo drugs for most cancers. The proportion of people with cancer in the U.S. who receive chemotherapy is 75 percent.

Cancer researcher Dr. J. Bailer said quite bluntly: "The five year cancer survival statistics of the American Cancer Society are very misleading. They now count things that are not cancer, and, because we are able to diagnose at an earlier stage of the disease, patients falsely appear to live longer. Our whole cancer research in the past 20 years has been a failure. More people over 30 are dying from cancer than ever before... (Yet) more women with mild or benign diseases are being included in statistics and reported as being 'cured'. When government officials point to survival figures and say they are winning the war against cancer they are using those survival rates improperly." [*New England Journal of Medicine*, September/October 1990]

Official cancer statistics simply omit African Americans, a group that actually has the highest incidence of cancers. They also don't include patients with lung cancer which is the most common cause of cancer-related death in men and the second most common in women. However, the statistical data include millions of people with diseases that are not life-threatening and are easily curable, such as localized cancers of the cervix, non-spreading cancers, skin cancers and *ductal carcinoma in situ* or DCIS – the most common kind of non-invasive breast cancer. Even pre-cancers, most of which never develop into full-fledged cancer, are nevertheless included to boost the dismal success rate of modern cancer therapy.

With a death rate that is actually 6 percent higher in 1997 than in 1970, there is nothing to suggest that modern cancer therapy is scientific, effective, or worth the pain, effort and vast expense. This trend has continued to this day, yet with a failure rate of at least 93 percent, medical cancer therapy cannot be considered a treatment at all, but rather a serious threat to societal health.

The Power of Belief

According to the laws of quantum physics, in any scientific experiment, the observer (a researcher) influences and alters the object of observation on a very fundamental level (observer-observed relationship). This fundamental principle of physics applies to you just as much. After all, your body is composed of molecules that are made of atoms; these atoms are composed of subatomic particles which, in turn, are made of energy and information. There is actually not even a trace of matter in what we consider physical creation. Although something may appear to be as solid and concrete as a rock, there is nothing solid about it; only your sensory perception makes it appear so.

Your thoughts also are merely forms of energy and information that influence other forms of energy and information, including the cells of your body. For example, if you are sad about something, your body posture changes and your eyes lose their luster. Eye cells, like all other cells in the body, respond to your thoughts, just as a soldier follows the orders of his superior. The bottom line is this: **If you believe strongly enough that you**

have cancer or if you are afraid of it, you face a significant risk of manifesting it in your body.

The placebo effect can work both ways. The belief that you have a deadly disease can be just as powerful as the belief that a certain medical drug can heal you. In an instant, the energy of your thoughts and beliefs delivers the information they contain to every cell in your body. The energy and information that make up the atoms, molecules, genes, cells, organs and systems in your body have no agenda of their own. They are certainly not malicious. All they do is follow orders. You manifest both what you like and what you do not like. In other words, you are what you believe. Furthermore, what you believe is determined by the way you see or perceive things. Clearly, your interpretation of cancer as a disease will likely turn it into a disease for you. Otherwise, cancer would just be a survival mechanism or a signal for you to take care of those aspects of your life that you have neglected thus far.

If you believe that cancer is a disease, you are more likely to be inclined to fight against it – physically, emotionally and spiritually. If you are strong-willed and the weapons you are using are powerful, you may be able to subdue this *enemy* of yours, at least for a while. In such a case, you will be proud of having *beaten* the cancer and, perhaps, you will praise the doctors or the medical treatment you endured for having saved your life. If you are weak and you use these same weapons in an attempt to destroy the cancer, you are likely going to succumb to what you would consider a malicious enemy. The doctor will express with regret that your body did not sufficiently *respond* to the treatment (the weapons), claiming that he tried everything and that nothing more could be done. He will neglect to inform you that the weapons he has put into your body can be deadly.

Chemotherapy is so poisonous that leaking a few drops of the drug onto your hand can severely burn it. If drops fall on a concrete floor, they can burn holes into it. Spilling any chemotherapeutic drug in the hospital or anywhere en route is classified as a major biohazard and requires specialists with spacesuits to dispose of it.

Just imagine the holes chemotherapy creates inside your blood vessels, lymphatic ducts and organ tissues when you undergo infusion after infusion! I have looked at the irises of patients (using iridology) who have gone through chemotherapy, and I saw the considerable erosion and damage of tissues throughout the body. Yes, this drug destroys cancer cells, but along with them, many of your healthy cells, too. Your entire body becomes inflamed. For this reason, your hair falls out when you undergo chemotherapy or radiation, and you cannot digest food anymore. Many patients develop anorexia – the loss of appetite or desire to eat. But this is not the only risk you can expect from modern cancer therapies. "Chemotherapy and radiation can increase the risk of developing a second cancer by up to 100 times," according to Dr. Samuel S. Epstein [*Congressional Record*, September 9, 1987].

Anticancer Drugs Make Tumors More Deadly

For the past 20 years, I have been making the *outrageous* claim that common cancer treatments, including chemotherapy medications, radiation therapy and angiogenesis inhibitors that are used to shrink cancerous tumors, are largely responsible for making them more aggressive and develop in other parts of the body (erroneously called metastases) as well. Over the years I have received a fair amount of ridicule, defamatory comments and outright death threats for publishing my unrelenting stance on the subject.

The National Cancer Institute states on its website: "Angiogenesis inhibitors are unique cancer-fighting agents because they tend to inhibit the growth of blood vessels rather than tumor cells. In some cancers, angiogenesis inhibitors are most effective when combined with additional therapies, especially chemotherapy." However, a 2012 study, which was supported by the National Institutes of Health (NIH), sheds new light on why the *effectiveness* of these cancer-fighting drugs is actually short-lived and can turn into a frightening scenario with possibly fatal consequences. This research shows that aggressive treatment (used for shrinking or removing even relatively small, slow-growing or encapsulated, harmless tumors) may create a situation where the entire body is riddled with highly aggressive cancers.

The groundbreaking study, published in the January 17, 2012 issue of *Cancer Cell*,[16] finds that a group of little-explored cells which are part of every primary cancerous tumor likely serve as important gatekeepers against cancer progression and metastasis. A relatively new class of

---

[16] *Cancer Cell*, Volume 21, Issue 1, 66-81, January 17,2012, http://www.cell.com/cancer-cell/retrieve/pii/S1535610811004478

anticancer drugs, known as angiogenic inhibitors, diminishes or destroys these cells, called pericytes, by cutting off the blood supply to the tumors.

Scientists and oncologists from around the world made the shortsighted assumption that by cutting off a tumor's life support system, consisting of a tumor's blood vessels, they could achieve a successful and permanent tumor regression. Little did they know that this would open a Pandora's box and create a cancer nightmare.

Cancer's Wisdom In Action

Seen from a holistic and truly scientific perspective, the above assumption is critically flawed. I have frequently made the argument that cancer is one of the body's final healing attempts to return to a balanced condition (homeostasis), and this noteworthy research clearly illustrates that cancer constitutes one of the body's most highly evolved and sophisticated protective mechanisms.

The study found that therapies which shrink cancer by cutting off tumors' blood supply may be inadvertently making tumors more aggressive and likely to spread. Said differently, to help prevent a cancer from getting out of control and invading other parts of the body, the body tenaciously and purposefully grows extra blood vessels. Why would the body do such a thing, you might ask?

Well, all cancer cells are normal cells that have turned anaerobic, meaning that they are so oxygen-deprived (due to congestion-caused oxygen deficiency) that they must mutate in order to survive and produce energy without having to use oxygen. To increase the oxygen supply to these congested cells and support the action by pericytes to prevent cancer progression and metastasis, the body **needs** to grow new blood vessels. In view of this, the currently applied medical approach of destroying these blood vessels is therefore counterproductive and must be considered dangerous. It destroys the very system the body uses to make sure that a particular cancerous tumor remains an isolated and curable event, and does not escalate into a widespread, uncontrollable and self-perpetuating disease process.

To make this very clear, cancer drugs don't just destroy cancer cells, but also cancer-protective cells and blood vessels transporting oxygen to both cancer cells and normal cells. Ionizing radiation and cancer drugs are outright carcinogenic and, thus, can cause new cancer cells to develop almost anywhere in the body.

Controlling Tumor Growth
Makes Cancer Spread More

There is no doubt that chemotherapy drugs, angiogenic drugs or radiation therapy can achieve significant tumor regression, but not without paying the hefty price of producing a multitude of new cancers. Besides the billions of corpses of dead cancer cells and pericytes this biological genocide leaves behind, there are also billions of inflamed or otherwise damaged cells and blood vessels that greatly increase the chances of developing any number of new, aggressive, deadly cancers.

Most of these cancers are too small, though, to be detected right away by diagnostic instruments, and doctors can get away with the proud expression, "We got it all," at least for a while. Yet within a year or two, these cancers almost inevitably become larger and detectable, and the same doctors then tell their patients that their cancer not only has *returned*, but has metastasized to other parts of the body.

The study spotlighted above provides us with the unexpected finding that may actually prove current cancer treatments, including chemotherapy, angiogenic therapy and radiation therapy, to be the greatest contributors to developing aggressive, terminal cancers and significantly lowering one's chances of survival.

In this investigation, senior author Raghu Kalluri, M.D., Ph.D., Chief of the Division of Matrix Biology at Beth Israel Deaconess Medical Center (BIDMC) and Professor of Medicine at Harvard Medical School (HMS), had actually intended to find out if the targeting of pericytes could inhibit tumor growth in the same way that other drugs inhibiting blood vessel growth to tumors can. After all, pericytes are an important part of tissue vasculature,[17] covering blood vessels and supporting their growth. What Kalluri and his team stumbled upon instead was both startling and extremely disturbing.

---

[17] The vessels and tissue that carry or circulate fluids such as blood or lymph through the body.

In an article titled, "Study Shows How A Group of Tumor Cells Prevent Cancer Spread – Paradoxical discovery finds that pericyte cells help prevent metastasis,"[18] Bonnie Prescottat, Beth Israel Deaconess Medical Center, Harvard Medical School, describes the dire implications of the study in some greater detail.

When applied to breast cancer, "Kalluri and his colleagues found that by depleting pericyte numbers by 60 percent in breast cancer tumors, they saw a 30 percent decrease in tumor volumes over 25 days," writes Prescott.

Since such significant tumor shrinkage will prevent or slow the growth of the targeted cancer, conventional medical *wisdom* dictates that this would be a favorable effect, and oncologists have hailed this approach to be a breakthrough in cancer treatment. However, the researchers also discovered that by destroying pericytes by 60–70 percent, the number of secondary lung tumors increased threefold, indicating that the tumors had metastasized.

"If you just looked at tumor growth, the results were good," says Kalluri. **"But when you looked at the whole picture, inhibiting tumor vessels was not controlling cancer progression. The cancer was, in fact, spreading.**

"We showed that a big tumor with good pericyte coverage is less metastatic than a smaller tumor of the same type with less pericyte coverage," says Kalluri, who corroborated these findings in multiple types of cancer by repeating these same experiments with implanted renal cell carcinoma and melanoma tumors, writes Prescott.

All of this questions the very argument pushed on unsuspecting cancer patients by medical professionals that treatment-caused tumor regression is a desirable objective. Just imagine if you were diagnosed with a cancerous tumor and your doctor told you that his proposed treatment could reduce the size of your tumor by 30 percent, but at the same time increase your chances of developing secondary tumors by a whopping 300 percent!

---

[18] http://www.bidmc.org/News/InResearch/2012/January/Kalluri_Cancer.aspx

Beware of Conventional Cancer Treatments

The history of conventional anticancer therapies is replete with cases where the treatment turned out to be far more devastating than the disease itself. This single piece of research provides us with the understanding that the body isn't reckless or irresponsible when it actually builds new blood vessels to support tumor growth. To the contrary, it is well equipped with the superb wisdom and physical means to pursue the best possible routes of survival, regardless of the circumstances such as toxicity, congestion and emotional stress.

Attacking the body's tumor cells is still an attack on the body, which is exacerbated when doctor and patient simplistically perceive cancer cells to be evil monsters that must be destroyed at any cost. Cancer diagnosis and treatment are severely stressful, violent acts against the body and will evoke a powerful fight-or-flight response that affects every part of the body. The death fright triggers continuous releases of stress hormones into the blood – powerful enough to shut down the digestive system and the immune system, and to constrict important blood vessels, including those that support the cancer-protective pericytes.

As this new study has demonstrated, the destruction of pericytes goes hand in hand with a dramatic increase in the number of secondary tumors in other parts of the body. The body is not a machine but a living being; it responds with emotions and biochemical changes to everything you think, feel and expose yourself to. Threatening the body on any level jeopardizes its healing abilities.

Cancer has a deeper meaning or purpose than purely random destruction, and ignorance about the true purpose of cancer is at the root of these misdirected cancer treatments. The body uses its own built-in survival and healing programs to keep cancer under control and to let the cancer do its job – this includes mopping up accumulated toxins and waste products, and keeping it from spreading or showing up in other parts of the body.

After examining 130 breast cancer tumor samples of varying cancer stages and tumor sizes, and comparing pericyte levels with prognosis, the scientists found that samples with low numbers of pericytes in tumors correlated with the most deeply invasive cancers, distant metastasis and 5- and 10-year survival rates lower than 20 percent.

To understand the exact mechanism behind the drastically increased risk of metastasis that follows drug treatment, I recommend you check out their study, which I consider to be one of the most important pieces of cancer research ever done. I am certainly not the only one to share this belief.

"These results are quite provocative and will influence clinical programs designed to target tumor angiogenesis," says Ronald A. DePinho, president of the University of Texas MD Anderson Cancer Center. And for Kalluri and his team, the emerging discoveries suggest that certain assumptions about cancer must be revisited. "We must go back and audit the tumor and find out which cells play a protective role versus which cells promote growth and aggression," says Kalluri. "Not everything is black and white. There are some cells inside a tumor that are actually good in certain contexts."

Cancer's Lessons To Us

To me, it makes no sense at all to use cancer-causing drugs and ionizing radiation to shrink malignant tumors in the short term, while causing existing cancers to become deeply invasive and deadly, and new cancers to show up in parts of the body distant to the original tumor. The shortsightedness of this approach seems obvious, and millions of people have fallen into the trap of gaining a little, but losing everything.

With regard to chemotherapy drugs, scientists at the University of Alabama at Birmingham (UAB) Comprehensive Cancer Center and UAB Department of Chemistry are currently (2012) investigating the suspected possibility that dead cancer cells left over after chemotherapy spark cancer to spread to other parts of the body (metastasis). "What if by killing cancer cells with chemotherapy, we inadvertently induce DNA structures that make surviving cancers cells more invasive? The idea is tough to stomach," said Katri Selander, M.D., Ph.D., an assistant professor in the UAB Division of Hematology and Oncology and co-principal researcher on the grant, in a statement to the media. Dead cancer cells have already been found to activate a pathway in the body mediated as a protein dubbed 'toll-like receptor 9', or TLR9, that is present in the immune system and in many kinds of cancers. "If TLR9 boosts metastasis, then researchers will work on finding targeted therapies that block or regulate this molecular pathway," Dr. Selander stated.

Angiogenic therapy has already been implicated with causing deadly metastasis, and chemotherapy is almost certainly following in this track for the same and additional reasons.

A few years ago, a leading oncologist in the U.S. contacted me and asked me if liver flushes could help his wife who suffered from terminal lung cancer. He told me that over six years they had tried all of the most advanced chemo drugs, to no avail. After each round of chemotherapy, more and more malignant tumors had developed in the lungs and spread to her liver and bones (now we know why). I told him that at this advanced stage, she had nothing to lose, but could turn the situation around by ridding the liver, blood and tissues of accumulated toxins. This would make tumor growth unnecessary.

The oncologist personally monitored and recorded the results of his wife's first liver flush. He reported back to me that she had released an astonishing amount of at least 2,500 gallstones which kept pouring out of her over a period of three days (something that is almost unheard of). Four weeks later, he informed me that the tumors in his wife's liver and bones had completely vanished and there was only one tiny speck of tumor remaining in her left lung. I recommended that she continue doing the liver flushes until all stones were gone. He also told me that she had become like a new person since she did the flush. A life-long constipation was gone and her skin appeared rejuvenated – no longer pale and grayish-looking. His wife said she had regained the energy she used to have 20 years ago, and the deep depression she had suffered from since her first cancer diagnosis had completely lifted.

I have personally seen cancer patients who successfully and naturally reversed their cancers, but were then talked into taking a round of chemotherapy just to be sure to *get it all*. They all died within a day or two of the first treatment.

The methods of modern medicine don't fight disease, they fight the body. Disease is the body's way of healing itself, and modern treatment is a sure way to impair or even destroy this ability.

Creating a Monster Where There Is None

All this raises a very important question: Could it possibly be that cancer is not a disease, but a healing mechanism of the body designed to remove something that does not belong there? If so, would it not make more sense to support the body in its natural drive to remove such obstructions rather than to suppress its effort with aggressive, destructive means? Most intelligent people would agree with this. For when the obstruction is gone, there would be no further need for the body to continue relying on such a desperate healing mechanism as cancer.

It is said that the proof of the pudding is in the eating. You will not know how the pudding tastes until you eat it. If you remove the causes of an illness and the illness disappears by itself, you will know for certain that there was no illness in the first place. There were only reasons that made the body do things it normally would not do. Whenever you prevent the body from conducting its normal activities, it has no other choice but to apply corrective measures that can at least alleviate the situation and restore some of its basic functions. But a truly healthy body cannot sustain cancer; it has no need to.

Sadly, most people in the Western hemisphere have never actually been through the learning experience of self-empowerment – that is, supporting the body while experiencing an illness and allowing it to heal itself, rather than fighting it with toxic treatments. If they fall ill, they immediately believe the body must be doing something wrong, whereas in reality it is doing something right to rectify a difficult situation they have created or allowed, for whatever known or unknown reason. If they hold on long enough to the belief that their body is making them sick, that misinterpretation of the real situation will turn into something that they eventually will experience to be true.

Furthermore, if many other people believe the same thing, it becomes an established *fact* we have to live with. Before long, an entire population knows this *fact* and behaves accordingly, with fear and apprehension. Their truth becomes a self-fulfilling prophecy, and natural instincts and common sense are thrown out the window.

Collectively, we have created an atmosphere that expects disease. Most people in the Western world turn to a doctor for every little problem they have. Even during pregnancy, the battery of checkups a woman and her growing fetus must undergo serve to program the mother and child for a life-long dependency upon doctors.

Now, it seems, we *must* have a doctor for the delivery, although billions of healthy babies have successfully been delivered without one. We also *need* a doctor to administer the various childhood vaccinations (another cause of cancer), to prescribe antibiotics for an ear or throat infection, to tell us whether we need to take out the tonsils or appendix, and to prescribe drugs for nervousness and attention deficit disorder because we live on sugar, food additives and fast foods, or are deprived of our parents' loving care and attention. Furthermore, a doctor *is* needed to tell us that we need statin drugs for an elevated cholesterol level, diuretic pills for high blood pressure, and an angioplasty to unclog our blocked arteries. The alarming list goes on almost indefinitely. And who really profits? Certainly it isn't the patient.

The masterminds of collective programming have succeeded in manipulating the food and medical industries for their own profit and control. No longer thinking for themselves, the majority of people have lost trust in their bodies' innate and instinctive healing ability. Instead, they turn to an industry that has no actual interest in keeping them healthy.

Many natural cures for cancer exist, more now than ever, but none of them is being researched, endorsed or promoted by those who claim to be the health custodians of the nation. The American Cancer Society, the National Cancer Institute, the American Medical Association (AMA), the Food and Drug Administration (FDA) and the major oncology centers all feel threatened by the successes of alternative cancer therapies. This is easy to understand, of course, given the 93 percent failure rate of conventional cancer therapies.

The world-renowned health researchers, Robert Houston and Gary Null, poignantly revealed the reasons behind the medical industry's cancer strategy: "A solution to cancer would mean the termination of research programs, the obsolescence of skills, the end of dreams of personal glory; triumph over cancer would dry up contributions to self-perpetuating charities... It would mortally threaten the present clinical establishments by rendering obsolete the expensive surgical, radiological and chemotherapeutic treatments in which so much money, training and equipment is invested... The new therapy must be disbelieved, denied, discouraged and disallowed at all costs, regardless of actual testing results, and preferably without any testing at all."

The prominent cancer researcher and Professor at the University of California (Berkeley and Davis), Dr. Hardin Jones, had this to say about the current cancer dilemma: "It is most likely that, in terms of life expectancy, the chance of survival is no better with than without treatment, and there is the possibility that treatment may make the survival time of cancer less." After analyzing cancer survival statistics for several decades, Dr. Jones, a Professor at the University of California, concluded that "...patients are as well, or better off, untreated." Dr. Jones' disturbing assessment has never been refuted. Dr. Jones has been quoted as follows: "My studies have proven conclusively that cancer patients who refuse chemotherapy and radiation actually live up to four times longer than treated cases, including untreated breast cancer cases."

When not treating cancer brings about better results than treating it, the question arises: Why then do our health agencies allow, encourage and even enforce treatments that have been proven to kill cancer patients prematurely? Perhaps the AMA has the answer to that question. One of the AMA's stated objectives and obligations is to protect the income of its members (medical doctors). The biggest income of AMA members is generated by treating cancer patients. On the average, every cancer patient is worth $50,000. If ever a cancer cure were officially recognized in this country (U.S.), it would threaten the income and livelihood of AMA members. The bylaws of the AMA practically prohibit the promotion of a cure for cancer.

After 60 years of intensive research and hundreds of billions spent on treatments for cancer that have killed thousands of patients, we are facing the collective challenge of our own survival. The only reasonable alternative to stop this fabricated monster is to learn the skills of healing ourselves. The other option will most likely bankrupt our country, endanger our livelihoods and lead us into the abyss of self-destruction.

Medical Predicaments

Every person with a sound medical background knows that the symptom of an illness is not, in itself, the real illness. Yet the majority of doctors today treat the symptoms as if they were the disease. Without knowing the causes of most of the over 40,000 listed diseases, medical textbooks nevertheless speak of *effective treatments* for these diseases. The disease agencies that were originally set up to protect the population against false claims of cures insist that only medical drugs can diagnose and cure diseases. Their agents seek out anyone who makes such claims using different methods than are being propagated by the medical industry and the drug cartels.

Accordingly, anyone who advocates a natural and harmless herb or food is mocked, vilified and may even risk prosecution. That prescription drugs have harmed countless people does not seem to encourage these agencies to go out and warn the masses to think twice before taking them. This would give the nearly one million people who die each year from the devastating side effects caused by prescription drugs a chance to save their lives.

Despite this, over-prescription is at epidemic levels. Nearly 1 in 2 Americans has used a prescription drug in the last month, exposing themselves to numerous side effects and enjoying few benefits.[19] A dose of healthy skepticism about prescription drugs and an openness to alternative medicine on the part of doctors would be a welcome step in healthcare practice. However, current trends suggest that such improvements won't be coming our way anytime soon.

You always create harmful side effects when you treat the symptoms of disease without removing its underlying cause(s). How scientific or reasonable can it be to treat a disease for which the cause remains obscure? How much medical expertise can a prominent oncologist claim if he treats your cancer without having a clue where it is coming from or why it has occurred? It's like putting a band-aid over a severed limb. It just doesn't make sense.

One of the key problems is that today's medical schools do not train their students to think for themselves when it comes to understanding the underlying causes of an illness. Medical doctors are required to follow a rigid treatment protocol, and if they deviate from it, this could easily cost them their license to practice. They may even end up in jail like so many doctors who, out of kindness and compassion, have offered unauthorized alternative treatments to their patients. Can we, therefore, reasonably

---

[19] *Archives of Internal Medicine*, June 13, 2011
See http://www.ncbi.nlm.nih.gov/pubmed/21670331

expect to find out from the medical doctors and the technologies they employ what really are the root causes behind our illness?

For the most part, we remain in the Dark Ages with regard to true healing. According to independent reports by the prestigious *New England Journal of Medicine*, a wing of the American Congress, and the World Health Organization (WHO), 85-90 percent of all medical procedures used by today's medical establishment are unproved and not backed up by scientific research. This includes almost every diagnostic procedure and treatment modality that is offered to you in your doctor's office or by your local hospital – most notably, the use of chemotherapy drugs and radiation.

If we cannot turn to medical doctors for true assistance and enlightenment in our quest for health and healing, could perhaps medical researchers bring us the answers we seek? This is just as unlikely. Most researchers are hired and sponsored by large drug corporations whose main interest lies in subduing and eliminating the symptoms of disease, not the disease itself. The main motivating force behind today's healthcare system, or shall I say, sickness care system, is the incessant need or greed to amass money, power and control. The desire to help humanity achieve health and vitality is shared only by those doctors and health practitioners who have genuine love and compassion for their fellow human beings.

Once again, it is sadly not in the best interest of the medical industry, including the pharmaceutical companies, to find a real cure for cancer or any other chronic illnesses, for this would make the treatment of disease symptoms obsolete. Removing the cause(s) of an illness almost never requires a separate approach that deals with the symptoms of the illness, for these would disappear on their own once the underlying causes are addressed. Unless used for emergencies, costly methods of medical intervention, such as allopathic drugs, complex diagnostic procedures, radiation and surgery, are unnecessary. They also deceive patients and are potentially harmful to their health.[20] The result is a permanent and ever-increasing source of income for drug companies, shareholders, medical institutions and medical practitioners.

If universal healthcare becomes a reality in the U.S., we will also experience a massive escalation of diseases and disease-related fatalities. Many people who currently cannot afford costly medical expenses or medical insurance tend to seek more natural, inexpensive ways of dealing

---

[20] For details, see *Timeless Secrets of Health & Rejuvenation.*

with illness; or else they don't seek any treatment at all. Given the high fatality rate among people receiving medical treatment, the risk of dying from no treatment at all is actually very slim.[21] (You can read more in my book, *The Amazing Liver and Gallbladder Flush* [2012], Chapter Three, in the section *Modern Medicine – Mankind's Greatest Killing Machine*.)

The no-treatment, low fatality risk, however, would be discouraged by *free healthcare*. When I lived in Cyprus in the 1980s, I witnessed an entire population that used to rely mostly on natural methods of healing for thousands of years suddenly become hooked on the modern medical system because it became freely available. Giving something away for free has always been an effective marketing tactic to make people do or buy what they otherwise would never do or buy. Offering free healthcare misleads the people of Cyprus, Germany, France, England and Canada, and it will do the same for the people of the United States, if implemented.

This is not to say that this trend is entirely the fault of the medical system. As long as people do not take responsibility for themselves, for their physical and emotional health, and for their dietary habits and lifestyle, we will have such a dangerous system in place. Millions of people experience devastating consequences resulting from medical treatments that are not warranted at all. Cancer patients, for example, tend to experience the most traumatic side effects because of the highly invasive nature of the treatments involved. The standard treatments for cancer are not meant to heal, but to destroy. The potential benefits of these treatments are not only questionable, but also, according to one of the most comprehensive documented studies, non-existent.

Can You Trust Chemotherapy?

Former White House press secretary Tony Snow died in July 2008 at age 53, following a series of chemotherapy treatments for colon cancer. In 2005, Snow had his colon removed and underwent six months of chemotherapy after his diagnosis. Two years later, he underwent surgery to remove a growth in his abdominal area, near the site of the original cancer. "This is a very treatable condition," said Dr. Allyson Ocean, a

---

[21] See the scientific evidence to that effect in Chapter Fifteen, *What Doctors Should be Telling You*, in my book *Timeless Secrets of Health & Rejuvenation*.

gastrointestinal oncologist at Weill Cornell Medical College. "Many patients, because of the therapies we have, are able to work and live full lives with quality while they're being treated. Anyone who looks at this as a death sentence is wrong." But of course, we now know, Dr. Ocean was indeed dead wrong.

The media headlines proclaimed Snow died from colon cancer, although they knew he didn't have a colon anymore. Apparently, the malignant cancer had *returned* (from where?) and *spread* to the liver and elsewhere in his body. But the truth beyond this *phantom* cancer was that the colon removal severely restricted his normal eliminative functions, thereby overburdening the liver and tissue fluids with toxic waste. The previous series of chemo treatments inflamed and irreversibly damaged a large number of cells in his body, and also impaired his immune system – a perfect recipe for growing new cancers. Now unable to heal the causes of the original cancer (in addition to the newly created ones), Snow's body developed new cancers in the liver and other parts of the body.

The mainstream media, of course, still insists that Snow died from colon cancer, thus perpetuating the myth that it is only the cancer that kills people, not the treatment. Nobody seems to raise the important point that it is extremely difficult for a cancer patient to actually heal from this condition while being subjected to the systemic poisons of chemotherapy and deadly radiation.

Before Tony Snow began the chemo treatments for his second colon cancer, he still looked healthy and strong. But after a few weeks of treatment, he started to develop a hoarse voice, looked frail, turned gray and lost his hair. These are the sort of symptoms that come from chemical poisoning, not cancer.

Do the mainstream media ever report about the overwhelming scientific evidence that shows chemotherapy has zero benefits in the 5-year survival rate of colon cancer patients?[22] Or how many oncologists stand up for their cancer patients and protect them against chemotherapy treatment, which they know can cause them to die far more quickly than if they received no treatment at all? Can you trustingly place your life into their hands when most of them would not even consider chemotherapy for themselves?

---

[22] Confirmation of deficient mismatch repair (dMMR) as a predictive marker for lack of benefit from 5-FU based chemotherapy in stage II and III colon cancer (CC): a pooled molecular reanalysis of randomized chemotherapy trials. (D. J. Sargent, S. Marsoni, S. N. Thibodeau, et al.)

What do they know that you don't?

The news is spreading fast that in the United States, physician-caused fatalities are on the rise each year. Perhaps many doctors no longer trust in what they practice, and for good reason.

"Most cancer patients in this country die of chemotherapy... Chemotherapy does not eliminate breast, colon or lung cancers. This fact has been documented for over a decade. Yet doctors still use chemotherapy for these tumors... Women with breast cancer are likely to die faster with chemo than without it," according to Alan Levin, M.D.

The research covered data from the *Cancer Registry* in Australia and the *Surveillance Epidemiology and End Results* in the U.S. for the year 1998. The current (as of 2012) 5-year relative adult survival rate for cancer in Australia is over 60 percent, and no less than that in the U.S. In comparison, a mere 2.3 percent contribution of chemotherapy to cancer survival does not justify the huge expense involved and the tremendous suffering patients experience because of the severe, toxic side effects resulting from this treatment.

With a meager success rate of 2.3 percent, selling chemotherapy as a medical treatment is one of the greatest scams ever committed. The average chemotherapy earns the medical establishment a whopping $300,000 to $1,000,000 each year, and has so far earned those who promote this poisonous *medication* over a trillion dollars. Medical doctors get $375,000 per patient for chemotherapy, radiation, x-ray, surgery, hospital stays, doctors and anesthesiologists, according to the U.S. Department of Commerce. To earn such a large amount of money so easily can be very tempting to any doctor. Meanwhile, a patient genuinely cured is a goldmine lost. It is no surprise that the medical establishment tries to defend this scam with everything it's got.

In 1990, the highly respected German epidemiologist, Dr. Ulrich Abel from the Tumor Clinic of the University of Heidelberg, conducted the most comprehensive investigation of every major clinical study on chemotherapy drugs ever done. Abel contacted 350 medical centers and asked them to send him anything they had ever published on chemotherapy. He also reviewed and analyzed thousands of scientific articles published in the most prestigious medical journals. It took Abel several years to collect and evaluate the data.

Abel's epidemiological study[23] should have alerted every doctor and cancer patient about the risks of one of the most common treatments used for cancer and other diseases. In his paper, Abel came to the conclusion that the overall success rate of chemotherapy was "appalling". According to this report, **there was no scientific evidence available in any existing study to show that chemotherapy can "extend in any appreciable way the lives of patients suffering from the most common organic cancers".**

Abel points out that chemotherapy rarely improves the quality of life. He describes chemotherapy as "a scientific wasteland" and states that even though there is no scientific evidence that chemotherapy works, neither doctor nor patient is willing to give up on it. The mainstream media has never reported on this hugely important study – of course this is hardly surprising, given the enormous vested interests of the pharmaceutical companies that help sponsor the media. An online search turned up exactly zero reviews of Abel's work in American journals, even though it was published in 1990. I believe this is not because his work was unimportant – but because it is irrefutable.

I must mention at this point that Dr. Abel's book on chemotherapy dates back to 1995, and is not considered up-to-date; moreover it only dealt with carcinomas, not with sarcomas.

However, his work on the inadequate benefits of chemotherapy with respect to carcinomas applies to the vast majority of cancers. Carcinomas are tumors made up principally of epithelial cells of ectodermal or endodermal origin. The solid tumors in nerve tissue and in tissues of body surfaces, or their attached glands, are examples of carcinomas. About 85 percent of cancers are carcinomas, including cervical, breast, prostate, skin and brain carcinomas.

Dr. Abel was fiercely attacked when he released his study. Like many great researchers, he may be very gun-shy now, too. For a scientist to keep his job and to continue receiving funding for new research, he must comply with the expectations of the medical industry, or at least keep his mouth shut. Patients have the right to be well-informed about the scientific basis of their treatment and should not hesitate to ask their oncologist to produce good comparative (randomized) studies showing that the planned treatment is really efficacious in terms of survival and/or quality of life.

---

[23] *Chemotherapy of Advanced Epithelial Cancer:* a critical review, Biomedicine and Pharmacotherapy, 1992; 46: 439-452

Accordingly, current data shows that chemotherapy has a mere overall 2.3 percent success rate in the United States and a 2.1 percent success rate in Australia. It's hardly worth calling a 2.3 percent success rate *successful* when doing nothing at all is significantly more so.

Many doctors go as far as prescribing chemotherapy drugs to patients for malignancies that are far too advanced for surgery, with the full knowledge that there are no benefits at all. Yet they claim chemotherapy to be an effective cancer treatment, and their unsuspecting patients believe that *effective* equals *cure*. The doctors, of course, refer to the FDA's definition of an *effective* drug; that is, one which achieves a 50 percent or more reduction in tumor size for 28 days. They neglect to tell their patients that there is no correlation whatsoever between shrinking tumors for 28 days and curing the cancer or extending life. **Temporary tumor shrinkage through chemotherapy has never been shown to cure cancer or to extend life.**

In other words, you can live with an untreated tumor for just as long as you would with one that has been shrunken or eliminated by chemotherapy (or radiation). Tumors themselves almost never kill anyone unless they obstruct the common bile duct or other vital passages. Certainly in primary cancer, the tumor is never health-endangering or life-threatening. And yet, it is treated as if it were the most dangerous thing on earth. All that progress made with regard to early tumor detection and successful shrinkage of tumors has not been able to increase the survival time of the cancer patient today from what it was 50 years ago. It is all too obvious that whatever standard medical treatment is used is the wrong treatment.

Besides, chemotherapy has never been shown to have curative effects on cancer. By contrast, the body can still cure itself, which it actually tries to do by developing cancer. Cancer is more a healing response than it is a disease. The *disease* **is** the body's attempt to cure itself of an existing imbalance. And, sometimes, this healing response continues even if a person is subjected to chemotherapy (and/or radiation). Unfortunately, as the previously mentioned research has demonstrated, the chances for a real cure are greatly reduced when patients are treated with chemotherapy drugs.

The side effects of the treatment can be horrendous and heartbreaking for both patients and their loved ones, all in the name of trustworthy medical treatment. Although the drug treatment comes with the promise to improve the patient's quality of life, it is just common sense that a drug that makes them vomit and lose their hair, while wrecking their immune system, is doing the exact opposite.

Chemotherapy's deadly poisons inflame every part of the body. It can give the patient life-threatening mouth sores. It attacks the immune system by destroying billions of immune cells (white blood cells). The drugs can slough off the entire lining of their intestines. The most common side effect experienced among chemo patients is their complete lack of energy. The additional drugs now given to many chemo patients may prevent the patient from noticing some of the side effects, but they hardly reduce the immensely destructive and suppressive effect of the chemotherapy itself.

And these effects have been touted by the medical community as proof of its effectiveness; indeed, chemotherapy can shrink or destroy some *cancerous* cells because that is what it does to *all* cells. But hasn't it occurred to chemotherapy advocates that wreaking havoc on the entire body is just making that patient miserable and setting them up for future illness?

What's more, many of those who tout anticancer drugs (if there can truly even be such a thing) are selective about those treatments which they advocate. For example, Canadian researchers at the University of Alberta discovered that the basic drug dichloroacetate (DCA), which is used for treating metabolic disorders, is effective in killing lung, breast and brain cancer cells without harming surrounding healthy tissue, by correcting lactic-acid, anaerobic environment-producing glycolosis.

So why isn't the medical industry or media interested? Quite simply, because the drug doesn't require a patent and therefore can't be upsold by major pharmaceutical companies to generate massive profits. It follows, then, that this profound discovery is likely to remain in obscurity.

It should be pointed out, however, that to reverse glycolysis with DCA, it is better to do this with cleansing the congested pathways of the body, to allow for proper cell oxygenation and tumor regression. Otherwise, you cannot be sure how the body reacts. In 2010 it was found that for human colorectal tumors grown in mice, under hypoxic conditions, DCA decreased rather than increased apoptosis, resulting in enhanced growth of the tumors. These findings suggest that at least in some cancer types, DCA treatment could be detrimental to patient health, highlighting the need for further testing before it can be considered a safe and effective cancer treatment. Besides, the treatment isn't effective in every person.

Therefore, while DCA is one of the rare examples of a pharmaceutical drug that may actually be effective for many patients, it is still far from being a panacea.

If you have cancer, you may think that feeling tired is just part of the disease. This rarely is the case. Feeling unusually tired is more likely due to anemia, a common side effect of most chemotherapy drugs. Chemo drugs can dramatically decrease your red blood cell levels, and this reduces oxygen availability to the 60–100 trillion cells of your body. You can literally feel the energy being zapped from every cell of your body – like physical death without dying. Chemo-caused fatigue has a negative impact on day-to-day activities in 89 percent of patients. Without energy, there can be little joy or hope, and all bodily functions become subdued.

One long-term side effect is that these patients' bodies can no longer respond to nutritional or immune-strengthening approaches to cancerous tumors. All of this may explain why **cancer patients who do not receive any treatment at all, have an up to four times higher remission rate than those who receive treatment.** The sad thing is that chemotherapy does not cure 96 to 98 percent of all cancers, anyway. Conclusive evidence, for the majority of cancers that chemotherapy has any positive influence on survival or quality of life, does not exist.

All in all, to promote chemotherapy as a real treatment for cancer is, to say the very least, extremely misleading. By permanently damaging the body, chemotherapy has become a leading cause of treatment-caused diseases such as heart disease, liver disease, intestinal diseases, diseases of the immune system, infections, brain diseases, pain disorders and rapid aging. This is in addition to the fact that it doesn't really do much to treat cancer, either.

Before committing themselves to being poisoned, cancer patients need to question their doctors and ask them to produce the research or solid evidence that shrinking a tumor actually translates to any increase in survival. If they tell you that chemotherapy is your best chance of surviving, you will know they are lying or are simply misinformed. As Abel's and other research have clearly demonstrated, there is no such evidence to be found in medical literature.

But of course, if an oncologist prescribes a course of chemotherapy to his patient who has pancreatic cancer, although it has been proven to be completely ineffective for this type of cancer, this irresponsible act actually leaves him protected against legal prosecution if the patient dies anyway.

Ironically, if the doctor didn't prescribe the toxic drug, he could be sued by relatives for medical malpractice.

The way the medical system is set up, it lures newly diagnosed cancer patients right into the chemo trap. If a patient were told he had to come up with $100,000 for one course of chemo treatment which would guarantee him a couple of more weeks to live than he otherwise would, he would think about it twice before giving his consent, thereby ruining the lives of his family. Not to mention the terrible side effects he would need to cope with during the last days of his life. But if health insurance pays for the treatment, it's a no-brainer for patients to immediately agree to this *life-saving treatment*, even if there is zero proof that it saves lives.

According to another study, "the failure to eradicate cancer may be as fundamental as a misidentification of the target."[24] In other words, though chemotherapy may be successful at annihilating chunks of tissue, it is unable to address the root of the problem. Why? Because the tumors that chemotherapy seeks to target and *cure* are merely the body's means of creating extra cells to cope with an existing problem. In other words, a truly healthy body will not sustain cancer, because it has no need to do so.

So What *Is* Cancer Exactly?

According to our current medical model, cancer is a general term that describes a group of 100 unique diseases that share one common factor: uncontrolled growth and spread of abnormal cells. Our body naturally produces more cells when it needs them. For example, every person who has done muscle training or exercised regularly knows that his muscles have become larger. However, if cells begin to divide without any readily apparent reason, they will form an excess mass of tissue which is considered a tumor. If the tumor is *malignant*, doctors refer to it as cancerous.

For as long as the basic underlying mechanisms leading up to cancer are not known and dealt with properly, cancer will remain a mystery disease. Cancer is a puzzling phenomenon that has falsely been labeled an *autoimmune disease*, a disease that allegedly turns the body against itself.

---

[24] See http://www.ncbi.nlm.nih.gov/pubmed/16027397

The truth is far from that. The body has been designed to sustain its life for as long as possible. Even the so-called *death gene* has only one purpose, which is to keep the body from self-destructing. Death genes are there to make sure cells die at the end of their normal lifespan and are replaced with new ones.

If the body is designed to live and not to destroy itself, why then would it suddenly allow the growth of extra cell tissue and kill itself? This does not make any sense at all. The main obstacle to finding real cures for cancer is that modern cancer treatment is rooted in the false assumption that the body sometimes tries to destroy itself. Medical students are trained to understand the mechanism of disease development, but they are left in the dark concerning the origins of disease.

Viewed superficially, to the students, an illness appears to be something destructive and harmful to the body. Seen from a deeper perspective, however, the same illness is but an attempt by the body to cleanse and heal itself, or at least to prolong its life. Since medical textbooks offer few insights into the true causes of illness, it is understandable that the majority of doctors today believe that the body has self-destructive, even suicidal, tendencies. Claiming to be non-superstitious and objective, they inadvertently admit that certain cells suddenly and mysteriously decide to malfunction, become malicious, and randomly attack other cells and organs in the body.

Based on this purely subjective and unsubstantiated belief, the doctor and his patient alike become almost obsessed with trying to protect the body from itself. Yet despite such undisputed notions of *truth*, none of this means that the body does, in fact, attempt or cause its own destruction. Would it actually astound you if I told you that cancer has never killed a person?

Wisdom of Cancer Cells

Cancer cells are not part of a malicious disease process. When cancer cells *spread* (metastasize)[25] throughout the body, it is not their purpose or goal to disrupt the body's vital functions, infect healthy cells and obliterate

---

[25] It has never been proven that cancer cells move around the body and indiscriminately form new colonies of cancer cells. Rather, new colonies may grow for the same reasons the previous ones did.

their host. Self-destruction is not the goal of any cell until it is old, worn-out and ready to be turned over, as many cells do on a daily basis. Cancer cells, like all other cells, know that if the body dies, they will die as well. A cancerous tumor is neither the cause of progressive destruction nor does it actually lead to the death of the body. There is nothing in a cancer cell that even remotely has the ability to kill anything. If you asked people walking in the street if they knew how cancer kills people, you would probably not get one definite, correct answer. Ask the same question of doctors and you may not get a much better result. You are unlikely to hear that cancer doesn't kill anyone.

Contrary to hearsay, what eventually leads to the demise of an organ or the entire body is the wasting away of healthy cell tissue, which results from a continued deprivation of nutrients and life force. **The drastic reduction or shutdown of vital nutrient supplies to the cells of an organ is not primarily a *consequence* of a cancerous tumor, but actually its biggest cause.**

By definition, a cancer cell is a normal, healthy cell that has undergone genetic mutation to the point that it can live in anaerobic surroundings (an environment where oxygen is not available). In other words, if you deprive a group of cells of vital oxygen (their primary source of energy), some of them will die, but others will evolve in a most ingenious way: the cells will become able to live without oxygen and will adapt to derive some of their energy needs from such things as cellular metabolic waste products. (I have discussed this further in the next chapter.)

This is somewhat similar to bacteria, which are divided into two main groups, aerobic and anaerobic,[26] meaning those that need to use oxygen, and those that can live without it. Aerobic bacteria thrive in an oxygenated environment. They are responsible for helping us with the digestion of food and with the manufacture of important nutrients, such as B vitamins. Anaerobic bacteria, on the other hand, can appear and thrive only in an environment where oxygen does not reach it. They break down waste materials, toxic deposits and dead, worn-out cells.

---

[26] There are some specialized bacteria that are both aerobic and anaerobic.

How Infection Can Prevent and Cure Cancer

Life on Earth would not be possible without infectious bacteria, fungi and viruses. Their existence and continuous interaction with humans and animals over millions of years have trained and evolved into what we refer to as the immune system, today. Our ability to live in harmony with our external environment is, in fact, rooted in our life-long relationship with these germs.

Even though we have many times the number of germs inside our body than we have cells, we have been taught to be afraid of them and fight especially those that are considered pathogenic (disease-causing). Nobody has told us, though, that acute infection can be a desirable event, even a necessary one, if we want to make it through life without incurring a major life-threatening illness.

Each new encounter with a germ and a possible, resulting infection further strengthen the immune system until it is fully developed and capable of living in complete harmony with the natural environment. This doesn't mean, though, that one must become sick in order to develop a healthy immune system. Most infections actually occur *silently*, without the person ever developing the symptoms of illness.

Since mass vaccination was introduced around the world, nearly every child is now being infected with different viruses by injection from the day of birth until at least age 15. Sometimes the child gets injected with three different viruses at the same time (through the mumps/measles/rubella vaccine). Vaccinations crudely interrupt or even inhibit the natural immunization program devised by nature itself. This unwise intervention can have unexpected and potentially devastating consequences throughout a person's life.

Ever since it was discovered that the presence of infectious agents, like E. coli bacteria in our gut, are a prerequisite for having a healthy gut immune system, some of us have begun to respect these germs as friends, not enemies. But isolating such germs from their natural environment, breeding them and manipulating them in a test tube, and then injecting them into the blood as vaccines, can turn these otherwise highly beneficial infectious agents into deadly weapons against which the body is defenseless.

A newborn animal or child can become blind by depriving it of light for an extended period of time. Likewise, a child's cellular immune system is rendered useless unless it becomes exposed to the germs that inhabit our environment.

Why Infections Can Save Lives

Infection is one of the greatest cures there can be. In fact, infection can prevent cancer and other illnesses, and, yes, cure them. In a 2005 epidemiological study covering over 151 previously conducted studies, researchers from the Department of Health Care and Epidemiology, University of British Columbia, found an inverse association between acute infections and cancer development [*Cancer Detection and Prevention*, 2006; 30(1):83-93. Epub, 2006 February 21].

According to the abstract of this study, entitled "Acute infections as a means of cancer prevention: Opposing effects to chronic infections?", exposures to febrile infectious childhood diseases were associated with subsequently reduced risks for melanoma, ovarian and multiple cancers combined, significant in the latter two groups.

Furthermore, epidemiological studies on common acute infections in adults, and subsequent cancer development, found these infections to be associated with reduced risks for meningioma, glioma, melanoma and multiple cancers combined, significantly for the latter three groups. Overall, risk reduction increased with the frequency of infections, with febrile infections affording the greatest protection. In other words, children who experienced all the typical childhood infections were most protected from developing cancers in adult life.

At a time when cancer is going to affect 1 in every 2 people, this finding should have made national news, and it should be taught at medical schools. National health policies should have been altered radically, but nothing ever happened. We are still being told that having mumps in children must be avoided at all costs. Never mind that the temporary inconvenience of a largely harmless infection could protect a person from developing a devastating form of cancer 20 or 30 years later, which, in turn, is typically attacked with potentially deadly methods of treatment (chemotherapy, radiation and surgery).

The discovery that acute infections are clearly antagonistic to cancer helps us understand why artificially induced fever has been successfully used for the treatment of cancer in European countries, especially in Germany. Of course, many doctors now treat fever as if it were a disease and often prescribe toxic pharmaceuticals to put out the *dangerous fire*. Yet, since fever is the body's natural way of healing and eliminating pathogens such as infectious viruses and bacteria, squashing it with medication practically prevents any effective healing in the body.

Fortunately, some good researchers now stand up for the body's innate healing tactics, which our mothers and grandmothers had known about all along. French microbiologist Dr. Andre Lwoff has discovered that fever cures even incurable diseases. One of the world's leading cancer specialists, Dr. Josef Issels, wrote along these lines: "Artificially induced fever has the greatest potential in the treatment of many diseases, including cancer." And Oxford professor Dr. David Mychles and his research team have independently proven the effectiveness of induced fever for treating disease, including cancer.

There is further historical evidence that infection prevents cancer in the population. For example, Rome used to be surrounded by swamps that bred malaria mosquitoes, infecting many in the city. The fever that Romans developed from time to time, though, kept their cancer rates well below the average found in the rest of Italy. Then the government decided to drain the swamps, but soon Rome's cancer rate increased dramatically to the normal rate in Italy.

The Magic of Nature

The WHO's official line is that infectious agents are responsible for almost 22 percent of cancer deaths in the developing world and 6 percent in industrialized countries. Viral hepatitis B and C are blamed for cancer of the liver; human papilloma virus infection is said to lead to cervical cancer; the bacterium Helicobacter pylori is held responsible for increasing the risk of stomach cancer. In some countries the parasitic infection schistosomiasis increases the risk of bladder cancer, and in other countries the liver fluke increases the risk of cholangiocarcinoma of the bile ducts. Preventive measures include vaccination and protection against infection and infestation. All this, of course, makes a lot of sense to almost everyone who hears it, unless they know a little about the magical ways of nature.

Destructive bacteria naturally increase in larger numbers wherever excessive waste matter accumulates and requires decomposition. Have you ever wondered why we have more bacteria in our body than we have cells? Most bacteria are produced inside the body, whereas relatively few enter it from the outside. The body also *grows* bacteria from tiny, indestructible colloids of life in our blood and cells. One of the world's most ingenuous medical researchers, Professor Antoine Béchamp (1816–1908), called these tiny cellular compounds microzyma. The German scientist, Dr. Günther Enderlein, who published papers on this research in 1921 and 1925, referred to them as protits. Protits are tiny dots in the blood and cells that you can see with any microscope. These dots or colloids of life are virtually indestructible and survive even after the body dies.

According to the phenomenon known as pleomorphism, these protits develop or change form in response to a changing condition (acid/base balance) of the blood or cell milieu. As the cell environment becomes acidified and toxic, the protits turn into microorganisms that are designed to break down and remove dead cells, toxins and metabolic waste products that the body is unable to remove.

If further destruction of dead, weak cells and other waste is required, the protits become viruses and, eventually, fungi. You may know how difficult it can be to get rid of a toenail/foot fungus. Fungi only go after dead, organic matter. The presence of congested and half-decayed or dead toe tissue practically forces the body to produce and/or attract more and more fungi to help decompose the lifeless parts of the foot.

As you might know, cancer cells are filled with all sorts of microorganisms. Allopathic medicine does not really explain how they get into the cells, unless they are viral. Most doctors assume that the germs come from the outside, but this assumption has been disproved and was even disputed by Louis Pasteur, the inventor of the germ theory.

As the brilliant scientists Béchamp and Enderlein demonstrated, these germs are created inside the cells in response to the presence of undernourished or poorly oxygenated cell tissue, or other toxic waste material that the body is unable to remove on its own. Their purpose is to decompose these damaged, weak cells. This microbial activity is commonly known as *infection*. Like cancer, an infection is not a disease. Rather, it is a sophisticated, combined attempt by the body and microbes to avert the suffocation and poisoning caused by accumulated toxic waste material in its tissues, the lymphatic system or the blood.

If you piled up kitchen garbage in one area of your house, it would attract a lot of flies and bacteria, and this would generate a foul-smelling odor. You would certainly not blame the flies and bacteria for the stench. They are just trying to digest some of the garbage. Likewise, those microbes that are attracted to or produced inside unhealthy cells are not part of the problem; they are part of the solution to the problem.

An infection, if properly supported by natural approaches of cleansing and nourishment,[27] can practically prevent the genetic mutation of aerobic cells into cancer cells. According to over 150 studies conducted in the past 100 or more years, spontaneous tumor regression has followed bacterial, fungal, viral and protozoal infections.[28] During episodes of fever, tumors literally break up, and the cancer cells are promptly removed via the lymphatic system and other organs of elimination.

During such a major infection, which is nothing but an appropriate healing response initiated by bacteria and the immune system, a considerable amount of toxic waste is broken down and removed from the body. This, once again, permits oxygen to reach the oxygen-deprived cells. Upon contact with the oxygen, the cancer cells die or otherwise mutate back into normal cells. The tumors have no more reason to be there, hence the occurrence of spontaneous remission of cancer in these patients. In some cases, brain tumors as large as the size of an egg have literally disappeared in this way within 24 hours.

Therefore, the standard approach of suppressing infection and its resultant fever among hospital patients stands responsible for the loss of millions of lives that could easily have been saved by letting the body's natural healing takes its course.

And it is a problem that begins in childhood. Parents are taught to greatly fear these natural processes and bring their children in to the doctor and pump them full of antibiotics at the slightest fever. Yet this

---

[27] See my book, *Timeless Secrets of Health & Rejuvenation.*
[28] Research paper by S. A. Hoption Cann, J. P. van Netten, and C. van Netten (July 2003) — Department of Healthcare and Epidemiology, University of British Columbia; Special Development Laboratory, Royal Jubilee Hospital and Department of Biology, University of Victoria, British Columbia, Canada.

fever is merely an indication that the child's immune system is strong and already doing its job [*Pediatrics,* June 2001 Vol. 107 No. 6, pp. 1241-1246].

There are over 100 studies suggesting that not only do germs *not* cause cancer, but also that infections may be a means of cancer prevention by strengthening the immune system. Vaccines and medicines that interfere with this process are largely responsible for the weak immune systems that allow, indeed desperately need, cancer to thrive as an emergency means of healing the body.

We can therefore conclude that infection is not something to be feared, but rather something to be embraced as part of the body's natural system of maintaining balance and ridding itself of toxins. Allopathic medicine's knee-jerk tendency to respond to any and all infections with antibiotics ultimately only makes our immune systems weaker and renders us vulnerable to greater illness down the road.

Germs Don't Cause Cancer

The germs involved in an infection become active and infectious only when waste matter has gathered or tissue damage has already occurred. This is true whether they are of a bacterial or viral origin, and whether they are generated within the body or introduced from the external environment. Destructive microorganisms simply have no business in a clean, well-circulated, oxygen-rich environment. There is nothing to be disposed of, and no immune response is necessary to protect the body.

Even if harmful germs were to enter cell tissue in a healthy body, they would do it no harm. A virus simply cannot penetrate into the nucleus of a well-oxygenated cell because exposure to oxygen would kill it. A well-oxygenated cell also produces powerful antiviral drugs, such as interferon. If for some reason a virus has made contact with a cell, but its presence is not beneficial to the body, the virus will be destroyed by the cell's natural defense mechanisms or the general immune system. Viruses do not help cells mutate into cancer cells, unless this is in the best interest of the body. We should not fall into the trap of misinterpreting this to be an act of self-destruction. **It is important to recall at this point that cancer is not a disease, but a healing mechanism that occurs only when all other protective measures have failed.**

There is profound purpose and intelligence at every level of physical creation, from the smallest of particles to the most complex star clusters in the large-scale universe. Just because many scientists and doctors prefer to see nature as behaving in a random, incoherent fashion does not mean it actually is chaotic and unpredictable.

Cancer is not as chaotic as the *experts* would have us believe. It has as much purpose and meaning as does a virus or bacterium. A virus only infects the nucleus of a cell that is on the verge of becoming anaerobic. To find virus material in cancer cells is, therefore, not proof that viruses cause cancer. In fact, viruses try to prevent the demise of the body. They are created for the body and by the body. It is completely normal for weak, deteriorating cells to transform their protit colloids into bacteria, viruses and fungi to help prevent more damage to the body than has already occurred, due to the accumulation of toxic waste matter.

Suppressing an infection with germ-killing medication destroys much of the germ population. However, it is the germ population that helps to stimulate a much-needed immune response to rid the body of cancer-causing toxins.

Modern vaccination programs are largely responsible for the significant deterioration of natural immunity among the vaccinated populations around the world. The body does not acquire real immunity to infectious diseases by exposing it to vaccines (antibody production alone does not create immunity). In fact, with each vaccine, the immune system becomes more depleted. The short-term gain of becoming symptom-free through the use of such magic bullet approaches can have serious repercussions in the long term.

The toxic waste and cell debris gathered in the body can act like a time bomb, but most people do not want to hear it ticking. They stick their heads in the sand, hoping that somehow the problem will simply go away. However, when the ticking becomes too unnerving and the patient experiences symptoms of disease, the resulting visit to the doctor may smash the clock; nevertheless, it still leaves the bomb intact. It remains just a matter of time before the bomb explodes. But without a warning mechanism, the strike will come as a nasty surprise.

On the other hand, allowing the body to receive assistance from helpfully destructive germs may dismantle the bomb entirely. The toxic secretions from these microbes prompt the immune system to launch a preemptive strike against potential cancer formation. A spontaneous remission of cancer is not a rare miracle. It happens in millions of people who unknowingly diffuse these *time bombs* through an infection, such as the simple cold or flu. This is how 95 percent of all cancers come and go without any notice or medical intervention.

Based on statistical information, we can estimate that treating cancer with suppressive methods such as radiation, chemotherapy and surgery reduces the chance of complete remission from 28 percent to 7 percent or less. In other words, medical treatment is responsible for the deaths of over 1 in every 5 cancer patients. Still think that chemotherapy is a good idea?

Oh, Those Bad Free Radicals!

You may wonder about those bad oxygen free radicals that everyone talks about. Isn't it true that they are behind most cancers and other diseases? If this is true, how can we defend ourselves against them, other than by removing them with such antioxidants as vitamin C?

Oxygen free radicals are typically responsible for causing many of man's common ailments, including cancer, hardening of the arteries and aging of the skin. Nearly everyone is aware of the term oxidative stress, and food supplements that boast antioxidant benefits abound. However, published research at the German Cancer Research Center (Krebsforschungszentrum) shows that these highly reactive molecules maybe a lot less harmful than once thought. According to the researchers, it is apparently not even possible to influence these oxidative processes through substances that act as antioxidants.

Oxygen free radicals are highly reactive oxygen molecules. They are involved in causing rust in iron and turning fats rancid. They are also found in arteries that have become occluded with plaque. Many researchers believe that free radicals are involved in the formation of cancer cells. However, like bacteria, free radicals have been given an unjustifiably bad reputation. Free radicals have existed since the beginning of life on Earth. **Why would they now lead to cancer in 1 out of every 2 people when just 100 years ago only 1 in 8,000 people suffered the same fate?** Did free radicals just become a lot more *vicious* in the past 100 years, ever so eager to oxidize us to death? The answer is a resounding "No".

Free radicals only oxidize and destroy what is already weak and potentially damaging to the body. They never attack healthy, vital cell tissue. Weak or worn-out cells and accumulated metabolic waste material – which the body's lymphatic system normally removes without a problem – become a hazard when they are trapped in the tissues and the free radicals are not doing their job. Increasing free radical activity and spreading infectious germs are therefore the next best alternatives to the body's own cleansing and eliminative efforts, especially when the body's immune system is already compromised. Thus, neither free radicals nor germs can rightfully be considered a *cause* of illness and aging. Since illness is actually a healing mechanism and aging is a form of advanced congestion in the body, free radicals must, in fact, be considered the beneficial *effects* of illness and aging.

The more often infections are *prevented* or suppressed through medical interventions, the less efficient the liver and kidneys, as well as the immune, lymphatic and digestive systems become in keeping the body's cell tissues free of harmful, noxious deposits.

Yet, not only do infections and free radicals act as cleansers; pain also serves as a healing aid. Pain is merely a signal that the body is actively involved in a healing response that includes repairing damaged tissues and cleansing itself. By suppressing pain with medication, you short-circuit the body's internal communication and healing mechanisms, and practically force it to hold on to, and eventually suffocate in, its own waste. Cancer is a natural consequence of dealing with such a distressing, unnatural situation.

Mutated Genes Do Not Cause Cancer

Cancer cells are normal, oxygen-dependent cells that have been genetically reprogrammed to survive in an oxygen-deprived environment. Why would a healthy cell nucleus, which contains the genetic makeup (DNA) of the cell, suddenly decide to give up its need for oxygen and turn itself into a cancer cell? This is a simple question that lies at the very core of the complex mystery surrounding cancer.

Those who know in their gut that the law of cause and effect applies to every natural phenomenon must wonder whether cancer is, after all, only the natural effect of an underlying, unnatural cause. To treat cancer as if it were a supernaturally malicious illness without removing its underlying cause is nothing but malpractice. It is clear that such an approach has potentially fatal consequences for most cancer patients. Instead of reducing cancer occurrence and cancer mortality, standard medical approaches used for treating cancer actually contribute to increasing both.

Blaming the genes doesn't help, since the genetic blueprint in a cancerous cell is no longer aligned with the original genetic blueprint (DNA) found in other normal cells of the body. However, its genes didn't suddenly decide or volunteer to be *mal-aligned* or malignant, as they call it. Genetic blueprints do not act on anything; but when the cell environment changes, they become altered or mal-aligned with the original blueprints.

According to American research,[29] the genes DNA-PK and p53 are essential components of the body's repair system. When they are intact, the cell is safe. But when either goes wrong, the cell divides and multiplies uncontrollably. DNA-PK normally repairs damaged genes. However, cancerous cells can also harness DNA-PK's power to repair themselves from damage caused by anticancer treatments. This makes these cells more resistant to the therapy, which may also explain why the orthodox cancer treatments, chemotherapy and radiotherapy, are such a failure.

The more intense the anticancer treatment is, the more *vicious* and powerful the cancer becomes. This, of course, dramatically reduces the chances for survival, just as repeatedly attacking bacteria with antibiotics makes them become resistant *superbugs*.

Now, p53 acts as a signaling system, sending out messages that stop damaged cells from dividing and forming tumors. This powerful gene is altered in about 80 percent of cancers. However, the focus of cancer research should not be on figuring out what kind of genetic mutation occurs, but on the changes in the body that necessitate it.

To repeat, genes do not just change without a reason. They only do so if they are forced to mutate in response to adverse changes in the cell environment.

---

[29] *Cancer Research*, 61, 8723-8729, December 15, 2001

Cancer: An Ingenious Rescue Mission

So what kind of extreme situation could possibly coerce a healthy cell to abandon its original genetic design and stop using oxygen? The answer is strikingly simple: lack of oxygen. Normal cells meet their energy needs by combining oxygen with glucose. *Cell mutation* occurs only in surroundings where little or no oxygen is available. Without oxygen, the cells have to find other ways to meet their energy requirements.

The second most efficient option for obtaining energy is through fermentation. Anaerobic cells (cancer cells) thrive in areas where plenty of metabolic waste products are trapped. These cells are capable of deriving energy from fermenting, for example, the metabolic waste product lactic acid. This is similar to a starving animal eating its own excrement.

By reusing lactic acid, the cancer cells accomplish two things. First, they derive energy for their sustenance. Second, they take this potentially dangerous waste product away from the immediate environment of the healthy cells. If cancer cells did not remove lactic acid from the cell environment, this extremely strong acid would accumulate and lead to fatal acidosis – destruction of healthy cells due to high levels of acidity. Without the presence of a lactic acid-metabolizing tumor, the lactic acid could perforate the blood vessel walls and, along with other waste material and contaminants, enter the bloodstream. The result would be blood poisoning and subsequent death.

The body sees the cancer as such an important defense mechanism that it even causes the growth of new blood vessels to guarantee that the cancer cells receive a much-needed supply of glucose and, therefore, are able to survive and spread. It knows that the cancer cells do not *cause*, but *prevent* death, at least for a while, until the wasting away of an organ leads to the demise of the entire organism. If the trigger mechanisms for cancer are properly taken care of – that is, if the body is properly balanced and can detoxify itself naturally – this outcome can be avoided.

Cancer is not an indication that the body is about to destroy itself. Cancer is not a disease; it is the final and most desperate survival mechanism the body has at its disposal. It only takes control of the body when all other measures of self-preservation have failed. To truly heal cancer and what it represents in a person's life, we must come to the understanding that what the body does when allowing some of its cells to grow in abnormal ways is in its best interest.

Chapter Two

Cancer's Physical Causes

Cancer, once again, is not a disease that strikes randomly and maliciously. Its increased occurrence in our era is merely our bodies' response to a lifestyle of chronic imbalance and toxic overload. This toxic overload takes many forms; therefore, it can be said that cancer has many causes. While I have already alluded to many of these, let us briefly review them:

- Chemical exposures, particularly pesticides and pollution
- Processed and artificial foods (as well as their often-poisonous packaging)
- Wireless technologies, *dirty* electricity and radiation from medical diagnostic technology
- Pharmaceutical drugs
- Lack of sunshine exposure and the use of sunscreens
- Obesity, stress and poor eating habits

Identifying the Origin of Cancer

To discover and understand the physical causes of cancer, you will first need to let go of the idea that cancer is a disease. You cannot have it both ways. Either you trust in your body's innate wisdom and healing abilities, or you don't. In the former case you are already encouraged by what your body is doing on your behalf, and in the latter case you are frightened by it. The perspective of what cancer means to you ultimately determines whether you will heal or continue to fight an uphill battle.

The commonly held belief that cancer is a disease represents a powerful force that nearly every cancer patient is confronted with. Although this belief is based on a misconception of what cancer really is, it nevertheless generates a preoccupation with being healthy, which, in turn, further strengthens the belief of disease. *Trying* to be healthy shows that there exists an imbalance on all levels of body, mind and spirit. A balanced, healthy person doesn't *try* to be healthy; he doesn't even think about it. He merely accepts and supports his body's own ability to regulate itself.

This is how spontaneous remissions occur. The body uses its maximum healing capacity when it is not preoccupied with stress, fear and harmful *treatments*. As always, there is something to be learned from every situation, including having cancer. A person's willingness to face, accept and learn from the issues that cancer brings up turns this *dis-ease* into a purposeful, potentially uplifting and sometimes even euphoric experience. During hundreds of interviews with cancer survivors over the past 30 years, I found that almost all of them shared one experience: it had caused the most important and positive changes ever in their lives.

In our modern societies, we learn to go more by superficial appearances and less by the concealed larger picture of things. It is the nature of life that for every symptom, an underlying cause exists. Yet, the cause lies hidden and may seem to be unrelated to the symptom. Purely mechanistic approaches to treating the body, as they are applied in the system of allopathic medicine, usually fall short in locating and healing these hidden causes. They will remain undetected unless we begin to view the body as a *process* that is organized by a superb combination of energy, information and intelligence, not just an assembly of different parts, as in a simple machine.

To treat the body as if it were composed merely of cells and molecules is akin to applying technology straight out of the Middle Ages to our present day world. Modern technologies and computers were derived from the principles of information and energy that came to light through the study of quantum physics. Yet with regard to understanding the nature of life and treating the human body, we still rely mostly on outdated and incomplete Newtonian principles. Understanding the way the human body operates becomes relatively easy once we apply the principles of quantum physics.

As consciousness, soul or spirit, you are the only true source of the energy and information that run your body. Your presence in the body and what you do, eat, drink, feel and think determine how well your genes are able to control and sustain your physical existence.

In other words, although genes appear to be in charge of essential functions in the body, as it has been proven by thousands of scientific studies, they are controlled by you. For example, research has shown that vitamin D, which your body produces in response to sun exposure, regulates over 2,000 genes which, in turn, regulate your immune system, digestion, repair and healing mechanisms, blood values, etc. Therefore, if you choose to avoid regular sun exposure, you inactivate these genes, thereby making yourself susceptible to multiple types of less ideal healing responses, including cancer. In the extreme case scenario, if you (the conscious presence) are no longer present in your body, the energy and information are withdrawn from every cell. We know this to be physical death.

Seen from a superficial point of view, you could conclude that death has turned the body into a disordered heap of useless particles. Of course, if you had a wider perspective of death, you would be able to see it as the beginning of new life; all the atoms that previously comprised these cells have simply relocated themselves to assemble once again in new forms, such as air, water, soil, plants, fruit, animals or other living beings. Life does not end with death; only the form changes. Furthermore, your consciousness remains unaffected by all of this because it is not physical and therefore cannot be destroyed.

Now, if you only partially withdrew your energy and purposeful connectedness from some parts of your body, would those parts not move into disarray and chaotic behavior? This is what medicine calls *disease*, when the body is no longer in ease or alignment with its typically orderly fashion. However, disease is only an illusion of perception. Like death, disease is nothing but the provider of new life. **Yet unlike death, disease offers us the opportunity to restore our life while remaining in this physical form.** Cancer only strikes when a part or parts of us are not alive anymore – physically, emotionally or spiritually. Cancer can resurrect these numbed, suppressed or congested areas, whether they are physical or non-physical in nature.

This resurrection, which begins with increased attention to these dead zones of our life, can occur in a number of ways. We may gradually become aware of how afraid or negligent we are of a particular body part, the body as a whole, our future or our past, nature, food, other people, the future of our planet, or other issues. Suddenly, we may begin to realize how deeply we have harbored intense negative emotions toward others or ourselves, or we may notice why we have allowed certain foods, beverages or drugs, such as painkillers, steroids and antibiotics, to contaminate our beautiful body. Cancer is a wake-up call, prompting us to take our life back when it no longer feels balanced or meaningful.

The *disease*, cancer, occurs only where channels or ducts of circulation and waste elimination have been consistently blocked for a long time. This chapter deals with the purely physical causes of cancer, although, to truly make sense of cancer, it must also be seen in the context of emotional and spiritual causes. All this is the subject matter of Chapters Three and Four.

Cancer's Progressive Stages

Since I am writing this book mainly for the layperson, I will avoid obscuring it with complex medical jargon and complicated references to scientific studies. Instead, I will explain in simple step-by-step terms how most cancers develop. You will see the common thread that connects the symptom, cancer, with its layers of origin. Together we will unravel the mystery of cancer by going through its progressive stages in reverse order. Please keep in mind that each cause is just another effect of yet another cause. Eventually, though, we will arrive at the root origin of cancer, which I will explain in Chapter Four.

I have mentioned before that a cancer cell is one that has lost the ability to fulfill its preprogrammed responsibilities of ensuring balance or homeostasis in the body. Instead of fulfilling its natural duty, such a cell has turned itself over to a new type of professional occupation that you could describe as *sewer worker*. It is not a coincidence or bad luck, but a necessity and blessing in disguise, that cancer cells grab hold of harmful by-products of metabolism and ingest them. As we shall see, this waste material has no means to escape the cell surroundings, except via the *hungry mouths* of cancer cells.

A common consensus among the majority of the medical and lay population holds that the gradual *degradation* of normal cells into cancer cells is due to random mistakes that the body somehow makes, perhaps because of hereditary reasons, often called genetic predisposition. This theory not only defies logic, but also the intrinsic purpose of evolution.

Every great discovery man has made has revealed that something seemingly useless or even harmful is actually imbued with meaning and purpose. The destruction of the blossoms of a fruit tree should not be mistaken as an act of self-annihilation; rather, it is the destructive force that brings nutritious fruit to life. Although the idea that cancer is a deadly weapon the body creates to destroy itself (an autoimmune disease) is based on medical tests, it does not reflect a high degree of scientific insight, and certainly defies all sense of wisdom and logic. Do we need a new, different interpretation of these tests to actually make sense of cancer and why it occurs?

As mentioned earlier, in 1900, only 1 in 8,000 people had cancer. Now, 1 in every 2 people can expect to develop some type of cancer at some stage in their lifetime. In the United States alone, nearly one million people die each year from a chronic illness, most of them from cancer. Cancer has surpassed heart disease as the number one cause of death. What is going on here? Nothing in the natural world suggests that this is normal. Not knowing what cancer really is has made it into a dangerous disease.

During every single day in your adult life, the body turns over about 30 billion cells. Out of these, an estimated 1 percent undergo a programmed genetic mutation and turn cancerous. Your immune system is programmed to detect these cells and destroy them. The body's *clean-up task force* is so efficient, perfectly timed and thorough that these anaerobic cancer cells stand no chance. Yet, it is essential for the body's own survival that these kinds of cancer cells are created every day; they make certain that the immune system remains stimulated enough to keep its defense and self-purification capability efficient and up-to-date.

This naturally raises the question of why the same immune system would refrain from attacking cancer cells that have mutated in response to dealing with severe congestion (as explained below). Let me ask the same question in a different way: Why does the immune system discriminate between these two kinds of cancers and decide to destroy one group of cancer cells while leaving the other unharmed?

This important question deserves an answer. The cancer we generally refer to as disease is not actually a disease at all; rather, it is an extended immune response to help clear up an existing condition of toxic congestion that suffocates a group of cells. Why in the world would the immune system try to hinder its own efforts to prevent certain toxic metabolic waste products from entering the bloodstream and killing the body? Given the circumstances, these cancer cells are far too precious and too useful for the body to eliminate them.

Even if they entered the lymphatic ducts and were transported to other parts of the body,[30] the immune system would still try to keep them alive for as long as they were useful. Cancer cells do not randomly spread throughout the body. They may grow in any place that is also congested and oxygen-deprived.

Both healthy and cancerous cells in the body are loaded with cancer-killing white blood cells, such as T-cells. In the case of kidney cancer and melanomas, for example, white cells make up 50 percent of the mass of the cancers. Since T-cells easily recognize foreign or mutated cell tissue such as cancer cells, you would expect these immune cells to attack cancer cells right away. However, the immune system allows cancer cells to recruit it in order to actually grow larger tumors and develop tumors in others parts of the body as well. Cancer cells produce specific proteins that tell the immune cells to leave them alone and help them grow.

Why would the immune system want to collaborate with cancer cells to make more tumors or larger ones? Because cancer is a survival mechanism, not a disease, by which the body uses the cancer to keep deadly carcinogenic substances and caustic metabolic waste matter away from the lymph and blood. In so doing, this prevents toxins from reaching the heart, brain and other vital organs. Killing off cancer cells would, in fact, jeopardize its survival.

It is important to know that the body attacks a cancerous tumor only after the congestion that has led to the tumor's growth in the first

---

[30] This is called *metastasis*. However, there is no evidence to show that metastasis really occurs. It is more likely that a *new* cancer develops in other parts of the body for the same reasons the first cancer developed.

place has been broken up. As mentioned in Chapter One, this would be the case, for example, following a major infection, such as the chickenpox or the flu. I will discuss other reasons for the occurrence of spontaneous remissions at a later stage in this book.

1. Congestion

So just what kind of congestion are we talking about here, and where is it coming from? Allow me to illustrate by using the following example: In a large city like New York, traffic may flow smoothly during normal hours or on Sundays, but at rush hour there are suddenly far more cars on the road than the city can handle. The resulting traffic congestion may force you to spend hours instead of minutes getting from your workplace to your home. Eventually, though, you will find your way home. This is what I call temporary congestion.

However, the situation would be different if there had been a major traffic accident due to ice and snow, and the roads leading to your home were now completely blocked. This accident affects every car waiting to move forward, although nothing is inherently wrong with the cars themselves. Equally affected are trucks that deliver goods to stores or take trash to landfills; mothers on their way home to feed their children; businessmen heading to the airport to catch a plane; and thousands of other commuters stranded for various reasons. The effect is the same for all involved – they are all equally unable to reach their destination. Unless someone removes the cause of the traffic congestion, they remain stuck among a vast number of exhaust-producing cars.

If someone were to come along and propose that the best way to clear the congestion would be to get a large bulldozer and push every car off the road, you would think he must be out of his mind. Yet, this is exactly how allopathic medicine deals with cancer. In cancer, a more or less permanent traffic jam has developed in the body, but this traffic jam has been caused by a holdup somewhere else. No longer can nutrients such as oxygen and glucose be delivered to their destinations, nor can cellular waste products be cleared away. Instead of using toxic drugs or surgical *bulldozers* to destroy or remove cells that have been affected by the traffic congestion, it would be a far wiser course of action to seek out the initial holdup that has led to the congestion in the first place.

We have already analyzed that normal cells turn cancerous when they do not get enough oxygen to do their metabolic work. Without cell metabolism, the body would turn cold and lifeless within minutes. To keep some sort of metabolism going without the use of oxygen, albeit far from ideal, the cells have to change (mutate) into anaerobic cells that are capable of utilizing accumulated metabolic waste products, and delivering at least some of the required heat and energy in the body. To blame and subsequently punish these cells for such an act of instinctive wisdom would be very shortsighted.

If you look for the underlying reason for this situation, it is the holdup that prevents oxygen and other nutrients from reaching the cells. There is basically only one such holdup, although it has two components – the thickening of the blood capillary walls and the congestion of the lymphatic ducts.

2. The Holdup

Please be reminded that we are trying to trace the origin(s) of cancer, step by step, moving from the symptom back toward the cause. The holdup or obstruction that causes a traffic jam is apparently due to the wreck of a car or truck; but, in reality, it is brought about by another factor, such as fatigue, distraction due to talking on a cell phone, speeding or drunken driving.

In the human body, such a *traffic jam* can be generated by thickened blood vessel walls, which prevent the proper passage of oxygen, water, glucose and other vital nutrients from the blood to the cells. Nutrients in the blood naturally pass through the blood vessel wall and gravitate to the cells through a process known as osmosis. After dropping off its precious cargo, the blood returns to the lungs, liver and digestive system to take up more of the same.

Some nutrients, such as water and oxygen, pass through the blood vessel walls freely, whereas others need assistance in the form of a carrier or guide. The hormone *insulin*, secreted by specialized pancreatic cells, plays such a role. It is released when any of several stimuli are detected. These include protein ingestion and presence of glucose in the blood.

Once injected into the blood by the pancreas, insulin takes up sugar (glucose) from the blood and transports it into muscle, fat and liver cells, where it is converted into energy (adenosine triphosphate or ATP) or stored as fat. This basic metabolic process, which is responsible for keeping the entire body alive and healthy, becomes disturbed once the blood vessel walls begin to thicken.

Why would the body allow its blood vessel walls to become thicker? The answer may shock you: to save it from suffering a heart attack, stroke or other form of sudden degeneration.

The most important fluid in the body is the blood, because it is what supplies oxygen to all of the body's tissues. If the blood gets too thick, the entire body begins to suffer oxygen deprivation. In thickened blood, platelets become aggravated and begin to stick together. This makes it difficult for the blood to pass through the tiny capillaries that supply the cells of the body with oxygen and other nutrients. If brain cells, nerve tissue or heart cells get cut off from the oxygen and nutrient supply, a whole range of acute and chronic disorders may result, including heart attack, stroke, multiple sclerosis, fibromyalgia, Alzheimer's disease, Parkinson's disease, cancer of the brain and many subsidiary problems throughout the body.

The Protein-Cancer Connection

The protein-cancer connection has become obvious ever since large-scale scientific studies, including the *China Study*, have demonstrated a virtual absence of cancer among people who don't eat animal proteins. Meat consumption in relation to cancer risk has been reported in over a hundred epidemiological studies from many countries with diverse diets. Based on Richard Doll and Richard Peto's work in 1981 [*Journal of the National Cancer Institute* 1981;66:1191–1308), it has been estimated that approximately 35 percent (range 10%–70%) of cancer can be attributed to diet, similar in magnitude to the contribution of smoking to cancer (30 percent, range 25%–40%). Recently, a large American study has provided strong evidence that the consumption of red and processed meats poses the greatest dietary risk of developing cancer.

In a National Institutes of Health (NIH)–AARP Diet and Health Study, researchers Genkinger and Koushik from the U.S. National Cancer Institute examined the health data of 494,000 participants. In this 8-year study [published in *PLoS Med.* 2007 December; 4(12): e345, and online 2007 Dec. 11. doi:10.1371/journal.pmed. 0040345], the researchers compared the rate of cancer occurrence among the 20 percent of participants who consumed the most red and processed meat[31] with the data on the 20 percent who ate the least.

The results of the study were dramatic. Participants who consumed the most red meat had a 25 percent higher risk of developing colorectal cancer compared with those who ate the least, and a 20 percent higher risk of developing lung cancer.[32] The risk of esophageal and liver cancer was increased by 20–60 percent. Higher meat intake also correlated with an increased risk of pancreatic cancer in men. In recent meta-analyses of colorectal cancer that included studies published up to 2005, summary associations indicated that red meat intake was associated with 28–35 percent increased risk while processed meats were associated with elevated risks of 20–49 percent.

The researchers indicated that 1 in 10 cases of lung or colorectal cancer could be averted by limiting red meat intake. According to the China Study and other cancer research considered during the past 60 years, cancer could actually become a rare illness if animal proteins were avoided altogether.

Other studies have found associations between meat consumption and the risk of bladder, breast, cervical, endometrial, esophageal, glioma, kidney, liver, lung, mouth, ovarian, pancreatic and prostate cancers. On the other hand, there are plenty of studies that point to the cancer-preventing effects of a plant-based or fruit and vegetable diet, including studies published in the *American Journal of Epidemiology* [July 15, 2007;166(2):170-80. Epub May 7, 2007] and *Archives of Internal Medicine* [December 10, 2007; 167(22):2461-8].

---

[31] Meat originating from a mammal, beef, lamb, pork and veal; and meats preserved by salting, smoking or curing.

[32] Lung and colorectal cancers are the first and second leading causes of cancer death, respectively.

The researchers of the NIH diet study suggested that meat contains a number of carcinogenic compounds, including some that are formed during cooking or processing (e.g., heterocyclic amines, nitrosamines). They also noted that meat contains other potential carcinogens, including heme iron (the type of iron found in meat), nitrates and nitrites, saturated fat, antibiotics, hormones and salts.

All of these substances have been observed to affect hormone metabolism, increase cell proliferation, damage DNA, encourage insulin-like growth hormones and promote damage of cells by free radicals – which can all lead to cancer. Children who eat processed meats increase their risk of developing leukemia by 74 percent, according to research published in the journal *BMC Cancer* [January 2009]. In adults, consumption of processed meats is known to increase the risk of pancreatic cancer by 67 percent and bladder cancer by 59 percent. A mere two bites daily increases likelihood of bowel cancer by 20 percent.

What Actually Happens When You Eat Meat?

One of the most blood-thickening agents is food protein, particularly from an animal source. Let us assume you eat a medium-sized piece of steak, chicken or fish. When compared to a carnivorous animal like a lion or a wolf, your stomach can produce only the relative amount of 1/20 of the hydrochloric acid needed to digest such a concentrated protein meal.

In addition, the relative concentration of the hydrochloric acid in cats or wolves is at least five times higher than in humans. A cat or wolf can easily eat and digest the bones of a chicken, whereas humans cannot. Most of the cadaver's protein, therefore, will pass undigested into the small intestine where it will either putrefy (80 percent) or enter the bloodstream (20 percent).

The liver is able to break down some of the absorbed protein, which forms the waste products urea and uric acid. This waste matter is passed on to the kidneys for excretion with the urine. However, with regular consumption of animal proteins, including meat, poultry, fish, eggs, cheese and milk, more and more intrahepatic stones are formed in the bile ducts of the liver.[33] This greatly reduces the liver's ability to break down these proteins.

Protein foods are among the most acid-forming and blood-thickening foods of all. Therefore, when a major portion of the protein ends up circulating in the blood, it will, of course, thicken the blood. To avoid the danger of a heart attack or stroke, the body will attempt to dump the protein into the fluid surrounding the cells (tissue fluid or connective tissue). This thins the blood and averts the imminent danger of serious cardiovascular complications, at least for the time being. However, the dumped protein begins to turn the intercellular fluid into a gel-like substance. In this condition, nutrients that are trying to make their way to the cells may be caught in the thick soup, which increases the risk of cell death due to starvation.

The body tries to avoid cell death by initiating another, even more sophisticated, survival response, which is next to ingenious. To remove the proteins from the intercellular fluid, the body rebuilds the protein and converts it into collagen fiber, which is 100 percent protein. (See **Illustration 1**) In this form, the body is able to build the protein into the basal membrane of the blood vessel walls. While accommodating the excessive protein, the basal membrane may become up to eight times as thick as is normal. Once the capillary walls are saturated with the protein or collagen fiber, the basal membranes of the arteries start doing the same thing. This eventually leads to a hardening of the arteries, which is the subject matter of Chapter Nine of my book, *Timeless Secrets of Health & Rejuvenation*.[34]

Now the body must face an even greater challenge. The thick walls of the capillaries (and, possibly, the arteries) have become an obstruction, blocking the nutrient supply to the cells. The blood vessel walls increasingly prevent oxygen, glucose and even water from penetrating the protein barricades, thus depriving cells of their bare nutrient essentials. Less glucose makes its way to the cells. As a result, cell metabolism drops to a lower level of efficiency and waste production increases, similar to a car engine that has not been tuned properly or given quality gas or oil.

---

[33] See *The Amazing Liver and Gallbladder Flush* for causes of stones in the bile ducts and gallbladder, and how to remove them safely and painlessly.
[34] This book discusses in depth the causes of heart disease, strokes and high cholesterol, and shows the reader how to remove these causes quickly and safely.

Thickening of Blood Capillary Wall

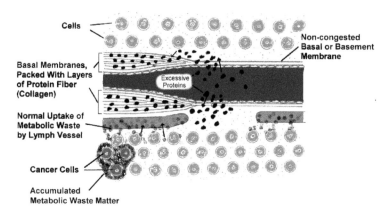

Hardening of Artery

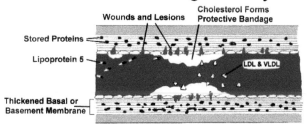

Illustration 1: When protein ends up circulating in the blood

In addition to congesting the blood vessel walls, another complicating factor comes into play. Part of the excessive protein is absorbed by the lymphatic ducts that accompany every blood capillary. These lymph ducts and their attached lymph nodes are designed to remove and detoxify the normal amounts of cell-generated metabolic waste products. They also take away the cellular debris resulting from the daily destruction of over 30 billion worn-out cells. Since cells are composed of proteins, much of the collected waste is already filled with old cell protein. Being forced to take up extra protein from ingested foods like meat, fish or milk simply overtaxes the entire lymphatic system and leads to the stagnation of lymph flow and fluid retention. Consequently, the congested lymph ducts are increasingly disabled as they attempt to take up the cells' metabolic waste products. This, in turn, leads to a higher concentration of metabolic waste material in the fluid surrounding the cells.

Lymph Node Removal for Breast Cancer –
Useless and Harmful

Surgical removal of lymph nodes and lymph vessels as part of standard medical procedure for breast cancer patients is not just useless, but also harmful, according to a study published in *The Journal of the American Medical Association* [JAMA.2011; 305(6):569-575.doi:10.1001/jama.2011.90].

In this groundbreaking study, 115 medical centers followed 891 women with early breast cancer and looked at the benefits of lymph node removal. The participants' median age was in the mid-50s, and they were followed for an average of 6.3 years.

The study found that in those women who had breast cancer that had spread to the lymph nodes, the removal of the nodes failed to increase their survival rate. After five years, 82.2 percent of the women who had the axillary nodes removed were still alive and in remission, compared to 83.9 percent of the women who did not get the operation.

Not only that, but lymph node removal also fuelled their chances of suffering serious harm. In fact, women in the study who had nodes removed experienced a 70 percent increase in complications compared with a 25 percent increase in women who did not. Such complications included infections, pain sensations and lymphedema.

What's astounding to the medical community, the researchers discovered that lymph node removal did not prevent the further spread of cancer to other lymph nodes. This clearly defies the hypothesis that lymph nodes harboring cancer cells are responsible for metastasis (spreading of cancer).

This is the rationale behind the common medical belief: "By removing a lymph node that contains cancer cells, these cells can no longer spread to other lymph nodes, or reach other parts of the body. Thus, the practice of removing lymph nodes is a reliable and effective preventive method against cancer metastasis." This sounds logical and reasonable to most medical doctors and their patients. However, the theory only makes sense if you also believe that cancer cells move around to infect other cells and make them cancerous, too. But, of course, this is just another hypothesis that lacks scientific backing.

As the above study clearly proves, the cutting out of lymph nodes that contain cancerous cells does nothing to prevent cancer from spreading.

What we must therefore conclude from this research is that, as previously discussed, cancer does not simply spread from one place to another.

I have always spoken out against removing those vitally important parts of the body's detoxification and waste removal system, which includes lymph vessels and lymph nodes. Breast cancer patients, especially, depend on an intact lymphatic system. And so I feel very encouraged by this team of researchers who had the courage to conduct such an important study and openly expose one of the oldest, cruelest and most rampant medical procedures as a scam.

With no difference in rate of survival or recurrence, removing lymph nodes is NOT justified. The research conducted "definitively showed that axillary lymph node dissection is not beneficial." Furthermore, "survival was independent of lymph node status," said the study authors. Why take women through such a taxing ordeal when there is no survival benefit?

In spite of the scientific evidence, medical centers, hospitals and doctors who either don't know about this research or choose to ignore it for reasons of financial gain, will continue to rip out women's axillary lymph nodes. In fact, some prominent institutions wouldn't even take part in the study, according to the authors. Surgeons particularly hope that the *bad* news (that lymph node surgery is unnecessary and harmful) will just go away in time, as it often does in the medical industry. Besides, the mainstream media didn't even report on this important study.

Women who had their axillary lymph nodes removed are more likely to suffer from a host of new health problems in the future. What's worse, the chance for a real cure of their cancer is greatly reduced, and a recurrence of cancer is more likely, because of it.

The author of an editorial accompanying the study, Dr. Grant W. Carlson, professor of surgery at Winship Cancer Institute at Emory University bluntly said: "I have a feeling we've been doing a lot of harm (by routinely taking out many nodes)." But since not many doctors and patients pay attention to this admission by the good doctor, the *war on cancer patients* will continue with full force.

Suffocation in Progress

The consequence of waste buildup in the cell environment is that cells not only become deprived of oxygen and other vital nutrients, but they also begin to suffocate in their own waste. The dramatic change of the cell environment leaves them with no other choice but to mutate into *abnormal* cells, given the circumstances.

Cell mutation does not occur because the genes of the cell had a bad day and decided to play malignant. Genes do not switch themselves on and off without a reason. Genetic blueprints have no control or power to do anything. They are merely there to help the cell reproduce itself. However, the genetic blueprint becomes naturally altered when the environment of the cell undergoes major changes. By drastically reducing the concentration of oxygen in the cell environment, the genes generate a new blueprint out of necessity. This enables the cells to survive without oxygen and instead use some of the metabolic waste products for energy. Mutated cells can take up, for example, lactic acid; and by metabolizing it, they are able to cover some of their energy needs. Although this abnormal type of cell metabolism has harmful side effects, by doing this, the body can avert, at least for a little while, the fatal poisoning of the affected organ or the blood. By keeping at least some of the oxygen-deprived cells alive through cell mutation, the organ is safeguarded against irreversible and sudden collapse and failure. **All of these adaptations make cancer a survival mechanism to keep the person alive for as long as circumstances permit.**

Cancer and Heart Disease – Same Causes

You may be interested to know that many of the factors which can lead to cancer are also important elements of cardiovascular disease. One of the most important of these is blood viscosity and the speed at which it flows. When the blood is too thick and flows too slowly, the patient is at a higher risk for clots, which are a known cause of metastasis.

Another issue that relates to both cancer and heart disease is plaque buildup in arteries. Conventional wisdom tells us this is a result of eating too much saturated fat, but this is not the case. A groundbreaking 1994 *Lancet* article reported that in an aortic artery clog, researchers identified over 10 different compounds in arterial plaque, but not a shred of saturated fat. They did, however, find that there was some cholesterol present, which is explained by cholesterol's known role as a healing salve for arterial abrasions, just like an internal scab. Yet, the cholesterol was not responsible for the clot, and the saturated fat was not even present.

This is so contrary to what has been taught for many years that you may question how this could possibly be the case. Yet once again, nature has been demonstrating this principle in the animal kingdom for millennia. A cat, for example, eats an almost exclusively meat-based diet, thereby consuming plenty of saturated fat and cholesterol. In this context, conventional wisdom would say they should be dying like flies of heart attacks; but they aren't.

It is worth mentioning at this point that only capillary and arterial walls can store excessive protein. Venules and veins, unlike capillaries and arteries, are responsible for taking up the metabolic waste product, carbon dioxide, and carrying it toward the lungs. They basically carry *empty-handed* blood, blood that has already *off-loaded* its nutrients and excessive protein, and passed these into the connective tissues. The blood is now ready to return to the lungs to take up oxygen, carbon, nitrogen and hydrogen molecules from the air. These four molecules make up all the amino acids in the body that are required for the building of cell proteins.[35]

As the blood passes through the digestive system, it takes up other nutrients needed for energy and cell nourishment, and perhaps proteins from an animal source. Concentrated proteins (as found, for example, in meat, fish, poultry, eggs, cheese and milk) are never stored in the walls of venules and veins, only in the walls of capillaries and arteries. Protein deposits in the basal membranes[36] of the capillaries and arteries injure and inflame the cells that make up these blood vessels.

To deal with these injuries or lesions, the body attaches protective plaque, including cholesterol, to the interior of the artery wall in order to prevent dangerous blood clots from escaping into the bloodstream and triggering a heart attack or stroke. Venules and veins, on the other hand, always remain free of plaque because their basal membranes are not exposed to the damaging proteins. For this reason, heart surgeons are able to take veins from the legs and use these as bypasses for

---

[35] More details about the protein self-sufficiency of the body can be found in the section on vegetarianism of my book, *Timeless Secrets of Health & Rejuvenation*.

[36] A normally very thin membrane that supports the cells comprising the blood vessel wall and keeps them in place.

arterial blockages. However, once put in the place of a coronary artery, a vein becomes just as exposed to excessive protein and, as a result, begins to develop protective plaque along its interior wall.

Cholesterol-containing plaque has gotten a bad name because not many physicians are aware of its real purpose. If more people knew that *bad* cholesterol (LDL) prevents bleeding of congested artery walls and, possibly, life-endangering blood clot formation, we might perceive *bad* cholesterol as life-saving cholesterol. By asking your doctor why the so-called *bad* cholesterol attaches itself only to arteries and not to veins, although it is present in both venous and arterial blood, you may stir some curiosity in him as to why cholesterol acts in this manner. He may discover that cholesterol is not the enemy here. In fact, the body uses LDL cholesterol in the healing of every wound, internal and external. LDL cholesterol is truly a lifesaver.

I bring up the topic of hardening of the arteries because heart disease and cancer are not so radically different. They share two common factors: blood vessel wall congestion and lymphatic blockage. Since heart cells cannot become cancerous, once they are deprived of oxygen for a certain period of time, they die of acidosis and simply shut down. We refer to this as a heart attack, although in reality there is no attack, just oxygen deprivation. In other parts of the body a similar oxygen-deprived environment will result in some cells that are able to continue living, but not without undergoing mutation into cancer cells. In other words, cancer of the tissues can only occur in the body if the circulatory system (including both the blood and lymph vessels) has suffered from congestion for a long time.

Death in Trans Fats

Protein is not the only reason for cancer-causing congestion to occur. Certain fats known as trans fatty acids, commonly known as *trans fats*, attach themselves to the cell membranes, thereby making it difficult for the cells to receive enough oxygen, glucose and even water. Oxygen-deprived, dehydrated cells become damaged and turn cancerous.

In particular, one's consumption of polyunsaturated fats as contained in refined and vitamin E depleted products, such as thin vegetable oil, mayonnaise, salad dressings and most brands of margarine, leads to a higher risk of cancer, particularly skin cancer. Since most animal protein foods also contain fats that are exposed to high heat during food preparation, or even contain added fats, as in fried chicken or fish sticks, the risk of cancer rises dramatically when these food items are combined and eaten regularly. The bottom line is that concentrated protein foods and refined fats hinder oxygen from entering the cells.

However, there are also certain fats that may be powerful weapons against cancer – one such fat in particular is extra virgin olive oil. According to *Archives of Internal Medicine* (1998), eating polyunsaturated fats increases the risk of breast cancer by 69 percent. By contrast, ingesting monounsaturated fats, as found in olive oil, reduces breast cancer risk by 45 percent. A study published in the science journal *BMC Cancer* reported that polyphenols, potent antioxidants found naturally in extra virgin olive oil, were effective in preventing the spread of breast cancer.

Indeed, the Mediterranean diet most associated with frequent consumption of minimally processed olive oil has often been linked to lower rates of several different cancers and heart disease. This is because olive oil has been shown to prevent oxidative damage, regulate platelet function (thereby preventing blood clots) and soothe inflammation.

This is, of course, in stark contrast to the results of consuming polyunsaturated fats, which attract many oxygen free radicals and become oxidized, turning rancid once exposed to air. Oxygen free radicals are generated when oxygen molecules lose an electron. This makes them highly reactive. Eating these aggressive fats causes them to attach to cell membranes in a manner similar to an oil slick in the sea, engulfing and suffocating birds and sea creatures. Therefore, the free radical activity in such fats has a severely damaging effect on cells, tissues and organs. While we depend on the body generating a certain number of oxygen free radicals to heal and keep our body clean, introducing oxidized fats into the body may flood it with these scavengers, thereby inflaming and damaging cells.

Oxygen free radicals can form in refined, polyunsaturated oils and fats once they are exposed to air and sunlight before consumption. The free radicals may also form in the tissues after the oils or fats have been ingested. Polyunsaturated fats are difficult to digest, since they are deprived of their natural bulk and are no longer protected against free radicals by their natural protector, vitamin E. This important vitamin, which is a powerful antioxidant, is being removed during the refining process. Eating a hamburger and French fries, for example, can flood your body with free radicals. However, blaming free radicals for causing damage in the body is like blaming the bullets for a shooting victim's injuries when, in fact, the person who pulled the trigger is responsible.

Saturated fats are solid and found in products such as lard and butter. They contain large quantities of natural antioxidants, which make them much safer against oxidation by free radicals. Since polyunsaturated fats are manufactured and do not exist in natural form, they are indigestible, and the body recognizes them as dangerous. Margarine, for example, is just one molecule away from plastic and therefore extremely difficult to digest. Free radicals, which are the body's natural cleansers, try to get rid of the fatty culprits that have affixed themselves to the cell membranes. When the radicals digest these harmful fats, they also damage the cell membranes. This is considered to be a main cause of aging and degenerative disease.

Research has shown that out of 100 people who consumed large quantities of polyunsaturated fats, 78 showed marked clinical signs of premature aging. They also looked much older than others of the same age. By contrast, in a study on the relationship between dietary fats and the risk for developing Alzheimer's disease, researchers were surprised to learn that the natural, healthy fats can actually reduce the risk for Alzheimer's by up to 80 percent. The study showed that the group with the lowest rate of Alzheimer's ate approximately 38 grams of these healthy fats every day, while those with the highest incidence of this disorder consumed only about half of that amount.

Another misunderstood component of the cancer debate is cholesterol, particularly *bad* LDL cholesterol. A study at Tohoku University, for example, suggests that this often-vilified form of cholesterol may actually be critical in the production of vitamin D from sun exposure, which, in turn, improves brain function. Furthermore, the statin drugs that are often prescribed to lower cholesterol levels may actually harm the heart.

Consequences of Free Radical Activity

Cells that are damaged by abnormal free radical activity are unable to reproduce properly, and this can impair major functions in the body, including those of the immune, digestive, nervous and endocrine systems. Ever since polyunsaturated fats were introduced to the population on a large scale, degenerative diseases have increased dramatically, skin cancer among them. In fact, polyunsaturated fats have even made sunlight *dangerous*, something that never would have been the case if foods hadn't been altered and manipulated by the food industry as they are done today.[37]

When polyunsaturated fats are removed from natural foods, they need to be refined, deodorized and even hydrogenated, depending on the food product for which they are used. During this process, some of the polyunsaturated fats undergo chemical transformations, which turn them into trans fatty acids (or trans fats), often referred to as hydrogenated vegetable oils. Margarine may be composed of up to 54 percent trans fatty acids, while a typical vegetable shortening can be 58 percent trans fats.

People who eat more trans fats from cheese, milk or processed foods may have a 48 percent increased risk of depression, compared with those who consume almost no trans fats. This is the conclusion drawn by researchers from the universities of Navarra and Las Palmas de Gran Canaria in Spain who studied the effects of trans fat consumption in 12,059 Spanish participants. The study, published in the journal *PLoS One* in January 2011, also shows that the effects of trans fats on mood may be more amplified in Americans, who eat more processed foods, a major source of trans fats, the authors wrote. The estimated consumption of trans fats by Americans is 6.2 times higher than by Europeans.

Also, people with current depression or a previous diagnosis of depression are 60 percent more likely to be obese, and twice as likely to smoke, as those who are not depressed, a large research study found. The study, which appeared in the March/April 2008 issue of the journal *General Hospital Psychiatry*, compiled data from more than 200,000

---

[37] See more details in my books, *Heal Yourself with Sunlight* or *Timeless Secrets of Health & Rejuvenation*.

adults in 38 states, the District of Columbia, Puerto Rico and the U.S. Virgin Islands.

In yet another study, conducted at Johns Hopkins University, researchers found that participants with a history of depression were four times more likely to develop breast cancer. The complete article can be found in the September issue of *Cancer Causes and Control* [2000;11;8:751-758].

In another large study published in 2003 in *Psychosomatic Medicine* [65, 884], researchers were able to establish an intriguing link between depression and pancreatic cancer in men.

Whether depression can actually cause cancer is still not clear, but it can certainly act as a co-factor, since depression suppresses the immune system and can lead to obesity and an increased likelihood of smoking, both of which are cancer risk factors.

You can detect hydrogenated vegetable oils in foods by reading the labels. Most processed foods contain them, including breads, crisps, chips, doughnuts, crackers, biscuits, pastries, almost all baked goods, cake and frosting mixes, baking mixes, frozen dinners, sauces, frozen vegetables and breakfast cereals. In other words, nearly all foods that are shelved, processed, refined, preserved and not fresh can contain trans fats. They inhibit the cell's ability to use oxygen, which is required for oxidizing foodstuffs to carbon dioxide and water. Of course, cells that are inhibited in completing their metabolic processes are likely to become cancerous.

Trans fats also make the blood thicker by increasing the stickiness of platelets. This multiplies the chances of blood clots and the build-up of fatty deposits, which can lead to heart disease. Researchers at Harvard Medical School, who observed 85,000 women over a period of eight years, found that those eating margarine had an increased risk of coronary heart disease. A Welsh study linked the concentration of these artificial trans fats in body fat with death from heart disease. The Dutch government appears to have already banned the sale of margarine containing trans fatty acids.

Why is an increased risk of heart disease so important in the consideration of cancer? Let me reiterate. It is because cancer and heart disease share the same causes. A heart attack occurs when a part of the heart muscle is deprived of oxygen and dies. Cancer occurs when a part of an organ or system in the body is deprived of oxygen and would die if the body's cells were not able to mutate and become cancerous. If the blockages leading up to oxygen starvation are not removed, either cancer or heart failure is most likely going to take the person's life. Oftentimes, cancer patients do not actually die because of the cancer, but due to a failing heart. In my experience with hundreds of cancer patients, I found that all of them also suffered from major cardiovascular problems.

It is not a new discovery that chronic oxygen deprivation of cells is behind cancer and other degenerative disorders such as heart disease. During the 1930s, Otto Warburg, M.D., discovered that cancer cells have a lower than average respiration rate compared to normal cells. He reasoned that cancer cells thrived in a low-oxygen environment and that increased oxygen levels would harm and even kill them. Winner of the 1931 Nobel Prize in Medicine, Dr. Warburg summarized the cancer problem in two short sentences: **"Cancer has only one prime cause. It is the replacement of normal oxygen respiration of the body's cells by an anaerobic cell respiration."**

Other scientists soon followed in Warburg's footsteps and had this to say:

"Lack of oxygen clearly plays a major role in causing cells to become cancerous." – Dr. Harry Goldblatt, *Journal of Experimental Medicine* (1953)

"Insufficient oxygen means insufficient biological energy that can result in anything from mild fatigue to life-threatening disease. The link between insufficient oxygen and disease has now been firmly established." – Dr. W. Spencer Way, *Journal of the American Association of Physicians* (December 1951)

"Oxygen plays a pivotal role in the proper functioning of the immune system; i.e. resistance to disease, bacteria and viruses." – Dr. Parris Kidd, Ph.D., Cell Biologist

"In all serious disease states we find a concomitant low oxygen state... Low oxygen in the body tissues is a sure indicator for disease... Hypoxia, or lack of oxygen in the tissues, is the fundamental cause for all degenerative disease." – Dr. Stephen Levine, renowned Molecular Biologist

"Cancer is a condition within the body where the oxidation has become so depleted that the body cells have degenerated beyond physiological control." – Dr. Wendell Hendricks, Hendricks Research Foundation

"Starved of oxygen, the body will become ill, and if this persists it will die. I doubt if there is any argument about that." – Dr. John Muntz, Nutritional Scientist

"He who breathes most air lives most life."
– Elizabeth Barrett Browning

3. Lymphatic Blockage

What is lymph and why is it so vitally important in the body? Lymph originates as blood plasma, which is packed with all sorts of *groceries*, including oxygen, glucose, minerals, vitamins, hormones, proteins, as well as antibodies and white blood cells. Blood plasma passes through the blood capillary walls and joins the tissue fluid that surrounds all the cells. Tissue fluid is also known as intracellular fluid, interstitial fluid or connective tissue. The cells take up nutrients from, and release metabolic waste products into, the tissue fluid.

About 90 percent of the tissue fluid returns to the blood stream where it again becomes blood plasma. The remaining 10 percent of the tissue fluid forms what is called *lymph*. With the exception of carbon dioxide, lymph contains all the metabolic waste produced by the cells, as well as pathogens, dissolved proteins and cancer cells (which are naturally generated as part of the normal turnover of cells). Lymph capillaries take up the lymph and remove this *trash*, thereby preventing suffocation and damage of cells.

The degree of nourishment, health and efficiency of the cells depends on how swiftly and completely waste material is removed from the lymph. Since most cellular waste products cannot pass directly into the blood for excretion, they must gather in the tissue fluid until they are removed by the lymphatic system. Lymph vessels carry this potentially harmful material into the lymph nodes for filtration and detoxification. Lymph nodes, which are strategically located throughout the body, also remove some fluid. This prevents the body from swelling and gaining excessive weight.

One of the key functions of the lymphatic system is to keep the tissue fluid clear of disease-causing toxic substances, which makes this a system of utmost importance for our health and well-being. Very few doctors, though, refer to it when they speak to their patients about the illness they are suffering from.

Practically every type of cancer is preceded by a major, ongoing condition of lymphatic congestion. Wherever lymph drainage is consistently the most insufficient, cancerous tumors manifest first. If more areas of the body are affected in this way, cancers may develop in multiple places. The lymphatic system works closely with the immune system in keeping the body free of harmful metabolic waste products, toxins, pathogens, noxious material and cell debris.

In addition to poor circulation of the blood, congested lymph ducts and lymph nodes cause an overload of harmful waste matter in the tissue fluid. Subsequently, this normally thin vital fluid thickens, thereby preventing proper nutrient distribution to the cells, which weakens or damages them. Cell mutation occurs when oxygen, carried by the blood to the cells, is continuously hindered from making its way through to them.

The most pressing question is: Where does lymph congestion begin? There may be several answers, but the most important ones relate to bile and diet. Restricted bile secretions in the liver and gallbladder, due to accumulated gallstones,[38] undermine the stomach's and small intestine's ability to digest food properly.

Undigested food is naturally subject to decomposition by destructive intestinal bacteria. This permits substantial amounts of waste matter and poisonous substances, such as the highly carcinogenic (cancer-causing) amines, cadaverines, putrescines and other breakdown products of fermented and putrefied food, to seep into the intestinal lymph ducts. Along with undigested fats and proteins, these poisons enter the body's largest lymphatic structure, the thoracic duct and its base, the cysterna chyli. The cysterna chyli is a lymph-dilation (in the shape of a sac or oval pool), situated in front of the first two lumbar vertebrae at the level of the belly button. (See **Illustration 2**) It extends itself to other smaller sac-like lymph vessels.

---

[38] See my book, *The Amazing Liver and Gallbladder Flush,* for details on stones in the liver and gallbladder and how to flush them out safely.

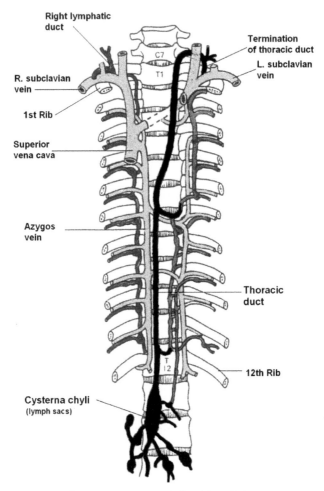

Illustration 2: Cysterna chyli and thoracic duct

Toxins, antigens and undigested proteins from animal sources, including fish, meat, poultry, eggs and dairy foods, cause these lymph sacs or pools to become inflamed and to swell (lymphedema). Once the cells of an animal die, which happens seconds after it is killed, cellular enzymes immediately begin to break down their protein structures. The heating/cooking/frying of animal proteins, such as eggs, fish and meat, coagulates (hardens) the proteins and tears apart their natural three-dimensional molecular structure. The resulting so-called *degenerate* proteins are not only useless to the body, but also actually become harmful unless they are promptly removed by the lymphatic system. Their presence naturally encourages enhanced microbial activity. Parasites, worms, fungi and bacteria feed on these pooled wastes. In some cases, allergic reactions occur. All this can severely impact the body's waste removal system, thereby preparing the ground for chronic lymphedema.

Lymphedema

When lymph congestion exists in the cysterna chyli, this crucial part of the lymphatic system can no longer properly remove the body's worn-out and damaged cell proteins. (Remember, the body has to remove 30 billion old cells each day.) This results in lymphedema. You can feel any existing lymphedemas as tender, hard knots by touching or massaging the area of your belly button while lying on your back. These knots are sometimes as large as a fist. Some people describe them as *rocks in the stomach*.

These *rocks* are a major cause of middle and low back pain as well as abdominal swelling, bloating and weight gain around the waist area. In fact, they are behind most symptoms of ill health, including heart disease, diabetes and cancer. Nearly all of the hundreds of cancer patients I have seen suffered from some degree of lymphedema, abdominal distension or bloating. The enlargement of the abdomen is usually accompanied by facial swelling (moon face), a double chin, puffy eyes and a thickening of the neck – indications of advanced lymphatic congestion.

Many people who have *grown a tummy* consider this extension of their waistline to be a harmless nuisance or a natural part of aging. They say that almost everyone has an enlarged tummy nowadays, and that this must be normal. They don't realize that they are breeding a living time bomb that may go off some day and injure vital parts of the body. Cancer almost always indicates the existence of such a time bomb.

Eighty percent of the lymphatic system is located at, and associated with, the intestinal tract, therefore making this area of the body the largest center of immune activity. This is no coincidence. The part of the body where most disease-causing agents are combated or generated is, in fact, the intestinal tract. Any lymphedema and other kinds of obstruction in this important part of the lymphatic system are due to an overload of intestinal toxic waste and can lead to potentially serious complications elsewhere in the body.

Wherever a lymph duct is obstructed, an accumulation of lymph exists at a distance to the obstruction. Consequently, the lymph nodes located along such a blocked duct can no longer adequately neutralize or detoxify the following: dead and live phagocytes and their ingested microbes, worn-out tissue cells, cells damaged by disease, products of fermentation, pesticides in food, inhaled or toxic particles, cells from malignant tumors and many of the millions of cancer cells generated each day by every healthy person.

Incomplete destruction of these things can cause the lymph nodes to become inflamed, enlarged and congested with blood. In addition, infected material may enter the bloodstream, causing septic poisoning and acute illnesses. In most cases, though, the lymph blockage occurs gradually over many years, without any *serious* symptoms other than swelling of the abdomen, hands, arms, feet, ankles, or puffiness in the face and eyes. This is often referred to as fluid retention, a major precursor of chronic illness. Many cancer patients suffer from one or several of these symptoms long before they are diagnosed with a cancerous growth.

Continuous lymphatic obstruction usually leads to cellular mutation. Almost every cancer results from chronic congestion in the cysterna chyli. Eventually, the thoracic duct, which drains the cysterna chyli and carries lymph upward toward the neck into the left lymphatic duct, is overburdened by the constant influx of toxic material and becomes clogged up, too. The thoracic duct connects with numerous other lymphatic ducts (See **Illustrations 2 & 3**) that empty their waste material into the thoracic *sewer canal*. Since the thoracic duct has to remove 85 percent of the body's daily-generated cellular waste and other potentially highly toxic material, a blockage there causes backwashing of waste into other, more distant parts of the body. This results in the swelling that is characteristic of local lymphedema, often found around the ankles.

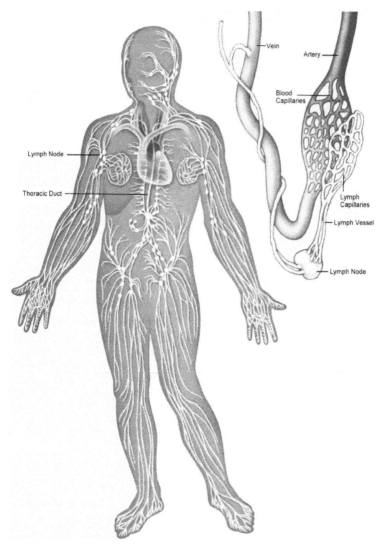

Illustration 3: Lymphatic system and lymph nodes

When the daily-generated metabolic waste and cellular debris remain trapped in an area of the body for some time, symptoms of disease start manifesting. The trapped waste can eventually become a trigger for abnormal cell growth. The following lists but a few typical examples of illness indicators that result directly from chronic, localized lymph congestion:

- Obesity
- Cysts in the uterus or ovaries
- Enlargement of the prostate gland
- Rheumatism in the joints
- Enlargement of the left half of the heart
- Congestive heart failure
- Congested bronchi and lungs
- Enlargement of the neck area
- Stiffness in the neck and shoulders
- Backaches
- Headaches
- Migraines
- Dizziness
- Vertigo
- Ringing in the ears
- Earaches
- Deafness
- Dandruff
- Frequent colds
- Sinusitis
- Hay fever
- Certain types of asthma
- Thyroid enlargement
- Eye diseases
- Poor vision
- Swelling in the breasts
- Breast lumps
- Kidney problems
- Lower back pains
- Swelling of the legs and ankles
- Scoliosis
- Brain disorders
- Memory loss
- Stomach trouble
- Enlarged spleen
- Irritable bowel syndrome
- Hernia
- Polyps in the colon
- Disorders of the reproductive system
- and many more….

If any of these symptoms (above) or a combination thereof persists for a number of years, cancer becomes a distinct possibility.

After collecting the lymph from all parts of the body, except the right side of the head and neck, right arm and upper right quadrant of the body, the lymphatic channel joins the left lymphatic duct. This duct returns the lymph to the circulatory system by draining into the left subclavian vein at the root of the neck. The subclavian vein enters the superior vena cava, which leads straight into the heart. In addition to blocking proper lymph drainage from these various organs or parts of the body, any congestion in the cysterna chyli and thoracic duct causes toxic materials to enter the heart and its arteries. This unduly stresses the heart, possibly enlarging it and causing irregular heartbeat and other complications. It also allows these toxins and disease-causing agents to enter the general circulation and spread to other parts of the body.

To emphasize once more, rarely is there a disease, including cancer, which is *not* due to lymphatic obstruction. It makes sense that if the main sewer pipe draining wastes from your home becomes clogged up, then all the smaller pipes draining the toilets, sinks, showers and bathtubs will get clogged up, too, and cause flooding. The obesity epidemic in the U.S. is largely due to (although not ultimately caused by) congested lymph systems that prevent bodily waste from being eliminated.

Lymph blockage, in the vast majority of cases, has its origin in a congested liver[39] as well as a detrimental diet and lifestyle. In the extreme eventuality, lymphoma or cancer of the lymph may result, of which Hodgkin's disease is the most common type.

Disease is naturally absent when blood and lymph flow is unhindered and normal. Both types of problems, circulatory and lymphatic, can be successfully eliminated through a series of liver cleanses and by following a balanced diet and lifestyle.

4. Chronic Digestive Problems

Prior to experiencing chronic lymph congestion, a person must have long-term difficulty with digesting food. Improperly digested foods become a breeding place for carcinogens – toxic compounds that can affect cellular behavior.

Four main activities take place in the alimentary tract of our digestive system: ingestion, digestion, absorption and elimination. The alimentary canal begins at the mouth, passes through the thorax, abdomen and pelvic region, and ends at the anus. When food is ingested, a series of digestive processes begin to take place. These can be divided into the mechanical breakdown of food through mastication and the chemical breakdown of food through enzymes. These enzymes are present in the secretions produced by the glands of the digestive system.

Enzymes are minute, chemical substances that cause or speed up chemical changes in other substances without themselves being changed.

---

[39] The causes of gallstones in the liver are fully discussed in my book, *The Amazing Liver and Gallbladder Flush.*

Digestive enzymes are contained in the saliva of the salivary glands of the mouth, the gastric juice in the stomach, the intestinal juice in the small intestine, the pancreatic juice in the pancreas and the bile in the liver. **It is important to know that digestive and metabolic enzymes (only those produced by the body itself) possess the most powerful anticancer properties of any substance in the body. Not producing enough of these enzymes has a clear-cut detrimental effect on cell health and can be considered directly responsible for cancerous growth in the body, regardless of the location.**

Absorption is the process by which tiny nutrient particles of digested food pass through the intestinal walls into the blood and lymph vessels for distribution to the cells of the body. The bowels eliminate as feces whatever food substances cannot be digested or absorbed. Fecal matter also contains bile, which carries the waste products that result from the breakdown (catabolism) of red blood cells and other harmful substances. In addition, a third of the excreted waste consists of intestinal bacteria. The body can only function smoothly and efficiently if the bowel removes the daily accumulated waste every day. Intestinal congestion arises when foods are inadequately digested. The natural consequence is the back-flushing of waste into the lymph, blood and upper parts of the body, including the stomach, chest, throat, neck, sensory organs and brain.

Health, once again, is the natural result of a balanced functioning in each of these major activities in the digestive system.[40] On the other hand, cancer and many similar survival (and healing) attempts arise whenever one or more of these functions are impaired. The presence of gallstones in the liver and gallbladder has a strong disruptive influence on the digestion and absorption of food, as well as on the elimination of waste. This increased toxicity in the body, coupled with its increasing inability to nourish itself through digestion, is what contributes to the progression of illness.

---

[40] How to fully restore all these functions of the digestive system is discussed in detail in my book, *Timeless Secrets of Health & Rejuvenation*. (See http://www.ener-chi.com/books/timeless-secrets-of-health-rejuvenation/)

5. Liver Bile Duct Obstruction

Gallstones (also known as intrahepatic stones) are not only found in the gallbladder, but also in the bile ducts of the liver. In fact, most gallstones are actually formed in the liver, and comparatively few occur in the gallbladder. An estimated 20 percent of the world's population will develop gallstones in their *gallbladder* at some stage in their lives. This figure, however, does not account for the many more people who will develop gallstones in their *liver* or who already have them.

During 30 years of practicing natural medicine, I have dealt with thousands of people suffering from all types of diseases. I can document that each person, without exception, has had considerable quantities of gallstones in their liver. Cancer patients and those suffering from arthritis, heart disease, liver disease and other chronic illnesses appear to have the most stones in their liver. Surprisingly, only a relative few of them report a history of gallstones in their gallbladder.

Gallstones in the liver are the main impediment to acquiring and maintaining good health, youthfulness and vitality. They are, indeed, one of the major reasons people become ill and have difficulty recuperating from illnesses, including cancer.

The liver has direct control over the growth and functioning of every cell in the body. Any kind of malfunction, deficiency or abnormal growth pattern of the cells largely results from poor liver performance. Due to its extraordinary design, the liver often seems to perform normally, with a blood test indicating balanced amounts of liver enzymes, even after it has lost up to 60 percent of its original efficiency. As deceiving as this may be to the patient and doctor alike, the origin of most diseases can easily be traced to the liver.[41]

All diseases or symptoms of ill health are caused by an obstruction of some sort. If a blood vessel is blocked and, therefore, can no longer provide speedy delivery of vital oxygen or nutrients to a group of cells, the cells will have to enforce specific emergency measures in order to survive. Of course, many of the afflicted cells will not survive the *famine* and will simply die off. However, other more resilient cells will learn to adjust to the adverse situation, by means of cell mutation, and will feed off trapped, toxic metabolic waste products and everything else they can

---

[41] See details in my book, *The Amazing Liver and Gallbladder Flush.*

grab from other cells. Although, in reality, such a survival response helps to prevent the body's immediate demise through possible septic poisoning and organ failure, we tend to label this as *disease*. In the case of cell mutation, cancer is the label that is applied.

The important question is how such a simple thing as obstructed bile flow can cause such complex diseases as congestive heart failure, diabetes and cancer.

Liver bile is a bitter, alkaline fluid of a yellow, brown or green color. It has multiple functions. Each one of these profoundly influences the health of every organ and system in the body. Apart from assisting with the digestion of fat, calcium and protein foods, bile is needed to maintain normal fat levels in the blood, remove toxins from the liver, help maintain proper acid/alkaline balance in the intestinal tract and keep the colon from breeding harmful microbes.

Bile prevents and possibly cures cancer and heart disease, the two leading causes of death! The importance of bile for maintaining good health has not been fully acknowledged, at least not by mainstream medicine. However, scientific evidence has been mounting that suggests the bile pigments bilirubin and biliverdin, which give color to bile, play an extremely important physiological role in humans.

According to a study published in 2008 in the prestigious medical journal *Mutation Research*, bile pigments possess strong anti-mutagenic properties.[42] The researchers state that in the past, bile pigments and bilirubin, in particular, were thought of as useless by-products of heme[43] catabolism (breaking down) that can be toxic if they accumulate. "However, in the past 20 years, research probing the physiological relevance of bile pigments has been mounting, with evidence to suggest bile pigments possess significant antioxidant and anti-mutagenic properties," the study concludes.

Doctors tend to make you panic if your skin color or eyes turn yellow (jaundice). They won't tell you that your body is actually in the process of getting rid of dangerous peroxyl radicals and a number of classes of mutagens (polycyclic aromatic hydrocarbons, heterocyclic amines, oxidants), all chemicals known to cause cells to become cancerous.

---

[42] Mutat Res., 2008 Jan-Feb;658(1-2):28-41. Epub, May 18, 2007
[43] Component of hemoglobin, the red pigment in blood

Sometimes the body appears to make you ill so that it can clean you out and make you truly healthy.

I consider this research finding to be one of most important discoveries in the field of medicine, something that the most ancient system of medicine – 6,000 year old Ayurveda – has known all along. Bile, unless trapped by stones in the bile ducts or by stones in the gallbladder, can prevent healthy cells from mutating into cancer cells. In fact, studies have found that people with higher concentrations of bilirubin and biliverdin in their bodies have a lower incidence of cancer and cardiovascular disease.[44]

According to Japanese research, the increased levels of bile pigments during jaundice can even resolve persistent difficult-to-control asthma due to acute hepatitis B.[45]

Naturally, these and similar findings raise the question whether what medical science considers to be diseases may actually be complex survival and healing attempts by the body. When treated and suppressed with pharmaceutical drugs, the body's healing efforts may be completely compromised. Instead of waging a drug war against the body, we might just as well support it by removing unnecessary, accumulated obstructions. Given the immensely important role that bile and its components play in the body, it makes perfect sense to keep the bile flow unhindered at all times.

Cleansing the liver and gallbladder of all accumulated stones helps to restore homeostasis, balance weight and set the precondition for the body to heal itself. The liver cleanse is also one of the best precautions you can take to protect yourself against illness in the future.

Unnatural Foods and Beverages

In the United States, the food industry produces over 40,000 different food products, the vast majority of which have no or very limited nutritional value. Highly processed, refined, *improved*, fortified, preserved, flavored, pre-cooked, genetically modified, gassed, radiated,

---

[44] Mutat Res., 2008 Jan-Feb;658(1-2):28-41. Epub, May 18, 2007
[45] Tohoku J Exp Med., 2003 March;199(3):193-6

microwave-heated and other altered foods have the common effect of starving human cells.

Cancer is the result of progressive famine on the cellular level. It occurs when the body no longer receives what it needs to grow according to its original design. To survive and prevent the organs from collapsing due to severe malnutrition and energy depletion, the cell nucleus is left with no other choice but to mutate and begin to function anaerobically.

An anaerobic cell is like a sick, homeless person who, alienated from the rest of society, lives off the decomposed and toxic foods that the affluent, healthy members of society have left behind as garbage. The nutritional value of the typical modern diet is nothing short of useless trash. Take for example, French fries or potato chips. Although they are known to contain carcinogenic fats, along with harmful additives and preservatives, millions of American children and adults consume them day after day in large quantities.

Try the following experiment: the next time you order French fries at McDonald's or a similar fast food restaurant, take some of them home with you, and leave them in an open space. You will discover that they will not decompose or even change color (unlike French fries made from fresh potatoes which will quickly shrivel up, turn grey and become moldy). Now, repeat the experiment with a hamburger. The hamburger will also last for years without deterioration. No bacteria will even try to decompose it. These and most other manufactured *foods* such as margarine, for example, are made to last forever, perfectly preserved so they can make it through the lengthy manufacturing and transportation process, and are *safe* for the consumer.

Are you wondering what kind of chemicals these foods must be saturated with to enable them to resist even bacteria and mold? Few consumers understand what exactly goes into them, although some of the preservatives are listed on the food labels (but often in print that is too fine to read). And what can the body possibly do to digest these chemical additives? Nothing at all.

If you are fortunate, they simply pass through the intestinal tract without being digested (diarrhea); it is more likely, though, that they have constipating effects and accumulate in the gut, as seen in the grossly extended tummies of those who eat such Frankenstein foods on a regular basis. Since ingesting these foods causes severe nutritional deficiencies, they also cause food cravings that can never be satisfied.

The food industry knows this *dirty little secret* and meets the ever-increasing demand for such *smart* foods by producing an even greater variety of mouth-watering products that especially cater to the obese or overweight. Eye-catching phrases include low cholesterol, fat free, low sodium, low calorie and sugar-free. Although these foods should be utterly unappealing to the taste buds, chemical food additives and flavors ensure they taste great. There are now thousands of different manufactured foods that fall into this category. Of course, the food labels contain no warnings that these chemicals are known carcinogens.

Most believe that if an American grocery store or restaurant offers a particular food, it must be good and safe. They also believe that using microwaves to cook their food is safe and harmless. I will discuss microwave ovens in Chapter Five, and there is also a lot of detailed information on this topic in my book, *Timeless Secrets of Health & Rejuvenation*.

Health agencies set up by the government to keep people out of harm's way have their own sinister agendas in allowing deadly drugs and technologies to be marketed on a massive scale. How many people are questioning the FDA as to why it allowed genetically engineered canola oil to sweep the American food and restaurant industry without prior testing? Public records show that the FDA knew about the Canadian research which showed mice fed with this oil developed fatal brain tumors. But the agency was not willing to give up the millions of dollars in *licensing fees* that the approval of canola oil brought with it.

Likewise, poisonous drugs like aspartame, Splenda and MSG are often hidden in the majority of the nation's bestselling manufactured foods and beverages because of FDA approval. These drugs are more addictive than heroin, caffeine and nicotine taken together. They make it nearly impossible for their *victims* to abstain from overeating. Their disastrous effects on the human body are well documented, and the FDA, the Centers for Disease Control and Prevention (CDCP) and the food industry have known about it for many years.

MSG is a particular problem when it comes to obesity. Recent research shows that those who regularly consume MSG are 30 percent more likely to be overweight or obese. To make sure you don't fall into the MSG-obesity trap, it's best to avoid all processed foods. And remember, MSG is highly addictive. It addicts you to the foods that contain it [*The American Journal of Clinical Nutrition,* June 2011; 93(6):1328-36].

The food industry has only one incentive: to make people consume more food. Helping us to eat healthy, sustainable food in moderation is just not on its priorities, because that means fewer profits. Therefore, by placing addictive drugs into the most popular foods and beverages, the food industry has created a society where the eating habits of the majority of its members have spun out of control. With 75 percent of the population overweight or obese, American society as a whole is afflicted by a *tumor* of massive proportions; the resultant ill health of the majority and skyrocketing medical costs go along with it.

This tumor eats up an ever-increasing portion of our national resources. In 2007, $2.3 trillion was spent on healthcare; that's 4.3 times the amount spent on national defense then. No other nation in the world spends 16 percent of its GDP on healthcare as the U.S. does – and, I may add, without any obvious benefits. In fact, there is no other society in the world with as many sick people as the U.S.[46]

Having established the fact that leaving the safeguarding of one's health to corporations or government agencies is a foolhardy approach, let us return to the core problem in any serious health crisis: cellular starvation. The cells of the body are not interested in utilizing anything that does not serve their growth. The carcinogenic grease of refined and overheated fats and oils, coloring agents, chemical additives, preservatives, pesticides and all such unnatural substances ends up plastering the cells' membranes with impenetrable layers of gunk.

This does not even include the billions of poison-filled nutritional supplements Americans consume each day, as if they were real food. Just think of how many vitamin pills the average American swallows day after day, year after year – pills that are loaded with binders, fillers, artificial colors, aspartame or other deadly sweeteners, to name just a few. If you had the chance to look at a microscopic picture of the cell of a newborn baby, you would see how transparent, thin and clean the cell membrane is. On the other hand, if you were to examine the cell membranes of a 65 year old person eating the typical American diet and

---

[46] Editor's note: The total national health expenditure in 2014 was $3.0 trillion.
See http://www.cdc.gov/nchs/fastats/health-expenditures.htm

being on medication for one ailment or another, you would find these to be dark, thick and distorted. It doesn't take much to turn such cells into cancer cells.

The cells of a malignant tumor are surrounded by a layer of fibrin[47] that is 15 times thicker than that which surrounds healthy cells. All cancer cells are damaged or wounded. The fibrin coating protects cancer cells against deadly phagocytes, killer lymphocytes and cytokines.

Naturally, cells that are compromised in this way are separated from their *community* – that is, from all the other cells in the body. These alienated cells are truly *homeless.* Homeless cells seem to be out of control, and so doctors attack them with lethal weapons designed to poison, cut or burn them. Their goal is to wipe them out, and they may not realize the serious consequences that attacking cancer cells can have on the surrounding colonies of cells. Those who do realize the probable damage to healthy cells may feel this is a risk they must take in order to kill the offending cells.

Doctors practically play *Russian roulette* with the lives of their patients when they put them on chemotherapy and/or radiation treatments. They can never predict or know whether the patient will survive the assault or die from it. Dimitris, a Greek medical doctor who had studied and practiced medicine in the U.S. for several years before returning to his native country, came to visit me in Cyprus to see if I could do something for his terminal liver cancer. During the following six months he dealt with and removed all the possible root causes of his cancer, and subsequently the liver tumor shrank from the size of an egg to a tiny speck. One day, a former colleague of his convinced him to take one course of the latest and most powerful chemotherapy drug that had just been approved for treatment by the FDA.

Dimitris became convinced that killing the last few cancer cells would guarantee that the cancer would not return, and so he flew to the U.S. for treatment. Three days later, he was flown back to Greece, inside a coffin. He had died from drug poisoning. I had warned him that when the body goes into a rapid healing mode as he did, stopping this process

---

[47] Fibrin is involved in the clotting of blood. It is a fibrillar protein that is polymerized to form a *mesh* that forms a haemostatic plug or clot over a wound site. Recent research has shown that fibrin plays a key role in the inflammatory response and development of rheumatoid arthritis.

with poisonous drugs could be fatal. During the healing phase, the body is many times more vulnerable to chemical poisoning than it is in the protection mode, which in this case is represented by a growing cancerous tumor. I have witnessed the same phenomenon in other cancer patients who also gave into the temptation of *finishing off* their last bits of cancer. Their decision turned out to be a fatal one.

It is extremely difficult for the body to protect itself against poisoning when it is trying to heal itself. To damage healthy cells in the process of destroying cancer cells through chemotherapy drugs or radiation is bound to breed new, more aggressive cancer cells. The only real chance of surviving cancer depends on the amount of support the patient musters to strengthen the body's own healing efforts.

The approach to treating cancer as a disease is not only fraught with dangers and needless suffering, but also fails to address the underlying issue of diet. By feeding our children and ourselves non-physiological foods such as mold-resistant French fries and hamburgers that thicken cell membranes and force cells to mutate in order to function in an anaerobic environment, we are creating diseases that will literally wipe out entire communities. This trend has already begun to take its course.

Our modern society suffers greatly from cancer. It is up to each one of us to make those choices that favor life over death. What we put in our mouth has a lot to do with how our society will survive. Considering the statistic that 1 in every 2 Americans will develop some form of cancer, and knowing that the prospects of avoiding cancer are worsening each year, it only makes sense that we stay away from manufactured foods (and other cancer-producing factors) as much as possible.

If you have cancer, your chances of recovery will increase dramatically when you eat only natural foods that have not been manipulated or altered by the food industry. I especially recommend that you consume only organically grown foods, ideally locally grown, during the recovery period. This allows the body to focus on healing, rather than forcing it to engage its already weakened immune system in battles with chemical additives and pesticides.

Changing your diet also greatly reduces your risk of developing cancer. Diet plays a critical role in bringing about a permanent remission if cancer has already occurred. In an estimated 60 percent or more of all malignant cancers, diet plays a leading role in its onset. An anticancer diet can effectively cut your cancer risk by two-thirds. The most successful cancer-preventing diet is still the vegetarian model.

Compelling demonstrations of how entire countries can be virtually cancer-free are provided in population studies. Thus far, over 200 studies have been done on cancer occurrence among different groups of people in the world. As it turns out, cancer rates are much lower in developing nations than in the U.S.

The average American diet, consisting of very fatty, protein-rich, highly processed food items, has almost nothing in common with the diet typically consumed by folks in developing countries. Fruits, vegetables, legumes and grains still form the standard diet of people living in most developing countries, although the Western influence of bringing unnatural and fast foods into their towns and villages is now making its way into the eating habits of these populations. With these newly introduced, and now *fashionable* eating habits, formerly unheard-of disorders like osteoporosis, skin cancer, heart disease, arthritis and other problems are becoming more and more common.

To save our nation from self-destruction, we have no option but to return to the foods that nature has designed for us to eat. This also means we need to avoid foods that nature does not create. No natural contract exists between our bodies and margarine, for example. Margarine is a laboratory *food* that a natural organism is not equipped to make use of. It is just one molecule away from plastic! Simply leave margarine somewhere in a warm, dark, moist environment where bacteria are plentiful, and you will discover that these bacteria will leave it alone. They treat this unnatural product as if it were actually plastic.

For millions of years, the human body relied for its sustenance on natural foods that grew around it, and so it is delusional to believe that our bodies can suddenly learn to subsist on the barrage of new, manufactured foods that have flooded our supermarkets and grocery stores. We don't even know whether a food such as corn, soybean products or potatoes is man-made (genetically engineered) or not.

Most manufactured foods contain some genetically modified food ingredients. In truth, food that is not grown by nature, cannot serve as food at all. The body has no connection to or recognition of man-made foods that no longer match the *signature* of real foods. Instead of nourishing the cells of the body, manufactured foods slowly starve them to death by accumulating in the organs and tissues. **Therefore, feeding the body exclusively with manufactured foods is basically suicidal. Eating the typical American diet consisting of red meat, fried foods, processed dairy products, refined grains and sugary desserts is, in fact, synonymous with unintentionally killing oneself.**

In an observational study, investigators examined the relationship between the dietary patterns of more than 1,000 people who had been treated for stage 3 colon cancer and their risk of colon cancer recurrence. The researchers found that those who followed a typical American diet were three times more likely to experience a recurrence of colon cancer than their counterparts who followed a mostly vegetarian diet, and they also were more likely to die. The study, which was reported in the *Journal of the American Medical Association (JAMA)*, is the first to address the effect of diet on recurrence in a population of colon cancer survivors. The researchers say the results strongly suggest that a diet consisting primarily of red and processed meats, French fries, refined grains, sweets and desserts increases the risk of cancer recurrence and decreases survival.

There is some good news, though, that certain foods can somewhat counteract the cancer-producing effects of the typical American diet. A Japanese study at Nagoya University showed that the pigment in purple corn impedes the development of cancer in the colon. The researchers divided animals into two groups, one of which received food mixed with a natural carcinogenic substance found in the charred parts of roasted meat and fish, and another group that also received 5 percent pigment of purple corn. In the group that was fed the carcinogen, 85 percent developed colon cancer, compared with only 40 percent that also received the pigment. Other studies showed that purple corn also prevents obesity and diabetes.

Deadly Cell Phones and Other Wireless Devices

An increasing number of medical researchers, environmental protection agencies, governments and individuals are concerned that wireless technology may be causing serious harm to people and the environment. Cell phones do cause cancer, according to published research:

- In 2007, Germany warned the population to avoid wireless devices. The Israeli government also banned the placement of antennas used for cell phone reception on residential buildings.
- In September 2007, based on its analysis of research conducted in 15 different laboratories, the EU's European Environment Agency (EEA) issued warnings to all European citizens advising them to stop using Wi-Fi and cell phones, citing fears that the ever-present use of wireless technology has the potential to become the next public health disaster on the level of tobacco smoking, asbestos and lead in automobile gas (as reported by The Bio Initiative Working Group).
- As reported on CBC (July 12, 2008), Toronto's department of public health advised teenagers and young children to limit their use of cell phones in order to avoid potential health risks. According to the advisory, which is the first of its kind in Canada, children under the age of eight should only use a cell phone in emergencies, and teenagers should limit calls to less than 10 minutes per day.
- As little as 10 minutes on a cell phone can trigger changes in brain cells linked to cell division and cancer, suggests a study conducted by researchers from the Weizmann Institute of Science in Israel, published in the *Biochemical Journal*. The changes they observed were not caused by the heating of tissues.
- **Regular cell phone use raises the risk of developing a brain tumor** for many users, according to a Finnish study published online in the *International Journal of Cancer*. The study, conducted by numerous researchers from many universities, found firm corollary evidence that using a cell phone causes the risk of getting a brain tumor called a glioma to rise by 40 to 270 percent[48] on the side of the head preferred for using the phones. This is the same type of brain tumor doctors discovered in Senator Ted Kennedy. Malignant glioma is the most common primary brain tumor, accounting for more than half of the 18,000 primary malignant brain tumors

---

[48] Those who used modern cellular (mobile) phones for more than 2,000 hours in their lifetime had the highest risk increase. Surprisingly, the risk was highest among people under age 20.

diagnosed each year in the United States, according to the National Cancer Institute.

- Prolonged cell phone use may damage sperm in male users, suggests a study by researchers at the Cleveland Clinic Lerner College of Medicine at Case Western Reserve University in Ohio. The discovery was made during an ongoing study of 51,000 male health professionals in the United States.
- Pregnant mothers, who use cell phones 2–3 times per day, are found to give birth to children with malfunctioning cells.
- Young children exposed to cell phone radiation are found to develop serious growth problems because they have thinner skulls than adults and nervous systems that are still developing, making them more vulnerable to the radiation.
- Despite the insistence of many (particularly the cell phone industry) that non-thermal radiation is biologically harmless, this is scientifically incorrect. Studies that prove the stress response of human cells when exposed to this type of radiation are well-known and peer-edited for accuracy.
- Scientists have found that microwaves transmitted by cell phones and other wireless devices can damage DNA, blood cells, nerve cells, eyes, and bone density; cause sleep disruptions; contribute to autism and Alzheimer's disease; lead to electromagnetic hypersensitivity; and, affect your heart rate and blood pressure.

In today's day and age, it is hard for cell phone users to imagine giving them up completely, but concerned individuals can help protect themselves in a number of ways. Using the cell phone only when reception is good, for example, minimizes the power your phone must use. Also avoid carrying the phone on the body, opting instead to keep it in a handbag. Whenever possible, keep calls short, keep the phone as far away from your head as possible, and keep it turned off when not in use. One cell phone may not be safer than another, but these simple steps can help to minimize the risk.

The media industry is the largest and most lucrative industry in the world, much bigger than oil. Almost every significant company is run, owned or heavily influenced by the 5-6 media giants. Cell phones make up a huge chunk of that. Any attempt to blame cell phones for the massive increase of cancers in the world is ridiculed and squashed by the mass media, just like cigarette smoking was, not too long ago.

Some people are okay with waiting until finally there is solid *evidence* that radio waves can cause cancer before they give up their beloved cell phones. Others continue using them, just as many continue smoking, although the risks for the latter are known. It is really up to each individual to decide what to do about it.

For me, personally, there is no question about it. I detect harmful energies from a distance, and certainly when they come as close to my body as a cell phone does. I use my cell phone very rarely, and if I do, it is just for a minute or two. I never felt comfortable with them, long before research began to indicate that they are not harmless at all.

On a different note, certain U.S. states and countries in Europe are banning the use of cell phones while driving. In England, where cell phone use is prohibited while driving, a new law will be implemented, prohibiting the use of hands-free phones as well. The government found that such phone use disorients the driver and increases the risk of accidents. The disorientation lasts for up to 10 minutes after use.

In comparison, a conversation with another person in the car showed no such adverse effects. This may indicate that it is not the conversation (using hands-free car phones) that interferes with concentration, reaction and focused attention, but rather the brain's exposure to harmful rays. You are still exposed to these rays 2 to 3 feet away from you.

Most users of cell phones and other wireless devices have no idea what low radiation can do to them, since it isn't tangible and only very few sensitive people experience a negative effect from them. Only when you stand in front of a radar device will you start perspiring and cooking from the inside out, just like food being cooked in a microwave oven. The heat is generated by the rapid movement of molecules (friction) and the breaking down of molecular bonds.

Each year, millions of birds are killed when they get too close to, or sit on, cell towers. And apparently, the same can happen to the human body when it is exposed to this type of radiation on a regular basis. After all, human cells are made of molecules, and molecular bonds are broken and destroyed when exposed to radiation. Strong radiation can literally burn off the entire skin of a person from the inside out. Weak radiation does this more slowly and less dramatically. But as you may know, x-rays, CT-scans radiation and microwaves accumulate, and you can never tell when the body responds with a healing crisis, such as cancer.

Many people are very unsuspecting, unconcerned or naive with regard to their health. The incidence of chronic disease has moved from 10 to 90 percent in just 100 years. It may not be just one thing that causes these degenerative diseases, but a combination of factors. And each factor becomes significant when combined with others.

Everyone must make their own choices and decide what is good for them and what isn't. There is no point trying to persuade someone, for this can cause resentment, which can be a much more serious cause of illness than radio waves or cigarette smoking.

I came across a simple device that can protect the body from the harmful rays and electromagnetic fields that almost constantly surround and bombard us (e.g., cars, computers, cell phones, electric appliances, cell towers, fluorescent lights, harmful chemicals in foods and the environment, and other common stress factors). The device works instantly, and it may have enormous implications for the health and well-being of individuals and families. In the past 12 years I have tested nearly a dozen methods or devices that supposedly protect against cell phone radiation, with disappointing results. However, I am extremely excited about this one. The product is called *Aulterra Neutralizer*.

The EM-Heavy Metal Connection

In 1993, the cell phone industry and U.S. government agencies gave the well-known American researcher, Dr. George Louis Carlo, a $28 million research grant to put to rest, once and for all, any concerns about risks associated with cell phones. Much to the benefit and relief of the industry, initial results covering three years of research indicated that there were no problems with cell phone use. However, by 1999, Dr. Carlo had gained significantly more evidence indicating a risk to DNA, eye cancers and brain tumors.

Following the discovery that cell phones can cause serious health conditions, including cancer, Carlo developed a theory that low frequency cell phone signals interfere with normal cell function. He found that cells exposed to cell phone radiation caused them to go into a protective/defensive mode – similar to what occurs during the fight-or-flight response – which prevents movement of nutrients and waste products through the cellular membrane. The inability to absorb nutrients weakens, damages or kills cells; and not being able to remove wastes outside cells results in a buildup of toxins.

This observation led Carlo to believe there was a close connection between the massive upsurge in usage of wireless technology and the dramatic increase in autism. He hypothesized that young children exposed to electromagnetic (EM) radiation are less able to process heavy metals ingested through air, food and water, and, as a result, begin to accumulate these in their tissues. If this happens to be the brain tissue, it causes neurological damage, including autism. In older people, such an accumulation of heavy metals in the brain can lead to damage of the DNA, multiple sclerosis and Alzheimer's disease. Mercury is already toxic at 1 in 1 billion-part quantities. That is about the same concentration of one grain of salt in one swimming pool. It is a well-established fact that mercury and other heavy metals such as lead are linked with neurological disorders like autism. In 2003, the *International Journal of Toxicology* released a study that showed the hair of autistic babies contained significantly less mercury and other heavy metals. Autistic babies are not able to excrete the toxic metals via the hair and the body's other natural waste removal outlets (hair is a waste product containing excessive proteins and minerals, among other things). Hence, these toxic metals remain trapped in their brains.

To prove the theory that EM radiation prevents autistic children from releasing toxic metals, Carlo and his colleague, Tamara Mariea, set up a trial with 20 autistic children. The study was reported in the November 2007 issue of the *Journal of the Australian College of Nutrition and Environmental Medicine*. The children spent a minimum of four hours, 2 or 3 times a week, in a clinic that was completely EM-free. They received no other treatment. Within three months, the children started to excrete heavy metals from their bodies.

If in fact EM radiation inhibits metal elimination from the body, then regular cell phone use can be blamed for increasing the chances of developing cancer. Many trace metals undermine the functions of a huge range of enzymes and proteins involved in cell signaling, life cycles, replication and cell death. Metals such as cadmium are known to be aggressively mutagenic, damaging DNA; elevated concentrations in

147

the body have been linked to prostate, renal and lung cancers. Similarly, raised levels of lead have been associated with myeloma (a cancer of plasma cells) and leukemia, as well as cancers of the stomach, small intestine, large intestine, ovary, kidney and lung.

Other metals, including chromium and zinc, have been associated with the more rapid progression of breast, colon, rectal, ovarian, lung, bladder and pancreatic cancers, and leukemia. Also nickel, antimony and cobalt are considered to be mutagens and have been linked to lung and nasal cancer.

Gum Disease and Cancer

When researchers looked at data collected between 1986 and 2002, they found that men with gum disease had a 63 percent higher chance of getting pancreatic cancer, even if they had never smoked. Scientists are not exactly sure why gum disease and cancer are linked, but some theorize that gum disease can increase inflammation which can be spread throughout the body. Other research has already linked gum disease to various diseases as well, including heart disease, stroke, diabetes, respiratory issues and lung infections.

American forefathers used brine to preserve their food and kill bacteria. The same germ-removing action of salt water can be harnessed to keep the gums free of infection. Millions of people have used warm salt water rinses to cure oral abscesses, gum boils, etc. Apparently, the warm salt water helps to draw excessive toxic fluid out of the gum tissue, thereby reducing swelling, alleviating pain and killing harmful bacteria. This allows the gums to heal and keep the teeth healthy, too. If used in an irrigating device, the warm salt water reaches all gum line crevices and periodontal pockets, which is important for complete reversal of gum disease and tooth decay.

Rinsing or irrigating the mouth with salt water several times a day is usually enough to prevent and reverse gum disease. For situations of advanced gum disease, however, you may also use Sanguinary, a herbal extract that has been used as a mouth rinse for centuries by native cultures.

Gum disease indicates the presence of large amounts of toxins in the body, especially in the alimentary canal which begins in the mouth and ends in the anus. In addition to the rinsing procedures mentioned above, it is also important to address the underlying causes, such as poor diet, dehydration, irregular lifestyle, congested liver and intestinal tract, and emotional stress.

Soladey's Dental Solution

I personally use a Soladey toothbrush to clean my teeth. Soladey has a patented design that is scientifically and clinically proven to significantly eliminate plaque more effectively than your regular toothbrush, without the use of toothpaste or dental floss. Soladey features a titanium oxide (TiO_2) metal rod, which is sensitive to light. It creates a natural ionic chemical reaction that separates the plaque from your teeth enamel and removes tobacco, coffee and other stains using the natural attraction of ions. You might have heard of a room ionizer that also produces ions. Plaque contains particles with a positive charge (positive ions). When the titanium rod reacts with light, it creates negative ions that attract the positive ions, like a magnet. The plaque just disintegrates and falls off your teeth, washing away when you rinse. Other stains are sucked right out of your teeth with this process.

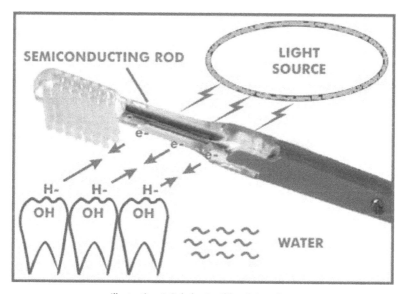

Illustration 4: Soladey toothbrush in action

149

There have been four clinical trials at four different dental universities in Canada and Japan, and they all found that the people who used Soladey had significantly less plaque on their teeth compared to the people who used the ordinary toothbrush. The research also showed an improvement in gingivitis. So Soladey works to protect your gums, as well as reduce plaque.

The scientific principles behind Soladey have been around since the 1970s and Soladey has now been sold in Japan for a few years, where it sells about two million brush units and five million replacement heads every year. Clinical studies on the effectiveness of Soladey technology to remove dental plaque have been conducted at Osaka Dental University, Nippon Dental University, Nihon University and the University of Saskatchewan in Canada. All institutes certify that Soladey is more effective in the removal of plaque and whitening of dental enamel than any regular bristle toothbrush on the market. (See Wellness Products http://www.ener-chi.com/wellness-products/ or http://www.ener-chi.com/wellness-products/soladey-ionic-toothbrushes/)

Sunscreens and Sunglasses – A Major Cause of Cancer

Unfortunately, the ultraviolet portion of sunlight is most easily eliminated by windows, houses, spectacles, sunglasses, sun lotions and clothing. And why is that a bad thing? Because ultraviolet light constitutes one of the most powerful natural medicines the world has ever seen. By the year 1933, researchers found there were over 165 different diseases for which sunlight proved to be a beneficial treatment, including tuberculosis, hypertension, diabetes and almost every type of cancer. To this day, no other treatment has shown such a wide range of benefits as sunlight.

Furthermore, sunscreens touted as necessary for good health are riddled with toxic chemicals, further compounding the problem. A 2008 study from the U.S. Centers for Disease Control and Prevention (CDCP) found that roughly 97 percent of Americans are contaminated with the chemical oxybenzone. This common sunscreen additive has been linked to allergies, hormone disruption, cell damage and low birth weights.

And the effectiveness of sunscreens in preventing skin cancer is highly questionable. "Sunscreens were never developed to prevent skin cancer," Zoe Diana Draelos, editor of the *Journal of Cosmetic Dermatology,* said in a 2010 report. "In fact, there is no evidence to recommend that sunscreens prevent skin cancer in humans." They prevent the skin from absorbing the sunshine it needs to produce essential vitamin D. Moreover, the toxicity of these commonly used skin creams makes them very dangerous.

It is becoming increasingly clear that not only do sunscreens *not* prevent skin cancer, but also the ingredients in many commercial sunscreens, such as retinol and retinyl palmitate, are photocarcinogenic and become toxic when exposed to sunlight – meaning they actually play a role in causing skin tumors and lesions. In fact, as tested by the Environmental Working Group, less than 8 percent of sunscreens are *safe and effective* according to their standards.

However, it is essential that people have regular exposure to the sun without using a sunscreen in order to maintain their levels of vitamin D. "But what about harmful UV rays?" you might ask. Gradual exposure to the sun on a regular, limited basis will help you develop a tolerance for it, even if you are prone to burning. You can also supplement with the natural antioxidant astaxanthin, which acts as a natural sunscreen that reduces oxidative damage caused by sun overexposure.

In my book, *Heal Yourself with Sunlight,* I cite scientific research which clearly shows that the sun cannot cause skin cancer even if it causes sunburn. There is no scientific research to date proving that the sun causes skin cancer. Skin cancer and damage from sunburn are two different things. Also, you cannot develop an allergy to the sun. However, as explained in the book, there are certain foods (i.e., strong acids like trans fats from eating fried foods, meat, melted cheese, chips, sodas, alcohol, etc.) and chemicals that when ingested, or are applied to the skin (such as carcinogen-packed sunscreens), the UV rays and acids or chemicals react with one another, which can lead to an inflammatory response. This can mimic an allergy and high sensitivity to the sun.

In my many years of working with the liver flushes, I also found that when the liver is packed with intrahepatic gallstones, one becomes very sensitive to the sun. The liver cannot detoxify the blood properly, which causes toxins to be removed via the skin, and this can interfere with melanin production. When the skin is exposed to the sun, it may redden and become inflamed. I lived in warm countries most of my life, including Cyprus for 15 years, as well as Africa and India. After I cleaned out my liver, all my sensitivities disappeared and I don't even burn when in the sun anymore. The more toxins make their way into the skin, the more likely it would burn.

Also, wearing sunglasses prevents the production of a brain hormone that regulates melanin production in the skin, which is supposed to prevent deep penetration of UV rays. Wearing sunglasses therefore causes UV-A rays to more thoroughly penetrate the deepest layers of the skin, damaging cells and mutating genes. This also interferes with vitamin D production, which is one of the most powerful preventive factors for all types of cancer, including cancers of the skin. Again, this has nothing to do with the sun, but rather with wearing sunglasses. People who live indoors nearly all the time have been shown to have the highest rates of skin cancer according to large studies conducted in England, U.S. and Australia. Besides, the cancers tend to show up in parts of the body that are almost never exposed to the sun.

Lastly, research also shows that UV radiation is actually lessening each year, not increasing. In some years it goes down by as much as 0.4 percent. This is more concerning, in that we actually will need more exposure to the sun than ever before in order to make the essential amounts of vitamin D to stay healthy. Thankfully, doctors are now warning that the old policy of vilifying the sun has caused an epidemic of rickets (bone deformities), cancers, heart disease, osteoporosis, multiple sclerosis, influenza and all other diseases linked with vitamin D deficiency.

The sun is considered the main culprit for causing skin cancer, certain cataracts leading to blindness and aging of the skin. Only those who take the *risk* of exposing themselves to sunlight find that the sun actually makes them feel better, provided they don't use sunglasses, sunscreens or burn their skin. The UV rays in sunlight actually stimulate the thyroid gland to increase hormone production, which in turn increases the body's basal metabolic rate. This assists both in weight loss and improved muscle development. Farm animals fatten much faster when kept indoors, and so do people who stay out of the sun. Therefore, if you want to lose weight or increase your muscle tone, expose your body to the sun on a regular basis.

Any person who misses out on sunlight becomes weak and suffers mental and physical problems as a result. His vital energy diminishes in due time, which is reflected in his quality of life. The populations in Northern European – countries like Norway and Finland, which experience months of darkness every year – have a higher incidence of irritability, fatigue, illness, insomnia, depression, alcoholism and suicide than those living in sunny parts of the world. Their skin cancer rates are higher, too. For example, the incidence of *melanoma* (skin cancer) on the Orkney and Shetland Isles, north of Scotland, is 10 times that of the Mediterranean islands.

UV light is known to activate an important skin hormone called solitrol. Solitrol influences our immune system and many of our body's regulatory centers. Additionally, in conjunction with the pineal hormone melatonin, Solitrol causes changes in mood and daily biological rhythms. The hemoglobin in our red blood cells requires ultraviolet (UV) light to bind to the oxygen needed for all cellular functions. Lack of sunlight can therefore be held co-responsible for almost any kind of illness, including skin cancer and other forms of cancer. Using sun protection protects only the multi-billion dollar sunscreen and cancer industry, not your skin or your life. Consider these remarkable scientifically proven facts regarding ultraviolet light:

- Improves electrocardiogram readings
- Lowers blood pressure and resting heart rate
- Improves cardiac output when needed (not contradictory to lower resting heart rate)
- Reduces cholesterol, if required
- Increases glycogen stores in the liver
- Balances blood sugar
- Enhances energy, endurance and muscular strength
- Improves the body's resistance to infections due to an increase of lymphocytes and phagocytic index (the average number of bacteria ingested per leukocyte in the patient's blood)
- Controls a gene that is responsible for producing a powerful broad-spectrum antibiotic throughout the body
- Enhances the oxygen-carrying capacity of the blood
- Increases sex hormones

- Improves resistance of the skin to infections
- Raises one's tolerance to stress and reduces depression

On the other hand, there is not a single scientific study which can prove that sunlight itself is responsible for causing skin cancers or other illnesses. There are always other factors present, such as acidosis of the tissues (due to eating an overly acidifying diet consisting of animal proteins, trans fatty acids and manufactured foods and beverages), most pharmaceutical drugs, an accumulation of heavy metals and harmful chemicals in the tissues, toxic blood, a severely congested liver, an unbalanced lifestyle and, foremost of all, sunglasses and sunscreens.

The human body was designed to absorb UV light for very good reasons, otherwise we would have been born with a natural sunscreen for UV light on our skin and in our eyes. One of the most important reasons is that UV radiation is necessary for normal cell division. Lack of sunlight disrupts normal cell growth, which can lead to cancer. Wearing sunglasses, including regular UV-reflecting spectacles and contact lenses, is largely responsible for certain degenerative eye diseases, such as macular degeneration. Most people who wear sunglasses on a regular basis report continuously weakening eyesight.

Depriving your eyes of adequate exposure to ultraviolet light can have serious consequences for your skin and even pose a risk to your life. Normally, as soon as the optic nerves of your eyes sense sunlight, your pituitary gland produces hormones that act as boosters for your melanocytes. Melanocytes produce melanin, the pigment that gives skin its natural color and protection against sunburn. When skin is exposed to the sun, melanocytes produce more pigment, causing the skin to tan, or darken, and your melanocytes start producing melanin on overdrive. However, when you wear sunglasses, this process becomes disrupted. Instead of kick-starting the melanocyte production to protect your skin against sunburn, your pituitary gland thinks it is getting dark outside and, thus, greatly reduces production of melanocyte-stimulating hormones. Subsequently, your skin produces less melanin, which causes it to be less protected and, in turn, become damaged.

The dramatically increased incidence of skin damage seemingly caused by the sun (but really by wearing sunglasses) is exploited by the sunscreen and cancer industry. The main reason the dermatology industry promotes sunscreen products is because it is heavily funded by sunscreen manufacturers.

It is worth noting at this point that the pharmaceutical and medical industries are comprised of large corporations whose primary objective is to make money. Being public companies, they are only obligated to their shareholders. Pharmaceutical companies, for example, make certain to design and produce only drugs that may temporarily relieve or suppress the symptoms of diseases, but never actually cure them. In fact, it is their written policy to turn down offers by independent researchers who have discovered highly effective remedies for such conditions as eczema, diabetes and cancer. For this business to thrive and be perpetually profitable, drug giants must ensure their products produce sufficiently harmful side effects in the patients who take them. Of course, the drug-caused disorders require further medical tests and treatments which benefit the entire medical industry. There is an entire arsenal of new drugs that are prescribed to treat the side effects produced by previously administered drugs.

In the example of sunlight above, by advertising the dangers of sunlight and promoting the use of sunglasses and sunscreens, the pharma/medical industry made certain that the number of skin cancers and numerous other health problems would increase. They then recommended the appropriate treatments to combat these diseases which, in turn, will lead to further escalations of these same diseases. These principles of psychological deception are known quite well to the industry and are applied to almost every so-called *disease*. The result is that nearly every person in the United States already has or will develop one or several serious illnesses at some stage in their life. Something as *harmless* as sunglasses or sunscreens has created a health disaster of unimaginable proportions.

As the health author of website *NaturalNews* reported, a CDCP study shows that 97 percent of Americans are contaminated with an extremely toxic sunscreen chemical called oxybenzone. This chemical is found in nearly 600 sunscreen products, including children's formulas. Most sun-blocking creams and lotions also contain avobenzone for broad-spectrum protection against short- and long-wave UV-A rays which are falsely considered to be the main culprits responsible for long-term skin damage.[49] Most sunscreens also contain a cocktail of a dozen or more cancer-promoting fragrance chemicals and numerous petrochemical-derived synthetic substances. Many of these carcinogenic chemicals are readily absorbed through the skin, much to the annoyance of the consumer who has to keep reapplying the *protective* sunscreens. (Sunscreens come in the form of lotion, cream, oil, ointment, stick, gel/jelly, spray, liquid and pad.)

The producers of these products claim that most of the harmful chemicals become degraded in the presence of sunlight and must therefore be safe for the consumer, a claim that is outright false since almost every person in America is contaminated by sunscreen chemicals (according to the U.S. Centers for Disease Control and Prevention). Avobenzone, butyl-methyoxydibenzoylmethane and oxybenzone particularly penetrate the skin very quickly. Other chemicals found in sunscreens include dixoybenzone, PABA and PABA esters, ethyl dihydroxy propyl PABA, glyceryl PABA, p-aminobenzoic acid, padimate-O or octyl dimethyl PABA, cinnamates (cinoxate, ethylhexyl p-methoxycinnamate, octocrylene, octyl methoxycinnamate), salicylates (ethylhexyl salicylate, homosalate, octyl salicylate), digalloyl trioleate and menthyl anthranilate. There is an almost complete lack of any adequate safety testing of these chemicals. Cosmetics contain them too, and the body absorbs them like a sponge.

Many heavily-used chemical sunscreens have a strong free radical-generating effect, which is believed to be the main reason behind skin cancer. To make it clear, while the body's own free radicals work is synchronized with its constant need for dealing with normal wear and tear, as well as the turnover of cells and detoxification, exposure of the body to large amounts of toxic chemicals causes serious oxidative cell damage. Scientists use such chemicals to start free radical reactions during chemical synthesis. These chemicals are so dangerous that those who handle them in a laboratory must keep them away from their skin. When combined with other chemicals and exposed to ultraviolet light, they then generate the copious amounts of free radicals required to bring about the desired chemical reactions. On your skin, however, such chemical reactions are anything but desirable.

---

[49] For details on how blocking out of some or all UV rays leads to damage of deeper skin tissue, see *Heal Yourself with Sunlight* or Chapter Eight of *Timeless Secrets of Health & Rejuvenation.*

One major study looked at how sunscreens could increase melanoma risk. Its team of researchers found that worldwide, the greatest rise in melanoma has occurred in countries where chemical sunscreens have been heavily promoted by the medical establishment and the pharmaceutical and chemical industries. Queensland now (as of 1992) has more incidences of melanoma per capita than any other place on Earth. The study was published by *American Journal of Public Health*, Vol. 82, No. 4, April 1992, pp. 614-15.

The question of why the incidence of skin cancer has increased so dramatically since the massive promotion of sunscreens should have raised a red flag among consumers. But, instead, it made them lather their skin with even more of these deadly chemicals. The mass media (financed largely by drug giants) made certain that the population would not hear about such important studies as the following ones.

Dr. Gordon Ainsleigh in California found that the 17 percent increase in breast cancer observed between 1981 and 1992 may be the result of the pervasive use of sunscreens over the past decade.[50] According to several studies, men who regularly use sunscreens have a higher rate of melanoma, and women using sunscreens have a higher rate of basal cell carcinoma.[51]

The medical industry's biggest argument in favor of using sunscreens is that they prevent skin cancer because they prevent sunburn, implying that skin cancers are caused by sunburn. But this is more a correlation than a cause-effect relationship. More recent studies done in England and Australia actually found much higher skin cancer rates among people who live mostly indoors compared with those who spend most of their time outdoors.

As Drs. Cedric and Frank Garland of the University of California have pointed out, there is no scientific proof that sunscreens protect against melanoma or basal cell carcinoma in humans [Garland, C.F., et al. "Could sunscreens increase melanoma risk?"*American Journal of Public Health*, 1992; 82(4): 614-615]. According to the Garlands, the increased use of chemical sunscreens is the primary cause of the skin cancer epidemic. A study by Drs. Mike Brown (Kate Law of the Cancer Research

---

[50] Ainsleigh, H. Gordon. Beneficial effects of sun exposure on cancer mortality. *Preventive Medicine*, Vol. 22, February 1993, pp. 132-40

[51] *Journal of the National Cancer Institute*, Vol. 86, No. 10, May 18, 1994, pp. 798-801; *International Journal of Alternative & Complementary Medicine*, 1994; 12(12): 17-19

Campaign) and Philippe Autier (European Institute of Oncology in Milan) reported that children using sunscreen returned from holiday with more skin moles – a possible sign of increased cancer risk. Whether or not sunscreens increase the risk of developing skin cancer, at least there is overwhelming evidence that sunscreens don't prevent skin cancer.

In February 1998, epidemiologist Marianne Berwick of Memorial Sloan-Kettering Cancer Center in New York presented a careful analysis of data on sunscreen use and skin cancer at the annual meeting of the American Association for the Advancement of Science. Sunscreens may not protect against skin cancer, including melanoma, she concluded. "We don't really know whether sunscreens prevent skin cancer. After examining the available epidemiological data and conducting our own large case-control population-based study, we have found no relationship between sunscreen use at any age and the development of melanoma skin cancer," said Dr. Berwick.

Although sunscreens do prevent sunburn, Dr. Berwick concluded that sunburn itself is not the direct cause of cancer. She argued that if people develop melanoma, it may be because they are genetically susceptible and likely to develop skin cancer regardless of the amount of sunlight exposure or protection from sunscreen.[52] Dr. Berwick objected to the universal blanket advice about using sunscreens during all time spent outdoors.

Dr. Berwick's previously conducted research (1996) found no relationship between a history of sunburn and the development of melanoma.

The American Academy of Dermatology (AAD), which is largely funded by sunscreen and skin care product companies, of course strongly condemned Dr. Berwick's research and called her a "number crunching scientist". I guess that's what scientists do — crunch numbers.

Now back to what sunscreens can actually do to you. They may not only be responsible for melanomas, but also for many other types of cancers and dysfunctions as well. What is most disturbing is that many commonly used sunscreen chemicals have strong estrogenic actions which may seriously affect sexual development in children and sexual

---

[52] For more details about the possible factors responsible for developing skin cancer, see *Heal Yourself with Sunlight* or *Timeless Secrets of Health & Rejuvenation*.

function in adults, and further increase cancer risks. Exposing your body to chemicals that can alter hormonal balance puts your health at great risk, to put it mildly.

It takes all of 30 seconds for the skin to absorb whatever is placed on it into the bloodstream. Of course, the sunscreen industry neglects to inform you that there is not much difference between drinking your sunscreen lotion and lathering it on your skin, except ingesting it would actually cause you much less harm because your digestive system would filter out most of the poison. The skin has no other option than to dump this cocktail of carcinogens right into the circulatory system, and from there into the liver, kidneys, heart and brain. I will leave it to your imagination what such a chemical assault means for these vital organs.

The Vitamin D Factor

Sunglasses and sunscreen agents are among the most health-endangering products that exist because they block absorption of ultraviolet rays which your body needs to produce vitamin D. Besides hindering the essential exposure of your eyes and skin to the rays of the sun, the use of sunscreens and sunglasses is largely responsible for the chronic vitamin D deficiency that plagues 80 percent of the American population. Vitamin D deficiency is associated with depression, prostate cancer, breast cancer, osteoporosis and almost every other degenerative disorder. "The elderly, who spend little time in the sun and use sunscreen agents frequently, may be at risk for vitamin D deficiency," according to a statement made by the Mayo Clinic.[53] Vitamin D deficiency is strongly associated with bone disease and fracture. Makes you wonder why so many elderly people suffer from bone disorders.

Research findings (published in the *Archives of Internal Medicine*, June 9, 2008; 168(11):1174-1180) join a growing body of evidence indicating that an adequate level of vitamin D, which you can obtain by spending an average of 20 minutes in the sun each day (dark-skinned people may need an hour or more), is crucial to maintaining good

---

[53] http://www.mayoclinic.org/drugs-supplements/sunscreen-agent-topical-application-route/before-using/drg-20070255

health. Men who are deficient in vitamin D were found to have more than double the normal risk of suffering a heart attack or dying even after all other possible risk factors, such as hypertension, obesity and high levels of blood fat, were excluded. Populations in northern countries (with less intense sunlight and lower levels of vitamin D) have a higher incidence of heart disease than sun-filled southern countries. In addition, more heart attacks occur in the winter months, when sunlight is scarce. Furthermore, low levels of vitamin D showed an increased risk of developing diabetes and dying from breast cancer.

A study conducted by scientists at the German Cancer Research Center Deutsches Krebsforschungszentrum, DKFZ, collaborating with researchers of the University Hospitals in Hamburg-Eppendorf, provides clear evidence that post-menopausal women with low blood levels of vitamin D clearly have a significantly increased risk of breast cancer. The study was released in April 2008 and published in the medical journal *Carcinogenesis*. Among other cancer-inhibiting effects, sunlight-induced vitamin D increases the self-destruction of mutated cells and reduces the spread and reproduction of cancer cells.

Sun exposure can help you prevent as many as 16 different types of cancer, including pancreatic, lung, breast, ovarian, prostate and colon cancers. Research has clearly shown that it can cut your risk by as much as 60 percent. On the other hand, lack of sun exposure and subsequent vitamin D deficiency kills more than one million people each year.

It is no coincidence that cancer rates are lowest in countries closest to the equator where people get proper sunshine exposure – a fact that has been known and verified since the 1940s. Subsequent research has strongly suggested that that vitamin D blood levels in the 50 to 80 ng/ml range are linked to significantly reduced cancer risk. Regular, unhindered sun exposure is essential to ensure adequate vitamin D. In colder climates and winter months, supplementation can also help ensure healthy levels.

Comparatively, the risk of being harmed by the sun is minimal. The most dangerous of skin cancers, which is melanoma, usually appears in parts of the skin where the sun barely reaches. If you have the opportunity for optimal protection, expose your entire body to the sun, including the private parts.

Milkweed sap is another well-known natural remedy for skin growths. Simply take a milkweed plant, break a leaf and apply the milky sap to the skin. Avoid direct contact with your eyes as this could cause serious stinging and possible damage to the cornea.

Happy and Healthy With Serotonin

Spending most of the time inside buildings – cut off from the UV light and other healing rays of the sun – creates an enormous challenge for the body, mind and emotions. Ultimately, all hormones in the body are regulated by the circadian rhythm (day and night cycle). The powerful neurotransmitter and intestinal hormone serotonin closely follows the movement of the sun in respect to the Earth. Peak secretion occurs during noon time when the sun's intensity is the strongest.

In the central nervous system, serotonin plays an important role as a neurotransmitter (hormone) in the modulation of anger, depression, aggression, body temperature, mood, sleep, sexuality, appetite and metabolism. In the gastrointestinal tract, which contains about 90 percent of the body's total serotonin, it is responsible for balanced digestive functions. In the blood, the major storage site is platelets, which collect serotonin for use in mediating post-injury vasoconstriction. Research suggests that serotonin plays an important role in liver regeneration and acts as a mitogen (induces cell division) throughout the body. Failed induction of cell division is a leading cause of cancer.

In addition, Italian research on mice conducted at the European Molecular Biology Laboratory in Monterotondo, Italy, found that defective signaling of serotonin in the brain may be at the root cause of Sudden Infant Death Syndrome (SIDS). This makes a lot of sense. Newborn babies who are being kept in dark rooms and rarely get out into the sun are deprived of vitamin D (purposefully not supplied by mother's milk) and produce little or no serotonin.

Worldwide, many more babies die of SIDS in one year than who die of cancer, heart disease, pneumonia, child abuse, cystic fibrosis and muscular dystrophy combined. The Italian research shows that the tested mice suffered drops in heart rate and other symptoms of SIDS, and many of the animals died at an early age. Low levels of serotonin in the animals' brainstems, which control heartbeat and breathing, may have caused sudden death, researchers said in the July 4, 2008 issue of *Science*. Since serotonin in humans controls about the same functions as in mice, researchers believe that the same phenomenon occurs in human infants.

The implications of the existing research conducted on serotonin are wide-reaching. Any prolonged imbalance of serotonin levels in the body affects the most basic functions in the body. Although fruits and vegetables contain serotonin, to digest these foods you need a healthy digestive system. The digestive system follows its own schedule, controlled by the serotonin cycle.[54] The serotonin cycle, in turn, follows the circadian rhythm. This makes sunlight the most powerful and natural sustainer of life and health. Sunlight is pure medicine, and it is free.

Precautions:

Plan to avoid unnecessary or prolonged exposure to sunlight, especially during the midday period in very hot climates, as well as protective clothing, sunglasses and sunscreen. Many drugs, such as LIPITOR®/atorvastatin, belladonna, furosemide, quinine, tetracycline and doxycycline may make your eyes and skin sensitive to sunlight. Medication, stimulants such as caffeine, nicotine and adrenaline, and recreational drugs such as cocaine and heroin can dilate the pupil, thereby allowing an excessive amount of light to enter the eye. This side effect may lead to the inappropriate use of sunglasses.

Highly acid-forming foods, including meat, eggs, cheese, fried foods and sugar, may also make your eyes and skin prone to sun damage. Accordingly, you may find you can never leave the house without sunglasses. It is a rather serious condition when the sun becomes so dangerous that you have to hide from it. The net result is that not getting enough sunlight lowers your vitamin D and serotonin levels, thereby increasing your risk of cancer and many other illnesses.

---

[54] See more details in the section, The Wonders of Our Biological Rhythms, Chapter Five of *Timeless Secrets of Health & Rejuvenation*.

Also be aware that most cosmetics contain UV-blocking chemicals. These include face creams, makeup products, moisturizers, lotions and anti-wrinkle creams.

If you feel you absolutely need a sunscreen product because you are unable to avoid the direct midday sun, make sure it has mostly natural, organic ingredients. Coconut oil, shea butter or aloe vera may also be sufficient for protection against sunburn.

Pharmaceutical Drugs

Some of the most powerful direct and indirect causes of cancer are pharmaceutical drugs. Most drugs consist of a combination of synthetically-derived chemicals that hook to the receptors of a cell in order to invoke or suppress specific responses that, for some reason, no longer occur naturally. Although this intervention on the cellular level sounds very logical and desirable, it can have serious consequences. It actually prevents your body from restoring its own natural responses when you try to determine the root causes of your health issues. After a while, your body will have no choice but to forsake the production of its own natural chemicals and become dependent on the drugs.

Most people know, for example, that cholesterol can be reduced naturally by maintaining a healthy diet and lifestyle. Yet many people refuse to do so and instead turn to statin drugs as *preventive* medicine in order to combat their cholesterol problems. These drugs are associated with a slew of health problems, including a heightened risk of developing diabetes, heart failure and high blood pressure, as well as preventing your body from creating its own vitamin D from sunlight.

Despite what Big Pharma propaganda will tell you, the body actually needs cholesterol to perform myriad functions, like producing cell membranes, hormones and bile acids to help you digest fat. The brain needs it to form memories. Now ask yourself if it makes any sense to use a drug that can *cause* heart disease as a preventive medicine for heart disease?

Say you refused to maintain your cholesterol level naturally and decided to take a statin drug as a *preventive* measure. The statin drug, in turn, gives you diabetes. There are plenty of drugs on the market to treat that, right? Yet many of these drugs, including metformin, sitagliptin and glipizide, have been linked to causing several forms of cancer, as well as anemia, muscle cramps, fatigue, memory loss and irregular heartbeat. These other side effects can also contribute indirectly to the development of cancer and should be avoided at all costs.

Diuretics prescribed for conditions such as hypertension, heart failure and edema cause the body to dehydrate itself, which can result in the loss of critical vitamins and minerals, and thicken the blood. They can also cause weight gain and depression. All of these common and well-known side effects can increase the likelihood of developing cancer down the road.

Another of the many directly or indirectly dangerous drugs on the pharmaceutical market are antidepressants. Many selective serotonin reuptake inhibitors (SSRIs) disturb the body's natural interactive cycles of serotonin/melatonin production, two of the body's most powerful brain hormones. As previously mentioned, serotonin[55] is associated with positive moods, appetite, sleep, muscle contraction and satiety; and melatonin is, among other things, a sleep-inducer, providing the body with deep and rejuvenating sleep.

By inhibiting the breakdown of serotonin in the body, these drugs disrupt the melatonin cycle and affect proper sleep induction. As the ongoing Nurses' Health Study[56] and other cancer research have shown, low melatonin levels in the blood greatly increase the risk of cancer. Melatonin controls a gene responsible for inducing normal cell death; low blood melatonin reduces that gene's activity, which in turn causes cells to live much longer than their normal lifespan. These uncontrolled cells become cancerous.

Interfering with the body's natural melatonin cycle is no small matter. In fact, the hormone can be an effective cancer treatment on its own. Numerous studies have suggested that melatonin can stop cancer cell growth in its tracks and keep it from spreading. In a study involving

---

[55] Most people believe serotonin to be a brain hormone only. However, approximately 80 percent of the human body's total serotonin is located in the digestive tract, where it is used to regulate intestinal activities. The remainder is synthesized in the central nervous system and blood.

[56] The Nurses' Health Study, established in 1976 by Dr. Frank Speizer, and the Nurses' Health Study II, established in 1989 by Dr. Walter Willett, are among the most definitive long-term epidemiological studies conducted on older women's health. The study has followed 121,700 female registered nurses since the mid-1970s to assess risk factors for cancer and cardiovascular disease (*Wikipedia*).

the brain cancer glioblastoma, for example, patients were given either radiation and melatonin, or just radiation. About 25 percent of the patients who took melatonin were still alive after a year, whereas all of the patients who were *treated* with radiation alone were dead. A similar Italian study on small-cell lung cancer produced similar numbers. Still more studies have shown that it is effective in treating pancreatic cancer.

It does this in a number of ways: first, it triggers cancer cells to destroy themselves, as well as directly kills them. It also inhibits tumor growth, reduces inflammation and blocks the effects of estrogen on cancer cells (especially important for hormonally-affected cancers like uterine and breast cancer). Perhaps most importantly, it stimulates the immune system.

So why is it that the medical establishment hasn't yet caught on to melatonin? It might have something to do with the fact that the drugs most commonly used to treat these cancers can cost upwards of $4,000 per month, whereas melatonin supplements cost only around $11 per month.

Antidepressants upset the most fundamental functions in the body, including the digestion of food and cell metabolism. Patients given the popular antidepressant paraoxetine (Paxil), for example, may suddenly feel much hungrier than usual and not feel full after eating. In view of this, they eat more and more, a sure way to gain weight and become obese. Obesity is considered the main risk factor for most chronic health issues, including heart disease, cancer and diabetes.

Some common antipsychotic drugs, such as olanzapine (Zyprexa), can bring about a weight gain of 30 pounds in a short period of time. These drugs boost dopamine, the hormone that causes food cravings. This class of drugs also decreases levels of leptin, a protein that suppresses appetite. In other words, those who take antidepressants may develop an unnaturally strong appetite that they cannot control by eating more. Think of the confusion and chaos this causes in the rest of the body, from producing more insulin and digestive juices, such as hydrochloric acid, bile and enzymes, to having to eliminate ever-increasing amounts of harmful waste material. Elevated insulin secretions alone increase the risk of cancer in the body.

Other drugs, such as hormone replacement therapy (HRT) and the contraceptive pill or injections, lead to weight gain in up to 70 percent of users, once again interfering with the body's most basic functions. They also increase breast cancer risk. While this risk is considerably elevated during use of hormone medication, it drops back to the original level within about five years after a woman has stopped taking hormones. This is the result of a study by the German Cancer Research Center in Heidelberg and the University Hospital of Hamburg-Eppendorf.

Besides breast cancer, taking HRT or contraceptives can cause uterine (endometrial) cancer, ovarian cancer, vaginal bleeding, stroke, dementia, blood clots, deep vein thrombosis (DVT) and heart disease. They also destroy beneficial bacteria in the digestive system, thereby affecting absorption of the vitamins B6 and zinc. Prolonged deficiency of these nutrients, among others, can increase the risk of cancer, as well as heart disease, insomnia, memory loss and irritability. As of June 2011, Bayer was facing 25,000 lawsuits for playing down in ads the horrific side effects caused by the world's best-selling birth control pill YAZ®. Just imagine, one little pill a day causing suffering and death among millions of young people.

Bone-building drugs also cause weight gain. Prednisone, cortisone and other steroids used to treat dozens of conditions, including asthma, lupus and cancer, frequently cause weight gain because they increase appetite and force the body to retain fluids. Steroids cause just as many disorders as the conditions for which they are used, including liver cancer, heart disease, depression, hostility and aggression, eating disorders, stunted height, risk of HIV, acne, and dozens more.

Tamoxifen is a popular drug prescribed to prevent breast cancer recurrence in women. The drug can cause weight gain of up to 25 pounds, enough to dramatically increase the risk of other cancers, heart disease and diabetes.

Many people, doctors and patients alike, perceive the ability of modern medicine to interfere with the body on the cellular level as a *medical miracle*. But this miracle has brought more destruction into the world than it has prevented or eliminated. We have created an endless, vicious cycle by treating diseases that then cause other diseases, which, in turn, require further treatment. This self-perpetuating system of disease generation is largely due to the *medical miracle* that promises quick relief of symptoms at the expense of long-term suffering and ailments, and possibly, even death.

The situation is at a point where even drug company executives are beginning to speak out. In 2003, a senior U.K. executive with GlaxoSmithKline, Dr. Allen Roses, admitted that less than half of the patients who take prescription drugs actually benefit from them. His final analysis was that 90 percent of these drugs only *work* for about 30 to 50 percent of patients who take them – that's less effective than the placebo! Meanwhile, their prices have soared by 50 percent in the previous three years, from $2.3 billion a year to an annual cost to the taxpayer of $7.2 billion.

Although nearly one million people die each year from the side effects of medical treatments or medical errors, it is difficult for most people to forsake the illusion of a cure when learned scientists, doctors, pharmacists, the government and the drug makers so convincingly promise them a quick relief from their disease symptoms. It takes great courage, as well as trust in yourself, in your body's innate wisdom and in nature, to heal what is only yours to heal. To heal cancer, the entire *you* must become whole again, including your physical, mental, emotional and spiritual self.

Beware of Popular Anticancer Drugs

One of the most popular anticancer drugs is AVASTIN®, produced by the drug maker Genentech. In 2007, the drug sold a whopping $3.5 billion, with $2.3 billion in the United States. One course of treatment with Avastin can cost $100,000 per year. If a drug sells this well, it must be a very effective medicine, or so you could believe. However, when you read the following statement made by Genentech (2008) on their website,[57] you may wonder why it is prescribed at all: "Currently, no data are available that demonstrate an improvement in disease-related symptoms or increased survival with Avastin in breast cancer." The answer may lie in the fact that Avastin produces some of the worst side effects a drug can, and that is good business. The thousands of doctors, hospital administrators and health agencies that endorsed this killer drug either fell for the scam, or welcomed it.

---

[57] http://www.gene.com/media/press-releases/11687/2008-11-23/avastin-plus-commonly-used-chemotherapie

Treatment with Avastin can result in the development of a potentially fatal **gastrointestinal (GI) perforation, a potentially fatal wound-healing complication, a potentially fatal hemorrhage,** fistula formation, strokes or heart problems (blood clots), hypertensive crisis (severe hypertension), posterior leukoencephalopathy syndrome (nervous system and vision disturbances), neutropenia (a reduced white blood cell count that may increase the chance of infection), nephrotic syndrome (a sign of severe kidney malfunction), congestive heart failure and many other bizarre symptoms or extreme illness.

Under great pressure, an FDA advisory panel recommended that the drug Avastin should not be used to treat breast cancer, because it fails to provide enough benefit (which is none) to outweigh the risks. An FDA review of the drug concluded that Avastin did not significantly lengthen the lives of patients. On the contrary, it killed a number of patients.

An article published in the *New York Times* (July 5, 2008) raised some troubling questions about this drug. It asks, "What does it mean to say the drug works? Is slowing the growth of tumors enough if life is not significantly prolonged or improved? How much evidence should there be before billions of dollars are spent on a drug? And when should cost be factored into the equation?" I will let a cancer patient answer that question:

In 2007, Jeanne Sather wrote on the then active website, Assertivepatient.com:

"Every three weeks, always on a Thursday afternoon, I amble on over to the cancer center for my IV treatment. (I also take Cytoxan, a chemo drug that comes in pill form, every day, plus a handful of other pills to help deal with the side effects and fringe benefits of being in cancer treatment – anxiety, high blood pressure, occasional depression, insomnia.) The total bill for each treatment session at the cancer center is something north of $20,000. The annual cost of my cancer care is more than $300,000. That's three hundred thousand dollars a year. Almost $30,000 a month to keep me alive….

Both Herceptin and Avastin are made by Genentech Inc., a San Francisco Bay Area company that is doing very well, thank you. The reason they are so expensive is that they are new, and there are no generic versions available. So Genentech can charge whatever it wants, without competition, for these life-saving drugs.

As a result of the high cost of Herceptin and Avastin, I am going to hit my lifetime max of $1 million on my health insurance before the end of 2007."

Beware of Arthritis Drugs

Do Arthritis Drugs Cause Cancer? This is the title of an article published in the *New York Times*, June 5, 2008. As stated in the article, the FDA had received reports of 30 cases of cancer among children and young adults treated with drugs for rheumatoid arthritis, psoriasis, Crohn's disease and other immune system diseases. The drugs involved are:

1. Enbrel, sold by Amgen and Wyeth
2. Remicade, sold by Johnson & Johnson and Schering-Plough
3. Humira, sold by Abbott Laboratories
4. Cimzia, sold by the Belgian company UCB

Because these drugs block part of the immune system, they naturally contribute to a higher risk of cancers and infections. The drugs' labels include a warning about a risk of lymphomas, which are cancers of immune system cells. The risk of developing cancer as a result of taking arthritis medication is also prevalent among adults. One study found that those given Humira or Remicade to treat rheumatoid arthritis had 2.4 times the cancer rate of those in control groups. The most common cancers resulting from these drugs are lymphomas, skin, gastrointestinal, breast and lung cancers. Tuberculosis is listed as a side effect, too. The question is whether it is better to live with psoriasis or arthritis, or to die from any of these other illnesses.

So who benefits from these drugs? You can draw your own conclusions. One year on Remicade costs about $12,000. The combined sales of Remicade, Humira and Enbrel in 2007 earned the drug makers $13 billion. You can easily heal the causes of arthritis, Crohn's disease and psoriasis through cleansing of the liver, kidneys and colon, eliminating animal protein from the diet and eating a nutritious vegetarian diet, while adhering to a balanced lifestyle. I suffered from rheumatoid arthritis over 35 years ago, and once I knew what caused it, I healed it quickly without any medical aid. I appeal to all parents whose children are afflicted with arthritis, Crohn's disease and similar disorders, to protect them against medical treatments designed to destroy their young and growing bodies. The *success* of these drugs is only measured by the degree of destruction or suppression of symptoms they can provide, but not by how much real healing they can induce.

Beware of Aspirin and Tylenol

Who would have thought that the *harmless* aspirin pills that millions of people swallow each day, every week, could actually cause one of the most serious cancers? A study at the Brigham and Women's Hospital (Boston, Massachusetts) of nearly 90,000 women, spanning 18 years of research, shows a 58 percent increased risk of pancreatic cancer when the participants took more than two aspirin pills a week. When the dosage exceeded 14 pills a week, the risk increased by 86 percent. Aspirin has even been linked to erectile dysfunction. According to an article entitled "Erectile dysfunction linked to aspirin and other NSAIDs" by Thomas H. Maugh II, *Los Angeles Times* (March 3, 2011), daily use of these drugs is associated with a 22 percent increase in the occurrence of erectile dysfunction.

Another over-the-counter painkiller, acetaminophen (the active ingredient in Tylenol, as well as other drugs including Excedrin and Theraflu), has been shown to increase risk of developing blood cancer when taken regularly for extended periods of time. A study by the University of Washington found that individuals who took the drug at least four days a week over the course of four years were twice as likely to develop certain blood cancers, including non-Hodgkin lymphomas, plasma cell disorders and myeloid neoplasms. This is on top of the already-existing FDA warnings that acetaminophen is extremely toxic to the liver.

Avoid The Drug Trap

It is becoming increasingly apparent that pharmaceutical drugs carry great risks. They kill at least 100,000 people in the U.S. each year. This figure could be much higher because only a fraction of drug-caused deaths are actually being reported by medical professionals. In nearly every case of death, the doctor issuing the death certificate writes down the name of the disease as the cause of death, instead of the drug that was used to *treat* the disease. If doctors suddenly stopped prescribing drugs today, thousands of lives would be saved tomorrow. This truth has been known for many years.

In 1976, Los Angeles County registered a sudden reduction of its death rate by 18 percent when many medical doctors went on strike against the increase of health insurance premiums for malpractice. In a study by Dr. Milton Roemer from the University of California, Los Angeles, 17 of the largest hospitals in the county showed a total of 60 percent fewer operations during the period of the strike. When the doctors resumed work and medical activities went back to normal, death rates also returned to pre-strike levels.

A similar event took place in Israel in 1973. Doctors staged a one month strike and reduced their daily number of patients from 65,000 to 7,000. For the entire month, mortality rates in Israel were down 50 percent. This seems to happen whenever doctors go on strike. A two month work stoppage by doctors in the Columbian capital of Bogotá led to a 35 percent decline in deaths. This practically makes the medical profession, together with hospitals, the leading cause of death.

Besides killing patients, pharmaceutical drugs can cause permanent damage to the immune system, liver, kidneys, heart, brain and other organs. Taking prescription drugs can also send you to the emergency room. A Vancouver, Canada study has documented that 12 percent of emergency room (ER) visits were the direct result of problems with a pharmaceutical drug. In addition, the length of stay for those admitted to the hospital was significantly longer. The study, reported by the *Canadian Medical Association Journal*, was carried out at Vancouver General Hospital, which has 995 beds and offers a wide range of services, including emergency care. The hospital treats 69,000 patients every year.

Pharmaceutical drugs are not designed to cure anything. They are designed to alleviate a symptom, which remains the body's way of dealing with an underlying, unresolved physical/emotional imbalance. Basically, these drugs are designed to prevent your body from healing itself. The mindset that you have to pop a pill in order to fix a headache or heartburn, because your doctor told you so, is responsible for your reluctance to find out what causes these symptoms. Once the pain is gone, the problem is gone; at least this is what most people believe and what many doctors preach. The problem with this mindset is that it ignores the fact that these symptoms are warning signs that you are doing, being exposed to, eating, or neglecting something that coerces your body into a healing response (symptom).

A symptom of pain or discomfort is not an illness, in itself, to be *cured* by a pill, wrongly called *medicine*. Real medicine supports and encourages the body to complete the healing process it has already begun (as indicated by the symptom). Pharmaceutical drugs are made to suppress the body's ability to heal, which reduces or eliminates the symptoms, but also fortifies the origins of the illness. This makes regular symptom-squashing (medical treatment) a leading cause of disease, including cancer. I recommend that you don't enter the drug trap; it only pushes you into a vicious cycle of dangerous drug addiction from which it is difficult to escape.

Chapter Three

Demystifying Cancer

If you want to want to beat cancer, accept and embrace it first.
If you want to be free of cancer, focus on being free.
If you want more laughter in your life, laugh more.
If you no longer wish to be afraid, do what you are afraid of.
If you want a better world, make it better.
If you see yourself a victim of some kind, change your perception.
If you want more peace in your life, spread more peace around you.

*There is only one **"do not"** you should know about:*
Do not focus your attention and energy on what you
do not want for yourself and others.
Instead, concentrate your thoughts on that which you do want. Health, joy,
abundance, freedom and peace
are among the choices we make in life,
not things that exist in separation from us.

Connecting the Pieces

Mary visited me when she was 39. A year earlier she had been diagnosed with advanced breast cancer. Her oncologist had prescribed the standard routine treatments for cancer – radiation and chemotherapy – but to no avail. Soon afterward, he advised her to undergo a mastectomy of her right breast. The operation took place shortly before her menstrual period began. Much to her relief, her doctors informed her that they *got all the cancer* and the situation was now under control. Little did her doctors know that, according to the science of chronobiology,[58] the risk of the cancer recurring is four times higher in women who undergo surgery one week before or during menstruation than for those who have surgery at other points in their cycle. While menstruating, a woman's immunity and iron levels are measurably lower. Her body is therefore not able to destroy all the cancer cells left over from surgery. Hence, the woman is at high risk for cancer cells developing in other parts of her body.

Not surprisingly, one year after her mastectomy, Mary began to complain of severe pain in her lower spine and left knee. Ten years earlier she had been diagnosed with cervical spondylosis[59] in her lower spine, caused by abnormal outgrowth and ossified cartilage around the margins of the joints of the vertebral column. This time, however, an examination revealed that she had developed bone cancer in her lower spine and left knee. The breast surgery and resulting suppression of the immune system had, as so often is the case, encouraged millions of cancer cells to develop in other, already weakened parts of Mary's body. Therefore, cancer cells began to grow in her lower spine where the resistance to cancer formation was particularly low.

Mary had also been suffering from severe menstrual problems for as long as she remembered. In addition, she had been diagnosed with anemia. However, despite taking iron tablets regularly for years, which caused her frequent nausea and stomach cramps, she remained anemic. She told me that her digestive system had "never worked properly", and constipation often lasted for as many as 3 to 5 days in a row. My examination revealed that her liver was filled with thousands of intrahepatic stones.

Mary also mentioned that she had received multiple antibiotic treatments over the years for all kinds of infections. It is a well-established fact that regular use of antibiotics sharply increases breast cancer risk. According to cancer research, the risk of breast cancer is twice as high among women who have taken 25 or more rounds of antibiotics of any variety over a 17-year period, in comparison with women who have used no antibiotics at all.

---

[58] Chronobiology is the science of *body clocks* attuned to the Earth's cycles and encoded in our cells. The human body is endowed with at least 100 such *clocks*, which are unrelated to our watch time. The circadian rhythm, for example, is responsible for numerous hormonal cycles that determine our hunger, moods, metabolism and rate of growth and aging. For more information, see *Timeless Secrets of Health & Rejuvenation*.

[59] Spondylosis is spinal degeneration and deformity of the joint(s) of two or more vertebrae.

Mary was brought up on a lot of candy, cake, ice cream and chocolate. A number of recent studies have linked a greater risk of breast cancer among women to a diet high in sugar (especially soft drinks and popular sweet desserts). Scientists now believe that the extra insulin released to process the simple starches and sugars found in these foods causes cells to divide, and estrogens in the blood to rise. Both of these factors (cellular division and blood estrogens) can contribute to cancer growth. Indeed, the insulin resistance that results from a lifestyle of excessive sugar intake can drive the mutations that create up to 80 percent of all cancers.

Another common factor in these situations is emotional stress, which triggers fluctuations in the body's levels of the hormone cortisone, and which is responsible for regulating many physiological processes, including anti-inflammatory responses and the metabolism of carbohydrates, fats and proteins. Researchers have also established that stress weakens the immune system and plays a direct role in the development of heart disease, upper respiratory tract infections, asthma, certain viral infections, autoimmune imbalances and even how wounds heal, according to a study at Carnegie Mellon University [October 10, 2007 issue of the *Journal of the American Medical Association*].

Moreover, stress can affect our daily habits in ways that make us progressively and cyclically unhealthier – turning, for example, to compulsive eating, drinking alcohol or smoking – which, in turn, makes us feel worse, and therefore more stressed. Taken together, emotional imbalance is, in itself, one of the most dangerous contributing factors to the development of cancer.

Cancer's Emotional Causes

Coming back to Mary's story, she had experienced a very sad childhood because her parents had great problems relating to one another. When I asked her, she could not remember even a single instance when there had not been tension between her parents. Being a very sensitive person at heart, she took everything more seriously than her more extroverted brother did, and consequently felt insecure, frightened and depressed. With a painful smile on her face, Mary said that she had always felt torn between her mother and father, and could not choose which one to favor.

Eating meals with her parents was particularly difficult. She was forced to sit and eat with them while being besieged by a very stressful atmosphere. Sometimes everyone would keep quiet, in an attempt not to arouse any new conflicts. Today she has a strong aversion to, and fear of, food, wolfing it down very quickly, often while standing or driving.

Mary also faces great difficulties at work. In her job as a teacher, she feels that her students are allowed to take their frustrations out on her, but she has to keep hers all inside. When she returns home, though, she shouts at her own children, which creates a lot of guilt in her. She wants to be a good mother, but believes she is not; she just doesn't know how to be kind to her children. Mary also told me that she never really wanted to be a classroom teacher; she always dreamed of becoming a gymnastics coach.

The frustration of not fulfilling her desires was a major cause of Mary's cancer. Right from the beginning of her life she was taught to conform to the social system, which for her meant that she always had to do what she was told. Deep within her, Mary had dreams that she could never fulfill because she did not want to stir up trouble or make other people think badly of her.

In order to keep the peace, Mary went along with what her parents demanded of her, but inside she was boiling with rage. When Mary walked into my office that morning, she gave me a beautiful smile which did not reveal the pain she was feeling. She had learned to conceal her inner world from the outer world. It was not so much the physical pain in her body that hurt her; it was all the bottled-up frustration, fear and insecurity that threatened the sensitive feelings of love and peace in her heart. The physical pain merely reminded her of the profound emotional heartache from which she had been suffering so long. Her endless attempts to suppress or hide her true inner feelings – through both childhood and adulthood – shaped a personality that eventually required a disease to bring it all to some kind of conclusion.

Torn between her parents for many years and trying to please both of them, Mary had never been bold enough to make a choice that would please herself and herself alone. The division within her heart sapped all her energy and happiness. The cancer started in her divided heart, reflecting all the unexpressed grief and frustration that had filled her early life.

It's All Psychosomatic, Isn't It?

This sounds farfetched, you might say. How can this be the case? Certainly, it might defy conventional wisdom, but that very *wisdom* has created a system of chronic sickness and ineffective, poisonous, costly, symptom-oriented medical treatment. Instead of continuing on this path, consider that just as placebos (which are basically designed to be medically *pointless*) have consistently been proven more effective than pharmaceutical drugs, so can underlying emotions have tremendous influence on one's physical body, for better or worse.

Whatever happens in our emotional body also occurs in our physical body, and vice versa. The real cancer is a trapped and isolated emotion, a feeling of *having no choice*. And likewise, being physically congested makes you emotionally trapped, too. Mind and body can never exist in isolation. What affects one, also affects the other; and this happens automatically and simultaneously.

Through the mind/body connection, any repressed feelings of wanting and deserving harmony, peace, stability and a simple sense of joy in life are translated into appropriate biochemical responses in the body. This effectively deprives the body's cells of all these positive qualities as well. Cells are not physical machines that have no feelings, no sense of 'I'-ness, no reaction to external changes or threats.

The emotional suffocation caused so much anger and frustration in Mary, that out of fear of not being loved or liked by others, including her parents, she targeted these negative emotions on her own body. Her *toxic* mind translated into a toxic body, and it threatened Mary's very survival. She threatened the health of the cells of her body by keeping her most important thoughts and feelings to herself.

Whatever you keep to yourself out of fear of being criticized or hurt, actually turns into poisons in the body. These poisons are so strong that if you cried and put your tears on a snake's skin, they would burn holes into it. I have actually seen this phenomenon demonstrated when I lived in Africa. Tears of joy, on the other hand, do not have any poison in them.

The constant stress that Mary experienced during dinnertime at her parental home had greatly impaired her digestive functions. Under stress or tension, the blood vessels supplying the organs of the digestive system become tight and restricted, preventing them from digesting even the healthiest of foods. Furthermore, to eat while you are emotionally upset suppresses the secretion of balanced amounts of digestive juices. Whenever you feel angry or upset, your bile flora (beneficial bacteria that keep bile balanced) are altered, which predisposes bile to coagulate. Constant emotional strain leads to stone formation in the bile ducts of the liver and in the gallbladder. The resulting curbed secretion of bile lowers Agni, the digestive fire.

Mary still associates the eating of her meals with the distress she experienced while sitting at her parents' dinner table. Her unconscious attempt to avoid everything that has to do with food and eating, programs her body to do the same. The body cannot properly digest and absorb foods that are eaten in a hurry. This led to the accumulation of large quantities of toxic waste in her small and large intestines. Chronic constipation and the poor absorption of nutrients, including fats, calcium, zinc, magnesium and vitamins, had increasingly depleted and weakened Mary's bone tissue, bone marrow and reproductive functions.

When the reproductive tissue, which maintains the genetic blueprint (DNA) of the cells, is starved of oxygen and nutrients, it is only a matter of time before normal and healthy cells begin to mutate their genes and divide abnormally in order to survive the *famine*. Normally, a host of immune cells, pancreatic enzymes and vitamins break down cancer cells in the body, wherever they appear.

However, most of the digestive enzymes are *used up* quickly when the diet is rich in animal protein, such as beef, pork, poultry, fish, eggs, cheese and milk, as well as sugar-enriched foods. Mary practically lived on these foods. Having suffered from poor digestion and constipation for most of her life, her body was virtually deprived of all of these natural antidotes to cancer cells. Cancers are much more likely to occur among those whose digestive functions are continually disturbed and who are deprived of a sense of emotional well-being, than in those whose digestive system is efficient and who generally have a happy disposition.

The spondylosis of Mary's lower spine signifies the weakening of her internal and external support system; it manifested in direct response to the lack of support and encouragement by her parents. Mary's body slumps forward while she sits, and looks half its size. She looks like a scared child, without confidence and trust. Her posture suggests that she is trying to protect her heart from being hurt again. In addition, her breathing is shallow and insufficient, as if she does not want to be noticed and possibly criticized or disapproved of by her parents. The knees serve as a support system for the entire body. A lifetime of *giving in* and *not standing up for herself and her desires* manifested as the knee problems she developed over the years.

Mary's Successful Remedies

Japanese research has shown that cancer patients whose cancerous tumors went into spontaneous remission, often within less than 24 hours, experienced a profound transformation in their attitude toward themselves before the sudden cure occurred. Mary needed to make several major changes in her life, one of which was to find a new job, even if this meant taking a pay cut. While Mary was still highly susceptible to stressful situations and chaotic noise, the edginess she felt at her school was hardly conducive to the healing process. She also needed to spend more time in nature, walk outside in the sun and on the beach, create paintings, listen to her favorite music, and devote some time to quietness and meditation every day.

In addition to following an Ayurvedic daily routine and diet, Mary began to use a number of cleansing procedures to rid her colon of stagnant, old fecal matter and to purify the blood, liver and connective tissue from accumulated toxins. The liver flush produced thousands of stones that had congested both her liver and gallbladder for at least 15–20 years.

The most important thing for Mary was to become more conscious about everything in her life. This included eating, emotional releases and listening to her body's signals for thirst, hunger and fatigue. She needed to become aware of her needs and desires and begin to fulfill them whenever possible. The most important realization she had to make was that she did not need to do anything that did not please her. Giving herself permission to make mistakes, and not judge herself if she made them, was essential therapy for her.

Mary's friends and family also needed to understand that she was at a very crucial stage of recovery where every positive thought and feeling toward her could serve as a tremendous support system, one that she had never experienced when she was young. She started to improve steadily six months after she adopted about 60 percent of my recommended advice. Today she feels that the *disease* has brought her a deeper understanding of life and has led to an inner awakening she had never experienced before. Free of cancer, Mary continues to improve and grow in confidence and self-acceptance.

Cancer – A Response to Rejection

Jeromy has Hodgkin's disease, which is the most common lymphoma. Lymphomas are malignant neoplasms of lymphoid tissue that vary in growth rate, also known as lymph cancer. Contemporary medicine cannot explain what causes the disease. Hodgkin's disease usually begins in adolescence or between 50 and 70 years of age.

When Jeromy was 22 years old, he noticed two enlarged lymph nodes in his neck. A few days later, he was diagnosed with Hodgkin's disease. In some people, the disease leads to death within a few months, but others have few signs of it for many years. Jeromy was one of them. Being a Kapha type,[60] he has a very athletic and strong body and is naturally endowed with a lot of stamina and physical endurance. His naturally slow metabolic rate can be considered responsible for the slow advancement of the illness.

Jeromy received his first chemotherapy treatment in 1979, soon after he was diagnosed with lymphoma, but there was no detectable improvement in his condition. In 1982, his doctors added multiple radiation treatments to the regular chemotherapy, but these produced severe side effects, including the loss of all body hair and Jeromy's sense of taste. His distress was considerable. Yet, despite numerous traumatic experiences caused by the various treatments during the following 14 years, Jeromy was not willing to give into depression and desperation. His

---

[60] See details about the Ayurvedic body types, *Vata, Pitta* and *Kapha,* in *Timeless Secrets of Health & Rejuvenation.* Of the three types, the *Kapha* type has the strongest bones and muscles.

strong fighting spirit permitted him to continue his work as general manager of a successful business enterprise.

Through the Ayurvedic pulse reading method and eye interpretation (iridology),[61] I was able to determine that from a very early age, Jeromy's digestive functions and lymph drainage had begun to decline rapidly. His liver showed the presence of a large number of intrahepatic stones. As it turned out, Jeromy had gone through a very traumatic experience when he was four years old, although at first he had difficulty remembering it. According to Jeromy, the most emotionally stressful event for him occurred at age 21, when his long-term girlfriend suddenly left him for another man. Exactly one year before she left, he discovered the lymph swellings in his neck. The rejection by his girlfriend was one of the most heart-breaking experiences of his life. Yet this experience merely triggered the memory of an even more painful rejection.

Fighting the Ghost of Memory

Jeromy was born in a developing country with an unstable political situation. When he reached the age of four, his parents sent him to a boarding school in another developing country, for his own safety. Unable to understand the reasons behind this move, he felt that his parents had stopped loving him and no longer wanted him around. All he remembered was the feeling of being cut off from what he considered his lifeline: the closeness with his parents. Although his parents believed that sending him away was in Jeromy's best interest, he suddenly lost the love of the most important people in his life, at an age when he needed it most. His little world had collapsed on this first *black* day in his life, and his body's main functions subsequently began to decline.

Jeromy spent much of his life trying to prove to his parents that he was worthy of their love. He was not aware, however, of his incessant drive to succeed in life. He proudly told me that he never gave up in life and that he refused to allow anything to get him down. One part of him never acknowledged that he was gravely ill. His physical appearance, except for being bald, did not reveal the battle his body was fighting. He invested all of his energy and time in his work, and he was very good at it.

---

[61] Diagnostic methods used to determine any existing imbalances in the body and mind.

To heal himself physically, though, Jeromy needed to become aware of the *rejected child* within him. He had buried that part of himself in the most hidden depths of his subconscious when he was four years old, and a second time when he was a young man and his girlfriend left him. This second rejection amplified the already deep hurt caused by what he considered a *rejection* by his parents.

The body stores all the experiences we have in some kind of invisible *filing cabinet system*. Accordingly, all the feelings of anger we have in life go into one file, sad events are placed into another, and rejections are deposited in yet a different file. These impressions are not recorded and stored according to linear time, but are compiled in terms of similarity. They feed the *ghost of memory* and give it more and more energy. Once a file is *filled up*, even a small event can trigger a devastating eruption and awaken the ghost of memory, thereby giving it a life of its own. This had happened in Jeromy's life.

The abandonment that Jeromy had experienced as a four year old reawakened in his awareness when his girlfriend left him. By ignoring or denying the fact that this rejection had ever taken place, he unconsciously directed his body to create the identical response, which was a cancer in the very system that is responsible for neutralizing and removing harmful waste in the body – the lymphatic system. Unable to get rid of the ghost of memory, which consisted of deep-seated fear and anger from feeling abandoned, Jeromy was also no longer able to free himself of dead, turned-over cells and metabolic waste products.[62] Both his liver and gallbladder had accumulated thousands of gallstones, which nearly suffocated him. His body had no choice but to give physical expression to the cancer that had tortured Jeromy's heart and mind for so many years.

Letting Go of the Need to Fight

All events in life that appear to be negative are, in fact, unique opportunities to become more complete and whole inside, and to move forward in life. Whenever we need to give ourselves more love, time and

---

[62] To be healthy, the human body has to remove over 30 billion dead, worn-out cells and a large amount of metabolic waste every day.

appreciation, but fail to fulfil these essential needs, someone or something in our life will push us in that direction. Feeling rejected by or being disappointed and angry with another person, highlights a lack in taking responsibility for the negative things that happen to us. Blaming oneself or someone else for an unfortunate situation results in the feeling of being a victim and is likely to manifest itself as disease. Moreover, if we cannot understand the accompanying message of our illness, we may even have to face death to appreciate life or living.

Cancer, in an unconventional sense, is a way out of a deadlocked situation that paralyzes the heart of a person. It helps to break down old, rigid patterns of guilt and shame that keep a person imprisoned and bound by a constant sense of low self-worth. The current medical approach does not target this major issue behind cancer, but the *disease process* does, provided it is allowed to take its course. Chemotherapy, radiation and surgery encourage a victim mentality in the patient and are unlikely to heal the root causes of this affliction. Miracle cures happen when the patient frees himself or herself of the need for victimhood and self-attack. When the person's inner sense of well-being and self-acceptance are strong, external problems fail to have a major disruptive impact. Therefore, removing the external problems in life alone may not be sufficient to induce a spontaneous remission; an accompanying inward change is also essential.

Jeromy needed to give himself the love and appreciation he did not feel he was getting from his parents. He also needed to make room for enjoyment and pleasure, taking time for himself, for meditation, for self-reflection, for being in nature and sensing the joy and energy it is able to evoke in us. Cancer cells are cells fighting to survive in a *hostile*, toxic environment. Letting go of the need to fight in life reprograms the DNA of the body, changing its course of warfare and eventual annihilation to one of healthy reproduction. Not needing to fight for their survival gives the cancer cells a chance to be accepted again by the entire *family* of cells in the body. Cancer cells are normal cells that have been rejected by what they consider home. They are deprived of proper nourishment and support. In their desperation to survive, they grab anything they can find to live on, even cellular waste products and toxins. This practically turns them into *outcasts*.

However, just as we want to be loved, cancer cells also need to know that they are loved. Cutting them out of the body through surgery, or destroying them with poisonous drugs or deadly radiation, adds even more violence to the body than it already has to deal with. To live in health and peace, we especially need to be friends with the cells of our body, including cancer cells. The saying, "Love thy enemy", applies to cancer cells just as it does to people. The cause of Jeromy's cancer was a lack of self-appreciation, a feeling of not being loved and wanted, of not feeling worthy or good enough. By waiting for his parents to show him their love, he effectively denied this love to himself. Jeromy came to realize that his disease was, in fact, a great blessing in disguise that could help him rediscover and love himself for the very first time.

If we could only see that what we call *disease* is a perfect representation of our inner world, we would pay more attention to what is going on inside, rather than try to fix something that does not really need fixing. Cancer, as hard as this may be to understand, has profound meaning to it. Its purpose is not to destroy, but to heal what is no longer whole.

Cancer – A Powerful Healer

Many years ago, a woman posted a message on my Curezone.com forum, Ask Andreas Moritz,[63] inquiring how she could support her twin sister who had just been diagnosed with cancer. She mentioned that her sister had rejected her, almost her entire life. She also told me that she was trying her best to be strong for her sister. I replied that being strong was not actually what her sister and she needed at this time.

This is what I wrote to her: "Cancer is most often caused by trying to be strong outwardly while not expressing or acknowledging the weakness and vulnerability that one feels inside. What your sister needs most from you now is to provide her with a mirror of herself. Show her how you really feel inside. Show her your own guilt, your poor self-worth, and your tears of constant rejection, so that she can start seeing these in herself and developing the courage to release the trapped emotions she has locked up inside her body. If you wish her to heal from this, show her all

---

[63] The forum is called *Ask Andreas Moritz* and is found on the health website *Curezone.com* where I have replied to thousands of questions from readers.

your weaknesses, and allow yourself to cry for her and for yourself. It will motivate her to do the same."

I continued explaining that her sister's cancer was merely an unconscious attempt to keep everything trapped inside, including foods, waste matter, resentment, anger, fear, and other negative feelings and emotions. "For this reason," I wrote, "to heal cancer, one must turn inside out and let the world see what one is hiding from (due to a false sense of shame and guilt). Guilt is a completely unjustified and unnecessary emotion because human beings are actually incapable of wrongdoing, although this is nearly impossible to understand when one does not recognize the larger picture of all things.[64] You can actually never cause someone else's problems unless the affected other person is allowing or requesting it (unconsciously) by direct decree of their Higher Self.[65] The guilt (of not loving or caring about her own twin sister) consists of powerful negative energies that started congesting and attacking the cells of her own body. Cancer is her chosen alternative way to break down the guilt in her heart – a way for her to bring to her conscious attention the false subconscious beliefs of past wrongdoing."

During conversations with cancer patients, I often raise the subject of death, which inevitably is something they face. I suggest to them that they cannot really die; nobody can. Physical death is only a tangible, real experience for those who are left behind. It is of little or no relevance for the Self of the person whose body passes away. In fact, there is not even a sense of loss of some kind, only a gain in expansion of joy, wisdom and love. Physical death does not touch the conscious being that beforehand resided in, and expressed itself through, the physical body. A snake that glides out of its old skin is not concerned about a part of its body dying and falling off.

As long as our sense of 'I' remains, which it always will, physical death cannot destroy us. In fact, death is a non-experience and, therefore, an illusion that is real only for those who rely on their physical senses to determine what they believe. When a loved one suddenly disappears from our lives as a result of physical death, we naturally grieve for him or her, are sad, or feel empty inside. Whereas the grief and sadness are real,

---

[64] See my book, *Lifting the Veil of Duality – Your Guide to Living Without Judgment*, to understand how *mistakes* and *wrongdoing* are learned negative concepts and beliefs surrounding experiences that could be immensely beneficial in our lives.
[65] Each person has a Higher Self guiding one's physical existence down to the minutest detail.

the reason for these emotions is not. The vanishing of someone occurs only relative to the observer. Nothing happens at all to the person who *disappears*; he remains who he has always been, only not in a physical body.

I have personally died several times (crossed over to the other side)[66] during bouts of severe illness or trauma. Once during my third bout of malaria in India in the early 1980s, I was clinically dead for a full eight minutes; I consciously experienced death as a birthing process where you become instantly identical with your own inner state of expanded consciousness and unadulterated joy. My father had the same experience, and neither of us had the sensation of dying. In reality, quite the contrary occurred: the intensity of being alive, awake and conscious of everything became so much more heightened, that the sense of dying was as remote as the faraway galaxies. By contrast, being pulled back into the sick physical body was rather like dying. When I buried my mother, it was a day of celebration, just the way she wanted it. Instead of feeling sorry for ourselves when a loved one dies, we can actually choose to honor and celebrate the departed soul by being happy for them. The only sadness and regret you may feel when you die physically is that the loved ones left behind don't share in your incredible joy and expansiveness of being truly free and alive.

Nothing in the self, or of the self, goes anywhere when someone goes through a death experience. "Accordingly," I wrote to this woman, "more important than continuing to live in her physical body is whether she manages to make peace with herself, because she will carry everything with her, except the flesh of the physical body. Whether she is ready to accept and embrace herself as she is, and thereby heal herself from the unconscious act of self-destruction, is completely up to her, and nobody can or should make that decision for her. As hard as it may be to understand, she is responsible for everything that is happening to her. The only thing you can do for her is to show her who *you* are and how *you* feel. This could be just the catalyst she needs in order to go through her own transformation. Telling her what to do is most certainly not what she

---

[66] During one episode of malaria in India, my soul or consciousness departed/detached from my physical body and *rose*, while I was completely aware of what was happening. I experienced no fear of dying and sensed no loss of any kind. I was in a state of incredible clarity that I could know anything if I wanted to. A doctor confirmed that my heart had stopped. I had a similar experience during a fainting spell. My heart stopped for five minutes before I returned to my physical body.

needs. By forgiving and, thus, healing yourself, you can be the best help to her, provided she has it in her to be open and ready to heal herself."

If you have a loved one who has cancer, you can play a very important role in his or her healing process. By opening up your own heart to him and sharing your own fears and perceived weaknesses, you are encouraging him to open up his heart to you as well. Allow the person to shed as many tears as he needs to, and do not try to pacify him and tell him, "It is all going to be okay." Let him have his experience of pain, despair, confusion, loneliness, hopelessness, anger, fear, guilt or shame. Cancer does not actually generate these emotions, but it may bring them up from the subconscious to more conscious levels of feeling and understanding. If the afflicted person knows that he or she can have all these feelings without having to hide them from you or push them right back inside, cancer can become a very powerful means of self-healing. Just staying by your friend's or family member's side without judging or trying to take away his pain will make you a better healer than any doctor could possibly be.

The Power of Resolving Conflict Situations

Unresolved conflict is most likely the starting point of any illness, including cancer. The body always uses the stress response to cope with the traumatizing effect of conflict. According to a study released by the *Journal of Biological Chemistry* on March 12, 2007, the stress hormone epinephrine changes prostate and breast cancer cells in ways that may make them resistant to cell death. The researchers found that epinephrine levels increase sharply in response to stressful situations and can remain continuously elevated during long periods of stress or depression. They discovered that when cancer cells are exposed to epinephrine, a protein called BAD, which causes cell death, becomes inactive. This means that emotional stress may not only trigger or contribute to the development of cancer, but also undermine or reduce the effectiveness of cancer treatments.

The German university professor, Ryke Geerd Hamer, M.D., originator of German New Medicine (GNM), discovered during routine CT scans of over 20,000 cancer patients, that each of them had a lesion in a certain part of the brain that looked like concentric rings on a shooting target or resembled the surface of water after a stone has been dropped into it. This distortion in the brain is known as *HAMER herd*. Dr. Hamer later found that these lesions resulted from a serious, acute-dramatic and isolating conflict-shock-experience in the patient. Whenever the conflict was resolved, the CT image changed; an edema developed, and finally scar tissue formed. Naturally, the cancers would stop growing, become inactive and disappear.

Simply by helping patients to resolve their acute conflicts and to support the body during this healing phase, Dr. Hamer achieved an exceptionally high success rate with his cancer therapy. According to public record, after 4 to 5 years of receiving his simple treatment, 6,000 out of 6,500 patients with mostly advanced cancer were still alive.

When I came across Dr. Hamer's work, I was thrilled because until then I felt basically alone in my life-long beliefs that cancer is a necessary way for the body to deal with an unnatural physical/mental/emotional situation. The first time I wrote about cancer as not being a disease was in the first edition of my book, *Timeless Secrets of Health & Rejuvenation*, back in 1995. Ever since I worked with cancers in 1981, I always told my patients that it wasn't the cancers that required treatment, but that *the whole organism* did. There is new research coming out which actually supports that, and is included in this updated edition of *Cancer Is Not a Disease*.

There is clear evidence that cancer requires a variable number of at least 2 or 3 risk factors to be in place before it can develop and allow the healing to begin. One of the most common of these co-factors is ionizing radiation, from routine x-rays, mammograms, CT scans, etc.

In fact, research shows that up to 75 percent of all cancers are caused by such radiation damage, although at least one other co-factor must be present, too. This can occur without any prior emotional or psychological conflict, and I can attest to that. Likewise, chronic vitamin D deficiency along with 1 or 2 more co-factors, such as a diet packed with trans fats, can also cause cancers such as melanoma. If permitted, the cancer can trigger a strong detox response in the body and disappear, but it may easily occur again if the person continues to avoid sun exposure. I also work with past-life trauma that manifests as serious conflict situations in this life. Without balancing these old accounts, a person may not be helped by the German New Medicine.

However, though I deeply appreciate his work and perspective, Dr. Hamer and I do have our differences. If Dr. Hamer exhibited the mental and physical state of health that his work purports to achieve, I would be tempted to accept all of it. What he eats and his lifestyle choices certainly have impacted his own health. So his idea that food has nothing to do with it doesn't ring true to me. I have been able to help millions of people regain their health through dietary adjustments alone. However, I am still very pleased to see that someone else shares the same or similar perspectives on cancer.

Chemotherapy drugs are known to create new cancers that are far more aggressive and fast-growing than otherwise possible, especially because the underlying causes are still in place. The drugs create so many gallstones in the bile ducts of the liver that, without cleaning them out, the body's immune system and healing capacity are so low that only the strongest people can survive such an ordeal. It's not a miracle when chemo drugs reduce the size of a tumor, and it can never get rid of all cancer cells, which is why in so many cases, the cancers *return*.

Research shows that Transcendental Meditation (TM) practice can tremendously reduce the need and expense of conventional healthcare. One study on elderly patients compared individuals over age 65 who practiced Transcendental Meditation with a control group of peers matched for age, sex and other factors. Researchers discovered that over a five year period, the group practicing meditation paid 70 percent less money to physicians than the control group. This is particularly inspiring because this age group accounts for disproportionately higher medical expenses compared to the population at large. The high cost of caring for the elderly is a major issue for many governments and healthcare insurance companies around the world [Herron, R.E. Cavanaugh, K. Can the Transcendental Meditation Program Reduce the Medical Expenditures of Older People? A Longitudinal Cost Reduction Study in Canada, *Journal of Social Behavior and Personality* 2005, 17: 415-442].

So why is meditation so drastically effective in reducing the need for conventional healthcare, even among the sickest and most vulnerable patients? Could it be that the common perception that our emotional well-being is separate from our physical health is profoundly false?

Cancer Is About 'Not Loving Yourself'

Many cancer patients have devoted their entire lives to helping and supporting others. Their selfless service can be a very noble quality, depending upon the motivation behind it. If they sacrifice and neglect their own well-being to avoid facing any shame, guilt or unworthiness within themselves, they are actually cutting off the very limb they are hanging on to. They are *selflessly* devoted to please others so that, in return, they may be loved and appreciated for their contributions. This, however, serves as an unconscious acknowledgment of *not loving oneself*. This may lock up unresolved issues, fears and feelings of unworthiness in the cellular memory of the organs and tissues in the body.

"Love thy neighbor as thou lovest thyself" is one of the most basic requirements for curing cancer. The true meaning of this phrase is that our love for others depends on the ability to love and appreciate ourselves. In other words, to be able to truly love someone without cords of attachment and possessiveness, one has to fully love and accept oneself with all the flaws, mistakes and inadequacies one may have. The degree to which we are able to care about the well-being of our body, mind and spirit determines the degree to which we are able to care about other people, too. By being critical of ourselves, or disliking the way we look, behave or feel, we close down our heart and feel unworthy and ashamed. To avoid exposing our shadow self (that part of our self we do not like) to others out of fear of rejection, we try to win over the love of others by pleasing them. This way, we assume we can receive the love we are unable to give to ourselves. However, this approach has little to do with love and fails to work in the long term.

Your body always follows the commands given by your mind. Such inner promptings as your thoughts, emotions, feelings, desires, beliefs, drives, likes and dislikes serve as the software with which your cells are programmed on a daily basis. Through the mind/body connection, your cells have no choice but to obey the orders they receive via your subconscious or conscious mind. As DNA research has proved, you can literally alter your DNA's genetic setting and behavior within a matter of a moment. Your DNA listens to every word you utter to yourself, and it feels every emotion you experience. Moreover, it responds to all of them.

You program yourself every second of the day, consciously and unconsciously. If you choose to, you can rewrite the program in any way you want to, provided you are truly self-aware. Once you know who you truly are, you cannot help but love, accept and honor yourself. You can no longer judge yourself for making mistakes in life, for not being perfect, for not always being how others want you to be. Seeing yourself in this light, you send a signal of love to your cells. The bonding effect of love unites differences and keeps everything together in harmony, including the cells of your body. When love, which should not be confused with neediness or attachment, is no longer a daily-experienced reality, the body begins to disintegrate and become sick.

The increase of love is the main purpose of our existence here on Earth. Those who love themselves are also able to love others, and vice versa. They thrive on sharing their full heart with other people, animals and the natural environment. People who accept themselves fully have no real fear of death; when their time comes to die, they leave peacefully without any regrets or remorse in their hearts.

Whenever we close our hearts to ourselves, we become lonely, and the body begins to become weak and diseased. It is known that widows and people who are socially isolated, or who have nobody with whom to share their deepest feelings, are the most prone to developing cancer.

Your body's cells are the most intimate *neighbors* you can have, and they need to feel your love and self-acceptance, to know that they are a part of you and that you care about them. Giving yourself an oil massage, going to sleep on time, eating nutritious foods and engaging in other healthy daily routines are simple, but powerful messages of love that motivate your cells to function in harmony with each other. They are also messages that keep the elimination of toxins flawless and efficient. There is nothing unscientific about this. You can visit a number of hospitals and ask the patients whether they felt good about their life prior to falling ill. The overwhelming response would be "No". Without being a medical researcher, you would have conducted one of the most important research studies anyone could ever do. You would have stumbled over the most common cause of ill health which is *not loving yourself* or, to use a different expression, *not being happy about how your life turned out*. Not being happy or satisfied in life is perhaps the most severe form of emotional stress to which you could possibly subject yourself. It is, in fact, a major risk factor for many diseases, including cancer.

Studies suggest that severe emotional stress can triple the risk of breast cancer. One hundred women who had a breast lump were interviewed before they knew that they had breast cancer. One in two who had the illness had suffered a major traumatic life event, such as bereavement, within the previous five years. The effects of emotional stress or unhappiness can severely impair digestion, elimination and immunity, thereby leading to a dangerously high level of toxicity in the body. Just ridding the body of cancer through *weapons of mass destruction* fails to remove the unresolved emotional pain behind it.

Chapter Four

Body Intelligence in Action

Cancer Cannot Kill You

Cancer, like any other disease, is not a clearly definable phenomenon that suddenly and randomly appears in some part(s) of the body, like mushrooms popping out of the ground. Cancer is rather the result of many crises of toxicity that have, as their common origin, one or more energy-depleting influences. Stimulants, emotional trauma, repressed emotions, an irregular lifestyle, dehydration, nutritional deficiencies, overeating, stress reactions, a lack of deep sleep, the accumulation of heavy metals (especially from amalgam tooth fillings), exposure to chemicals and inadequate sunlight are among the factors that hinder the body in its effort to remove metabolic waste, toxins and 30 billion turned-over cells each day. When these dead cells accumulate in any part of the body, this naturally leads to a number of progressive responses that include irritation, swelling, hardening, inflammation, ulceration and abnormal cell growth. Like every other disease, cancer is but a toxicity crisis. It marks the body's final attempt to rid itself of septic poisons and acidic compounds that have accumulated because the body was not able to properly remove metabolic waste, toxins and decomposing cells.

Cancer always manifests as the result of an already toxic state in the body. It is never the cause of a disease, but rather a reaction to a far advanced, unhealthful physical condition. Treating cancer as if it were the cause of a disease is like cleaning a dirty cooking pot (the toxin-infested body) with muck (the slew of poisons contained in the chemotherapy cocktail). Obviously, using toxic substances to treat a body that is already struggling to survive due to an overload of toxins will never bring about the desired result of a clean, well-functioning body. Of course, you can throw away the pot and thereby solve the problem. But when it comes to preparing a new meal, you will face an even bigger problem: you have nothing to cook your food in. Similarly, by killing the cancer we almost always kill the patient, too; perhaps not right away, but gradually.

Despite huge efforts and expenditures by the medical establishment (for whatever reasons), mortality rates from cancer have not decreased in over 50 years. Although surgery can certainly help neutralize or eliminate a lot of the septic poison kept in check by a tumor mass, and in a good number of cases improve the condition, neither surgery nor the other two main treatment procedures (chemotherapy and radiation) remove the cause(s) of cancer. What happened to Tony Snow can happen to anyone. A cancer patient may return home after a *successful* treatment, relieved and obviously *cured*, but continue to deplete his body's energy and gather toxins as he did before (by eating the same harmful foods and living the same taxing lifestyle). The immune system, already battered by one traumatic intervention, may not make it through a second one. However, if the patient dies, it is not actually the cancer that has killed him, but rather its untreated cause(s). Given the extremely small remission rate for most medically treated cancers (7 percent), the promises made to cancer patients that by destroying their tumors they will also be cured are deceptive, to say the least. Patients are rarely being told what turns a normal, robust cell into a weak, damaged, abnormal cell.

Tumor cells are cells that *panic* due to a lack of food, water, oxygen and space. Survival is their basic genetic instinct, just as it is ours. To survive in such an acidic, unsupportive environment, the defective cells are forced to mutate. They begin devouring everything they can get hold of to sustain themselves, including toxins. They leach more nutrients, such as glucose, magnesium and calcium, from the tissue fluid than they would need to if they were normally growing cells. To produce the same amount of energy as a healthy cell makes, a cancer cell requires 15 times the amount of glucose. Cancer cells need to ferment glucose, which is a very inefficient and wasteful method of producing cellular energy, similar to the burning of fossil fuels on this planet. Their healthier neighboring cells, however, begin to waste away gradually in the process, and eventually an entire organ becomes dysfunctional due to exhaustion, malnutrition or wasting. Cancerous tumors always look for more energy to divide and multiply cells. Sugar is one of their favorite energy-supplying foods. Craving sugar can indicate excessive cell activity, and many people who eat lots of sugar end up growing tumors in their body.

It seems obvious that cancer cells must be responsible for the death of a person; this is the main reason that almost the entire medical approach is geared toward destroying them. However, cancer cells are far from being the culprits, just as blocked arteries are not the real reason for heart disease. In fact, cancer cells help a highly congested body survive a little longer than it would without them. What possible reason could the immune system have to ignore cancer cells that cluster together to form a tumor mass – cells that it could easily destroy? The only reasonable explanation is that these cells are doing a critical job in a body filled with toxic waste.

Nature provides a clear example of this when one considers the function of poisonous mushrooms. A mushroom is the fleshy, spore-bearing fruiting body of a fungus. Would you call such a poisonous mushroom *vicious* or *evil* just because it could kill you if you ate it? No. In fact, those mushrooms in the forest attract and absorb poisons from the soil, water and air. They form an essential part of the ecological system in our natural world. Although the cleansing effect produced by these mushrooms is hardly noticeable, it allows for the healthy growth of the forest and its natural inhabitants. In fact, the survival of the entire planet depends on the existence of mushrooms.

Likewise, cancer cells are not at all vicious; in fact, they serve a similarly good purpose of absorbing some of the toxins in the body that would otherwise kill the person immediately. It is never the primary choice of normal, healthy cells to suddenly become *poisonous* or malignant, but it is the next best choice they have to avoid an immediate catastrophe in the body. If the body dies, it is not because of cancer, but because of the underlying reasons that led up to it.

To continue to do their increasingly difficult job, these tumor cells need to grow, even if it is at the expense of other healthy cells. Without their activity, an organ may suddenly lose its already weakened structure and collapse. Some of the cancer cells may even leave a tumor site and enter the lymph fluid, which carries them to other parts of the body that also suffer an equally high degree of toxicity or acidosis. The spreading of cancer cells is known as metastasis. However, cancer cells are programmed to settle only in the *fertile* ground of high toxicity (acidity), a milieu in which they can survive and continue their unusual rescue mission. They have mutated to be able to live in a toxic, non-oxygenated environment where they help to neutralize at least some of the trapped metabolic waste, such as lactic acid and decomposing cellular debris.

Given these circumstances, it would be a fatal mistake by the immune system to destroy these *estranged* cells that are doing a vital part of the immune system's work. Without the tumor's presence, large amounts of septic poison, resulting from the accumulated corpses of decomposing cells, would perforate the capillary walls, seep into the blood and kill the person within a matter of hours or days. It is important to remember that cancer cells are still the body's cells. If they were no longer needed, one simple command from the DNA would stop them from dividing wildly.

Tumors cannot kill anyone (unless they obstruct a vital pathway). We have already established that cancer cells contain no weapons to destroy anything. In addition, the vast majority of cells in a tumor are not cancerous at all. Cancer cells are unable to form tissues; only healthy cells can. A tumor could not exist without normal cells holding it together. If accounted for, the number of cancer cells contained in a prostate or lung tumor, for example, would be too insignificant to endanger the life of a person.

Tumors act like sponges for the poisons that circulate and accumulate in the blood, lymph and tissue fluids. These poisons are the real cancer, and they continue circulating unless a tumor filters them out. By destroying the tumor, the real cancer remains and keeps circulating until a new tumor is generated (called *recurrence*). By adding poisons in the form of chemotherapy drugs, antibiotics, immune-suppressants, etc., the real cancer (consisting of poisons) continues to spread and becomes ever more obstructive and aggressive. By removing the only outlet for these poisons, which is a tumor, the real cancer now begins to destroy the body. In other words, the treatment and neglecting to remove the real cancer (poisons) from the body are what kill the patient. Cancer cells don't endanger a person's life, but whatever causes them does.

To repeat, cancer cells inside a tumor are harmless; cutting out, burning or poisoning a tumor does not prevent the real cancer from spreading. Unless the real cancer is being addressed by cleansing the body and restoring normal digestive, eliminative functions, the growth of cancer cells continues to play an important role in the body's natural attempt to heal and survive.

The body has to exert a lot more effort to maintain a tumor than to eliminate it. If it were not forced to use cancer growth as one of its last survival tactics, the body would not opt for this final attempt at self-preservation – final, because it could very well fail in its attempt to survive against the odds. As mentioned before, most tumors (about 90–95 percent) appear and disappear completely on their own, without any medical intervention. Millions of people walk around with cancers in their body and will never know they had them. There is no cancer treatment that can even remotely compete with the body's own healing mechanism, which we unfortunately label as *disease*. Cancer is not a disease; it is a very unusual, but apparently highly efficient mechanism of survival, healing and self-protection.

We ought to give the most developed and complex system in the universe – the human body – a little more credit than it has so far received, and trust that it knows perfectly well how to conduct its own affairs, even under the grimmest of circumstances.

The Body's Desperate Attempt to Live

Nobody wants to be attacked by anyone; this also applies to the cells of the body. Cells only go into a defensive mode and turn malignant if they need to ensure their own survival, at least for as long as they can. A spontaneous remission occurs when cells no longer need to defend themselves. Like every other disease, cancer is a toxicity crisis that, when allowed to come to its natural conclusion, will spontaneously relinquish its symptoms.

Of the 30 billion cells that a healthy body turns over each day, at least 1 percent are cancer cells. Does this mean, however, that all of us are destined to develop cancer, the disease? Certainly not. These cancer cells are products of a *programmed mutation* that keep our immune system alert, active and stimulated.

The situation changes, though, when due to constant energy-depleting influences, the body can no longer deal adequately with the continual presence of worn-out, damaged and cancerous cells. The result is a gradual accumulation of congestion in the intercellular fluids. This can affect both the transportation of nutrients to the cells and the elimination of waste from the cells. Consequently, a large number of the corpses of dead cells begin to decompose, leaving behind a mass of degenerate protein fragments. To remove these harmful proteins, the body builds some of them into the basal membranes of the blood vessels and dumps the rest into the lymphatic ducts, which leads to lymphatic blockage. All of this disrupts the body's normal metabolic processes and alienates some groups of cells to such a degree that they become weak and damaged. Out of these cells, a number undergo genetic mutation and turn malignant. A cancerous tumor is born, and the toxicity crisis has reached its peak.

With the correct approaches, a tumor as big as an egg can spontaneously regress and disappear, regardless of whether it is in the brain, the stomach, a breast, or an ovary. The cure begins when the toxicity crisis stops. A toxicity crisis ends when we cease to deplete the body's energy and remove existing toxins from the blood, bile ducts, gastrointestinal tract, lymphatic vessels and tissue fluids. Unless the body has been seriously damaged, it is perfectly capable of taking care of itself. Medical intervention, on the other hand, reduces the possibility of a spontaneous remission to almost zero because of its suppressive and debilitating effects. Only those individuals with a strong physical and mental constitution can survive the treatment and heal themselves.

Most cancers occur after a number of repeated warnings. These may include:

- Headaches that you continually stop with painkillers[67]
- Fatigue that you keep suppressing with a cup of coffee, tea or soda
- Nervousness that you try to control through nicotine

---

[67] Find out what causes pain and what happens when you suppress it in the section, Painkillers—The Beginning of a Vicious Cycle, Chapter Two, of *Timeless Secrets of Health & Rejuvenation*.

- Medicines that you take to ward off unwanted symptoms
- Seasonal head colds that you don't have time to let run their course and pass on their own
- Not giving yourself enough time to relax, laugh, and be still
- Conflicts that you keep avoiding
- Pretending that you are always fine when you are not
- Having a constant need to please others, while feeling unworthy and unloved by them
- Possessing low self-confidence that makes you strive constantly to prove yourself to others
- Rewarding yourself with comfort foods because you feel undeserving

All of these and similar symptoms are serious risk indicators for developing cancer or other illnesses.

There are no fundamental physiological differences between the development of a simple cold and the occurrence of a cancerous tumor. Both are attempts by the body to rid itself of accumulated toxins, but with varied degrees of intensity. Taking medical drugs in an attempt to ward off a head cold or an upper respiratory infection, before giving your body the chance to eliminate the accumulated toxins, has a strongly suffocating effect on the cells of the body and a depressing effect on your self-worth. It coerces the body to keep large amounts of cellular waste products, acidic substances and, possibly, toxic drug chemicals in the tissue fluid (connective tissue) surrounding the cells. By repeatedly undermining the body's efforts to cleanse itself, the cells are increasingly shut off from their supply routes of oxygen and nutrients. This alters their basic metabolism and eventually affects the DNA molecule itself. The bottom line is that you are no longer feeling connected with yourself.

Located in the nucleus of every cell, the DNA makes use of its six billion genes to mastermind and control every single part and function of the body. Without the adequate supply of vital nutrients, the DNA has no choice but to alter its genetic program in order to guarantee the cell's survival. Mutated cells can survive in an environment of toxic waste. Soon they begin to draw nutrients from other surrounding cells. For these nutrient-deprived cells to survive, they also need to subject themselves to genetic mutation, which leads to the spreading or enlargement of the cancer. Cancerous growths are anaerobic, which means that they develop and survive without the use of oxygen.

Nobel Prize winner Dr. Otto Warburg was one of the first scientists to demonstrate the principal difference between a normal cell and a cancer cell. Both derive energy from glucose, but the normal cell utilizes oxygen to combine with the glucose, whereas the cancer cell breaks down glucose without the use of oxygen, yielding only 1/15 the energy per glucose molecule that the normal cell produces. It is very obvious that cancer cells opt for this relatively inefficient and unproductive method of obtaining energy because they no longer have access to oxygen. The capillaries supplying oxygen to a group of cells, or to the connective tissue surrounding them (usually both), may be severely congested with harmful waste material, noxious substances such as food additives and chemicals, excessive proteins, or decomposing cellular debris. Thus, they are unable to deliver enough oxygen and nutrients.

Because their oxygen and nutrient supply is blocked, cancer cells have an insatiable appetite for sugar. This may also explain why people with constant cravings for sugary foods have a higher risk for developing cancer, or why cancer patients often want to eat large amounts of sugar and sweets. The main waste product resulting from the anaerobic breakdown of glucose by cancer cells is lactic acid, which may explain why the body of a cancer patient is so acidic, in contrast to the naturally alkaline body of a healthy person.

To deal with the dangerously high levels of lactic acid and to find another source of energy, the liver reconverts some of the lactic acid into glucose. In doing so, the liver uses 1/5 the energy per glucose molecule that a normal cell can derive from it (glucose), but that's three times the energy a cancer cell will get from it. To help feed the cancer cells, the body even grows new blood vessels, funneling more and more sugar toward them. This means that the more the cancer cells multiply, the less energy is available to the normal cells; hence, the sugar cravings. In a toxic body, the concentrations of both oxygen and energy tend to be very low. This creates an environment where cancer spreads most easily. Unless the toxins and the cancer's food source are eliminated, and oxygen levels are sharply increased, the wasteful metabolism associated with cancer becomes self-sustaining and the cancer spreads further. If death occurs it is not caused by the cancer, though; it is due to the wasting of body tissues and final acidosis.

Genetic mutation is now believed to be the main *cause* of cancer. Yet in truth, it is only an *effect* of cellular famine and nothing more or less than the body's desperate, but often unsuccessful, attempt to live and survive. Something similar occurs in a person's body when he uses antibiotics to fight an infection. Most of the infection-causing bacteria that are being attacked by the antibiotics will be killed, but some of them will survive and reprogram their own genes to become antibiotic-resistant. Nobody really wants to die, and this includes bacteria.

The same law of nature applies to our body cells. **Cancer is the final attempt of the body to live, and not, as most people assume, to die.** Without gene mutation, those cells in the body that live in a toxic, anaerobic environment would simply suffocate and expire. Similar to bacteria that are attacked with antibiotics, many cells, in fact, succumb to the flood of toxins and die, but some manage to adjust to the abnormal changes of their natural environment. These cells know that they will eventually die, too, once their final survival tactics fail to keep the body alive.

To understand cancer and treat it more successfully than we currently do, we may have to radically alter our modern views about it. We may also have to ask what its purpose is in the body and why the immune system fails to stop it from spreading. It is just not good enough to claim that cancer is an autoimmune disease that is out to kill the body. Such a notion (of the body trying to commit suicide) goes against the core principles of physical life. It makes so much more sense to say that cancer is nothing but the body's final attempt to live.

By removing all excessive waste from the gastrointestinal tract and any harmful deposits from the bile ducts, connective tissues, lymph vessels and blood, the cancer cells will have no choice but to die or to reverse their faulty genetic program. Unless they are too damaged, they certainly can become normal, healthy cells again. Those anaerobic cells and seriously damaged cells that cannot make the adjustment to a clean, oxygenated environment may simply die off. By thoroughly cleansing the liver and gallbladder of gallstones and other toxins, the body's digestive power improves considerably, thereby increasing the production of digestive enzymes. Digestive and metabolic enzymes possess very powerful anti-tumor properties. When the body is being decongested through major cleansing and given proper nourishment, these powerful enzymes have easy access to the cells of the body. Permanently damaged cells or tumor particles are easily and quickly neutralized and removed.

Many people in the world cure their own cancers in this fashion. Some are aware of this because their diagnosed tumors went into spontaneous remission without any form of medical treatment, but most will never even know they had cancer because they never received a diagnosis. After passing through a bout of the flu, a week of coughing up bad-smelling phlegm, or a couple of days with a high fever, many people eliminate massive amounts of toxins and, along with them, tumor tissue. Cancer research on gravely ill patients at M.D. Anderson Cancer Center in Houston, Texas revealed a promising treatment to kill cancer cells by giving them a cold; that is, injecting tumors with a cold virus. It may still take a while, though, before researchers discover that catching a few colds can do the same job. Therefore, without interfering with the body's self-repair mechanisms, a person may experience a spontaneous remission of cancer, easily and with relatively minor discomfort.

Prostate Cancer

Risky Treatments

One study found that over three quarters of men diagnosed with prostate cancer or at risk for its development are treated aggressively, even though most prostate cancers are slow-growing and will never pose a threat to a man's life. And many of these aggressive treatments have serious side effects, not the least of which is incontinence and impotence. The study therefore recommended that the wisest course of action is a method of *active surveillance*, where the condition is monitored and only treated if it worsens.

Furthermore, because PSA tests that identify prostate cancer or its risk work by identifying a particular inflammation that can result from a number of other factors, these tests are notoriously unreliable. Doctors screen for prostate cancer by measuring levels of the prostate specific antigen (PSA), a marker of prostate inflammation. Many patients are then told to get prostate biopsies, oftentimes to discover they do not have cancer. It should be noted that these invasive screenings and treatments make patients vulnerable to later infection or complications, not to mention dangerous superbugs increasingly found in hospitals.

And why take the risk? Chances are, the vast majority of these cases will clear up on their own.

There is indeed enough scientific evidence to suggest that most prostate cancers disappear by themselves if left alone. A 1992 Swedish study found that of 223 men who had early prostate cancer but did not receive *any* kind of medical treatment, only 19 died within 10 years of diagnosis. Considering that one-third of men in the EC (European Community) have prostate cancer, but only 1 percent of them die (not necessarily from the cancer), it is very questionable to treat it at all. This is especially the case since research has revealed that treatment of the disease has not decreased mortality rates.

Moreover, survival rates are higher in groups of men whose *treatment* consists merely of watchful waiting, compared with groups undergoing prostate surgery. In the Trans-Urethral Resection Procedure (TURP), a quarter-inch pipe is inserted into the penis, to just below the base of the bladder, and the prostate is then fried with a hot wire loop. Far from being a safe procedure, one study found that a year after undergoing this surgery, 41 percent of the men had to wear diapers because of chronic bladder incontinence, and 88 percent were sexually impotent.

Even the screening procedure for prostate cancer can have serious consequences. According to a number of studies, more men who are screened with the prostate specific antigen (PSA) test die from prostate cancer than those who are not tested. An editorial in the *British Medical Journal* sized up the value of the PSA test with this comment: "At present, the one certainty about PSA testing is that it causes harm." A high enough positive PSA test is typically followed by a prostate biopsy – a painful procedure that can result in bleeding and infection. Evidence suggests that a large number of these biopsies are completely unnecessary. In fact, they may be life-endangering. Each year, 98,000 people die in the U.S. because of medical testing errors, PSA tests included.

Another serious problem with PSA tests is that they are notoriously unreliable. In a 2003 study undertaken by the Memorial Sloan-Kettering Cancer Center in New York City, researchers found that half of the men with PSA levels high enough to be recommended for a biopsy had follow-up tests with normal PSA levels. In fact, doctors at the Fred Hutchinson Cancer Research Center (FHCRC) in Seattle estimated that PSA screening may result in an over-diagnosis rate of more than 40 percent. To make matters worse, a disturbing study finds that fully 15 percent of older men whose PSA readings were considered perfectly normal had prostate cancer – some with relatively advanced tumors. (See References and Links.)

There is a much more reliable test than the PSA. The lesser known Anti-Malignin Antibody Screening (AMAS) blood test is very safe, inexpensive, and more than 95 percent accurate at detecting cancer of any type. Anti-Malignin antibody levels become elevated when any cancer cells are present in the body, and they can be detected several months before other clinical tests might find them. You can learn more about the AMAS test, and the scientific documentation supporting it, at the website http://www.oncolabinc.com/.

If men learned how to avoid a buildup of toxins in the body, prostate cancer could perhaps become the least common and least harmful of all cancers. Aggressive treatment of early prostate cancer is a controversial issue, but it should be controversial for every type of cancer, at whatever stage of development, especially when simple approaches such as cleansing of the organs of elimination, a balanced, decongesting diet and regular exposure to sunlight can provide the body with what it needs to ward off cancer.

There are a few other natural remedies for prostate enlargement that are worth knowing about. Nettle root extract, for example, has been proven more effective than conventional pharmaceuticals for men dealing with prostate enlargement.

Walnuts and pomegranates also contain compounds that help inhibit prostate cancer cells from interacting with testosterone and spreading. Increasing your intake of omega-3 and lowering your cholesterol level through regular exercise and a healthy diet can also be very beneficial.

Another natural remedy is one that is often decried by health professionals, but can be helpful in some ways. In the past I have only written about the negative effects of coffee, but I must admit that this isn't the whole truth. In fact, there are incredible positive benefits, especially in men. Although drinking coffee can cause dehydration and its many serious side effects, for those who still stay hydrated, coffee can be a life saver.

Research conducted by Harvard School of Public Health (HSPH) scientists suggests that coffee (caffeinated or decaffeinated) can reduce your risk of lethal prostate cancer by up to 60 percent, as well as prevent a host of other illnesses, including Parkinson's disease, type 2 diabetes, gallstones, liver cancer and cirrhosis. It has also been demonstrated to help prevent breast cancer. This is because it contains many natural antioxidant compounds that can reduce inflammation and regulate insulin. Green tea has similar effects with less caffeine than the average cup of coffee.

Avoid all dairy products (except unsalted butter). A Harvard study published in 1998 found a 50 percent increase in prostate cancer risk and a near doubling of risk of metastatic prostate cancer among men consuming high amounts of dairy products. The researchers attributed the high cancer risk from dairy consumption to the high total amount of calcium intake. High calcium levels in the body are known to increase the risk of cancer. Another Harvard study, published in October 2001, looked at dairy product intake among 20,885 men and found those consuming the most dairy products had about 32 percent higher risk of developing prostate cancer than men consuming the least.

Excessive calcium intake may cause the following complications:

- Kidney stones
- Arthritic/joint and vascular degeneration
- Calcification of soft tissue
- Hypertension and stroke
- Elevated VLDL cholesterol
- Gastrointestinal disturbances
- Mood and depressive disorders
- Chronic fatigue
- Mineral deficiencies, including magnesium, zinc, iron and phosphorus
- Interference with vitamin D's cancer-protective effects

About Prostate Enlargement

Prescription drugs for an enlarged prostate encourage testosterone-to-estrogen conversion. This can greatly increase cancer risk. Men who take them have even grown female breasts. Also beware of estrogen-mimicking foods, including soy products and others, that both men and women are advised to eat. There are better ways to prevent prostate enlargement. In a study published in the *British Journal of Urology International*, researchers from the University of Chicago reviewed the results of nearly 20 trials that tested Permixon, a commercial extract of saw palmetto. The results were overwhelmingly positive, including improved urine flow, reduction of urinary urgency and pain, improved emptying of the bladder, reduction in size of the prostate gland after two years and significant improvement in quality of life. In one trial, saw palmetto extract produced positive results similar to the drugs, but without the sexual dysfunction that accompanied drug use. Permixon is manufactured in Europe and not yet available in the U.S., but there are other supplements available here that are just as effective. Look for prostate products that contain beta-sitosterol, such as 'Prostate Care' by Healthy Choice Nutritionals, which is even more powerful than saw palmetto.

A Chinese study showed that drinking five cups of green tea daily may slow prostate cancer growth. The study was published online on October 7, 2003 in the *International Journal of Cancer* (Volume 108 Issue 1, pp. 130-135). More recent research (Japan Public Health Center-based Prospective study, 2007) showed that men could cut their risk of developing prostate cancer by half. Other research showed that black tea also has profound benefits, in that it reduces prostate enlargement and prostate cancer in men who drink just five cups a week. Black tea may also prevent prostate cancer.

A powerful remedy consists of drinking the juice of broccoli that has been boiled in 16 to 20 ounces of water. Drink half of the juice on an empty stomach in the morning and the other half in the early evening. Repeat every day until cancer or prostate enlargement is gone. Results should be noticed within a week.

The product 'Healthy Prostate & Ovary' is a blend of Chinese and Vietnamese herbs that are traditionally known to be supportive in promoting the health of ovary, prostate, breast and other organs and tissues. It also supports detoxification and production of energy, and enhances the body's immune response mechanisms. It contains extracts of astragalus (root), water plantain (root), crinum latifolium (leaves), bitter melon (fruit), papaya (leaves), and soursop (leaves). Apparently Vietnamese men and women taking crinum latifolium leaves rarely suffer from ailments of the reproductive system. In the U.S., this product is sold by NutriCology.

If red blotches appear on the penis, massage it with pure aloe vera gel, twice daily. Many prostate problems are due to trapped urinary deposits/crystals in the penis and disappear when removed by the gel. You should notice a clearing of the skin irritation within a few days.

For prostate enlargement, I strongly recommend doing a series of liver flushes and one or several kidney cleanses.[68]

Why Most Cancers Disappear Naturally

Every toxicity crisis, from a complex cancer to a simple head cold, is actually a healing crisis that, when supported by cleansing measures, leads to a swift recovery. However, if interfered with by symptom-suppressive measures, a usually short-lived *recovery* may easily turn into a chronic disease condition. Unfortunately, cancer researchers do not dare or do not care to find a natural cure for cancer; this is not what they are trained and paid for. Even if they did stumble over a natural cure, it would never be made public.

Indeed, there are occasional attempts made by prominent doctors and researchers to publish the success of alternative cancer therapies in medical and scientific journals. These attempts are almost always dismissed as *quackery*, in spite of the incredible successes of many of these so-called *quack* doctors. For example, Dr. Robert Good, President of Sloan Kettering Institute, a teaching hospital for Cornell Medical College, and a three-time Nobel Prize nominee, was unable to publish despite his impeccable track record, simply because what he hoped to publish was *too controversial* and confronted conventional wisdom.[69]

---

[68] For step-by-step instructions, see my book, *The Amazing Liver and Gallbladder Flush.*
[69] Editor's note: While the author was aware of this doctor's work in 2011, no information about this physician was found in the public domain at the time of publishing this book (in 2016).

You may wonder why there aren't any scientific studies on alternative cancer therapies published in medical journals. The answer becomes obvious when you read statements like this one, written in 1978 by an editor of a leading medical journal in response to Dr. Good's request to publish alternative findings: *"Don't you see this is all a fraud?"* You could only imagine the response by the scientific medical community if they were told that many cancers actually vanish without any treatment at all.

One of the most common and over-treated of all cancers is breast cancer. The majority of doctors either don't know or don't inform their patients that one of breast cancer's most common forms, *ductal carcinoma in situ* (DCIS), is rarely invasive, not easily detectable, and essentially has no symptoms. It's not surprising then that DCIS diagnoses skyrocketed only with the advent of diagnostic mammography. DCIS is best *dealt with* through watchful monitoring and lifestyle changes – yet the mere diagnosis of this *threat* is enough to convince unsuspecting women that their only option is costly, aggressive and harmful radiation, chemotherapy, surgery and other conventional cancer *treatments* that can then create problems for the patient that did not previously exist.

Meanwhile, the medical industry refuses to distinguish between truly invasive forms of breast cancer and DCIS, continuing to insist that conventional medicine is *saving lives* through early detection and unnecessary treatment of this generally harmless condition. Unfortunately for the medical establishment, however, it is much more likely that the 96–98 percent 10-year survival rate of DCIS patients is not due to their *expertise*, but simply to the benign nature of DCIS.

Rose Papac, M.D., a professor of oncology at Yale University School of Medicine, once pointed out that there is little opportunity these days to see what happens to cancers if left untreated. "Everyone feels impelled to treat immediately when they see these diseases," says Papac, who has studied cases of spontaneous remissions of cancer. Being stifled with fear, and in some cases being paranoid about finding a quick-acting remedy for the dreaded illness, many people don't give their body the chance to cure itself, but instead choose to destroy what does not need to be destroyed. This may be one of the main reasons why spontaneous remissions only occur in relatively few cancer patients.

On the other hand, numerous researchers have reported over the years that various conditions, such as typhoid fever, coma, menopause, pneumonia, chickenpox and even hemorrhage, can spark spontaneous remissions of cancer. However, official explanations of how these spontaneous remissions relate to the disappearance of the cancer are non-existent. Because they are unexplained phenomena, seemingly having no scientific basis, they are not used for further cancer research. Consequently, the scientific community's interest in discovering the mechanism for how the body cures itself of cancer remains almost non-existent. These *miracle cures* seem to happen most frequently in certain types of malignancies: kidney cancer, melanoma (cancer of the skin), lymphomas (cancers of the lymph) and neuroblastoma (a nerve cell cancer that affects infants).

Considering that most of the body's organs have eliminative functions, it stands to reason that liver, kidney, colon, lung, lymph and skin cancers are more likely to disappear when these major organs and systems of elimination are no longer overloaded with toxins. Likewise, malignant tumors do not develop in a healthy body with intact defense and repair functions. They only thrive in a specific internal environment that encourages and promotes their growth. Cleansing such an environment, by whatever means, can make a tremendous difference with regard to healing cancer.

A toxicity crisis like pneumonia or chickenpox, unless suppressed or combated, removes large amounts of toxins and helps the cells to *breathe* freely again. Fever, sweat, loss of blood, mucus discharge, diarrhea and vomiting are additional outlets for toxins to leave the body. After breaking down and removing the toxins in an unhindered way, the immune system receives a natural and much-needed boost. A renewed immune stimulation based on reduced overall toxicity in the body can be sufficient to do away with a malignant tumor that no longer has a role to play in the survival of the body. The undesirable chickenpox, pneumonia, fever or other such symptoms may actually be *a gift from God* (to use an unscientific expression) that could save a person's life. Refusing to accept the gift could cost the ill person his life.

Many people die unnecessarily because they are prevented from going through all the phases of an illness. Illnesses are nothing other than the body's many attempts to create outlets for trapped poisonous substances. Blocking the exit routes for these poisons, which happens when symptoms are being treated away, can suffocate the body and stop its vital functions. The body has an innate tendency and capacity to heal itself. Medical treatment should be limited to supporting the body in this effort rather than interfering with it. The existing medical model is based on suppression and intervention, not on assistance and support. This principle applies especially to modern vaccination programs and other rarely considered factors.

Chapter Five

Other Major Cancer Risks

Toxic Lives

We are well aware that we live in a world that is more toxic today than ever before. Between fluoride in the water, mercury in dental fillings, BPA in containers, pesticides on our food and our increasingly inactive lifestyles, we also know that this heightened toxicity probably isn't doing our bodies any favor.

Fluoride

Fluoride has long been promoted as a cure for cavities. Yet this potent neurotoxin and industrial pollutant is not as beneficial as five decades of dental propaganda has led us to believe. Americans spend upwards of $50 billion every year on fluoride cavity treatments. A study suggested that the protective layer left on tooth enamel by fluoride is a mere six nanometers thick – that is, 10,000 times thinner than a strand of hair. Whether this negligible amount of fluoride will actually protect enamel is highly doubtful.

What's more, there is absolutely no evidence that fluoride ingestion through water provides any benefit to your teeth. Yet fluoride is a toxin that, once ingested, can cause serious health problems. It is linked to reduced IQ in children and brain damage. Forty percent of American children also show signs of dental fluorosis, which indicates an overexposure to this toxin.

Over time, fluoride can accumulate in the body's tissues and can lead to other serious health issues, such as increased lead absorption, disrupted synthesis of collagen, hyperactivity and/or lethargy, muscle disorders, arthritis, dementia, bone fractures, lowered thyroid function, inhibited formation of antibodies, genetic damage and cell death, disrupted immune system, infertility and even bone cancer. A reverse osmosis system is the most reliable way to remove fluoride from your water.

The real cause of tooth decay is an excess of acids created by the sugar as it is metabolized by bacteria. Interestingly, many cultures that do not practice conventional dental hygiene still do not suffer tooth decay, because they do not consume the vast amounts of sugar that are commonplace in the American diet, where the number one source of calories is high fructose corn syrup.

Chemicals in Our Kitchens and Bathrooms

Researchers have discovered that almost all pregnant women carry numerous chemicals in their bodies, including some that have been banned since the 1970s. Many of these toxins are widely found in products we use daily – in our kitchens, in our bathrooms, in our offices, and to feed and groom ourselves. Through analysis of some 160 different chemicals, scientists detected polychlorinated biphenyls (PCBs), organochlorine pesticides, perfluorinated compounds (PFCs), phenols, polybrominated diphenyl ethers (PBDEs), phthalates, polycyclic aromatic hydrocarbons (PAHs) and perchlorate in the blood and tissues of virtually every woman studied.

Polychlorinated biphenyls (PCBs): This industrial chemical has been responsible for cancer and impaired fetal brain development. Though it has been banned in the U.S. for decades, it continues to pollute the environment.

Organochlorine pesticides: These are mostly insecticides (including DDT) that are common in modern conventional produce and the food supply. In the body, they break down slowly and can accumulate in fatty tissues. They have been linked to neurological damage, birth defects, Parkinson's, respiratory illness, immune system dysfunction, hormone disruption and, of course, cancer.

Perfluorinated compounds (PFCs): These chemicals are used in non-stick cookware. Research has linked them to lower birth weights among newborns, which puts them at risk for developmental problems.

Phenols: These are found in many personal care products and household detergents. They can damage the heart, lungs, liver, kidneys and eyes, as well as disrupt your endocrine system.

Polybrominated diphenyl ethers (PBDEs): These are flame retardants used in TVs, computers, sofas and other things you use around the house. They disrupt hormone release and can also negatively impact learning and memory.

Phthalates: These endocrine disrupters are found in many vinyl floors, detergents, some plastics, personal care products such as soap, deodorant and hair spray, plastic bags and food packaging, toys, and even blood storage bags and intravenous medical tubing.

Polycyclic aromatic hydrocarbons (PAHs): These potent carcinogens are released when substances such as gasoline or garbage are burned.

Perchlorates: These salts derived from perchloric acid are used in defense and pyrotechnics industries. Because they are water soluble, many areas of the world are experiencing widespread environmental contamination. They can disrupt hormone production and thyroid function, as well as trigger developmental problems in fetuses.

Bisphenol-A (BPA): This is an endocrine disrupter that can especially damage developing fetuses. Found in many plastics, it is increasingly coming to the forefront of consumer consciousness as being a dangerous toxin. In recent years, companies have begun to provide BPA-free alternatives in response to consumer demand for safer products. Natural health advocates have also been warning about **styrene**, a chemical additive used in products such as disposable coffee cups and foam take-out containers. The U.S. Department of Health and Human Services (HHS) has long been pressured by the chemical industry to ignore the risks posed by these toxins, and only recently faced the music and added them to its list of known carcinogens.[70]

As can be expected, the chemical industry quickly denounced this development, claiming that exposure to BPAs and styrene poses no significant danger. Even the American Cancer Society has not urged the public to stop using canned foods, plastic bottles and containers or

---

[70] http://ntp.niehs.nih.gov/go/roc12

foam food packaging, though they are riddled with these dangerous carcinogens.[71]

The extent to which these various chemicals have permeated the environment is truly alarming. One study performed by the Environmental Working Group examined blood samples from newborn babies and found on average 287 toxins (including mercury, pesticides and PFCs) in their systems. Fetuses, infants and children are especially vulnerable, which has contributed to the rising rates of birth defects, asthma, serious allergies and neuro-developmental disorders.

Sodium Benzoate

Another particularly dangerous chemical that is found virtually everywhere these days is sodium benzoate. Used as a preservative in many foods, it is a carcinogen that promotes cancer and kills healthy cells. While low levels of benzoic acid are naturally found in many fruits, this chemical version is synthesized in a lab from a reaction of benzoic acid and sodium hydroxide.

Unfortunately, it also happens to be one of the cheapest and most effective mold inhibitors on the market and, true to form, the FDA insists that the levels used in preserving food are *safe*. Shockingly, this toxin can be found even in foods that are labeled *natural*. It is particularly dangerous when combined with vitamin C or E, as this results in the creation of benzene, a known cancer-causing agent. It chokes out nutrients and deprives cell mitochondria of oxygen. If allowed to congest tissues, it can cause Parkinson's disease, neurological degeneration and premature aging. No amount of sodium benzoate is truly safe, and a gradual accumulation of this toxin can greatly increase one's risk of developing cancer.

Mercury

A study by the U.S. Geological Survey found mercury in every fish sample from across the United States. Increasing mercury concentrations are not only being found in fish, but are also appearing

---

[71] Editor's note: This may have changed or is in the process of changing, as of 2016.

in other species that consume them, even in remote areas of the planet. According to the CDCP, eating fish just two or more times a week has been found to raise mercury levels more than seven times beyond those who don't eat fish as often.

People can also be exposed to mercury through dental fillings and vaccinations. Mercury is a potent neurotoxin that is simply not safe, and should be avoided as much as possible. Infants and fetuses are particularly vulnerable, and when exposed to it can develop mental retardation, cerebral palsy, deafness and blindness. As summed up by Mayo Clinic pediatric neurologist Dr. Suresh Kotagal, "There is really no place for mercury in children."

Alcohol, Aluminum and Breast Cancer

Breast cancer risk increases in response to excessive estrogen production, because increased estrogen in the body can increase free iron levels. Iron is normally bound within the blood (called transferrin) and cells (ferritin) – however, increased estrogens in the body that result from consumption of soy, certain medications, various plastics and other toxins, as well as that naturally produced by fat cells, can release iron from its bound form, causing serious inflammation and free radical damage.

Alcohol consumption and aluminum absorption (from antiperspirants, vaccines, food containers, etc.) can also increase free iron levels. One study found that even moderate alcohol consumption of 3–6 drinks a week increased breast cancer risk by 15 percent. Heavy drinkers who consumed 30 or more drinks per week increased their risk by 50 percent. One of the study's researchers, James Garbutt, M.D., of the University of North Carolina in Chapel Hill, said, "What is important about this study is that it followed women over time and confirmed and extended the link between alcohol consumption and breast cancer. Given that many women drink alcohol in our society, this is an important observation and one that women should be aware of."

A Sedentary Life Can Kill

The sedentary lifestyle is more common than ever in the West. It's not unusual for people to spend their days sitting at a desk and their nights sitting in front of a television, instead of engaging in meaningful physical activity. Health experts are increasingly warning that an immobile life can be just as dangerous to us as cigarettes. As New York St. Luke's-Roosevelt Hospital Center cardiologist Dr. David Coven said, "Smoking certainly is a major cardiovascular risk factor and sitting can be equivalent."

Research consistently links chronic inactivity with myriad health issues, such as heart disease, obesity, diabetes, cancer and premature death. However, even moderate exercise (such as 30 minutes of brisk walking) can work wonders in combating this issue. It can help you keep your weight under control, as well as relieve stress, anxiety and depression.

And this problem isn't limited to working adults – children are also not getting enough exercise, and are therefore facing many of its consequences earlier in life than previous generations. Between larger homework loads, video games and too much TV time, kids are gaining weight earlier and setting themselves up for a lifetime of health problems.

Any amount of activity is better than nothing. Go for a walk, ride a bike to work, or swim in a pool. Don't let the sedentary lifestyle of our modern world lead to health problems that could be easily prevented.

Vaccinations – Ticking Time Bombs?

In addition to suppressing vulnerable immune systems, vaccines are well-known to inflict the body with a cocktail of toxic substances such as aluminum. Indeed, the amount of aluminum exposure that results from these vaccines, including anthrax, hepatitis and tetanus vaccines, well exceeds even the FDA's often questionable standards. One study found that newborns receive aluminum doses that are 20 times the safety limit (5 mg/kg/day), and by six months of age that dose rose to 50 times the limit.

Aluminum accumulates in tissues and can displace iron from its protective proteins. This, in turn, dramatically increases the risk of breast cancer as well as other iron-related diseases, such as liver degeneration, neurodegenerative disease, diabetes, heart failure and atherosclerosis.

Another vaccine campaign against 'swine flu' (H1N1) has backfired, as 12 different countries claim that this vaccine causes narcolepsy, an extreme chronic fatigue disorder whose sufferers can fall asleep suddenly and without warning. Finland, for example, reported that children vaccinated for H1N1 were 900 percent more likely to develop narcolepsy than non-vaccinated children. Yet the World Health Organization (WHO) continues to hype these questionably beneficial (but nonetheless highly profitable for Big Pharma) vaccines, including GlaxoSmithKline's Pandemrix. Moreover, this is hardly the first time the WHO has manufactured *pandemics* in order to stoke fear and generate huge cash flow for drug companies. GSK, for example, raked in upwards of $1.4 billion as a result of the 2010 *swine flu* scare.

The suppression of children's diseases through unnatural immunization programs can put the children at high risk for eventually developing cancer. Chickenpox, measles and other natural self-immunization programs (wrongly called *childhood diseases*) help endow a child's immune system with the ability to counteract potential disease-causing agents more efficiently and without having to go through a major toxicity crisis.

With more than 550,000 annual cancer deaths in the United States alone, the justification for mandatory immunization programs in this country is highly questionable. The standard approach to establishing immunity, which is unproved and unscientific, may undermine and override the body's own far superior programs of self-immunization. The body gains natural immunity through exposure to pathogens and, occasionally, a healing crisis, which naturally eliminates cancer-producing toxins. Vaccines, on the other hand, suppress natural immunity and replace it with fake immunity.

By design, all vaccines depress immune functions. Taken together, the cocktail of toxic chemicals and metals, along with the viruses and the foreign DNA/RNA from animal tissues in the vaccines, impair the immune system. Many of the vaccines contain neurotoxins and actual carcinogens. This is what is being pumped into a healthy body:

aluminum, thimerosal, formaldehyde, carbolic acid (phenol), the antibiotics neomycin, streptomycin and a variety of other drugs, the solvent acetone, glycerin (which can cause death), sodium hydroxide, sorbitol, hydrolyzed gelatin, benzethonium chloride, methylparaben and other chemicals known or suspected of causing cancer [Conscious Rasta Report vol. 3, no. 9: *Epidemic*].

The vaccines especially reduce polymorphonuclear neutrophils (PMNs),[72] lymphocyte viability, neutrophil hyper-segmentation and white cell count – all essential factors for maintaining a normal, healthy immune system and, thus, keeping track of daily cell mutations. It is insane to sacrifice naturally acquired immunity with a state of temporary, incomplete immunity against one or several diseases, including innocuous childhood diseases.

Vaccines also rob the body of vital immune-enhancing nutrients, like vitamin C, vitamin A and zinc, which are essential to build or have a strong immune system. The poisons contained in vaccines don't allow a young child to develop a healthy immune system, making it susceptible to many illnesses in the future. So are there safe vaccines?

"The only safe vaccine is the one that is never used." This statement is from James Shannon, former Director of the National Institutes of Health. Children are the most vulnerable because their immune systems are practically defenseless against the poisons in the vaccines. They have a lot against them since their mothers are *not* passing on immunity to them in the breast milk (because they themselves were vaccinated and no longer produce antibodies). Children die at a rate eight times faster than normal after a DPT shot. James R. Shannon of NIH understood this when he said: "No vaccination can be proven safe before it is given to children."

Former U.S. President George W. Bush once famously said: "I haven't got a flu shot and I don't intend to." Does even Mr. Bush know something the rest of us don't?

Researchers at the University of Chicago Medical Center say that 98 million Americans who took polio shots in the 1950s and 1960s may get a deadly brain cancer from the inoculations. Dr. Jonas Salk, revered as the pharmacological god who invented the polio vaccine, has since been

---

[72] PMNs are our body's defenses against pathogenic bacteria and viruses.

exposed as a medical criminal who performed illegal experiments on mental patients in his pursuit of this profitable vaccine.

Another vaccine *un-success* story: In mid-2011, the U.K. scrapped pneumonia vaccines after finally facing the music that they don't work.

Another leading virologist and inventor of 8 of the 14 routinely recommended vaccinations, longtime Merck employee Maurice Ralph Hilleman, admitted that vaccines pose a risk for cancer and other viruses, including HIV and AIDS.

Ultimately, whether manufactured vaccines directly or indirectly cause cancer is irrelevant. In neither case are they truly beneficial. It is important to know that conventional immunization programs can prevent the body from developing a potentially life-saving healing crisis. All these different vaccines administered to millions of children and adults every year profoundly affect the body's ability to heal itself. The injected vaccines contain large protein molecules that clog up the lymphatic vessels and lymph nodes, and cause metabolic waste products and turned-over, dead cells to become trapped in the tissue fluids. The same effect undermines the efficacy of immune cells circulating in the lymph.

The Vaccine-Autism Link Is Now Clear

Whether vaccines can so severely damage the body that it causes autism is still being discussed. However, a study entitled "Scientists fear MMR link to autism" found measles virus in 70 out of 82 autistic children tested. Most importantly, none of them were wild measles strains. They were all strains from *safe* MMR (measles, mumps and rubella) vaccinations. The study seems to confirm the findings of British doctor Andrew Wakefield, who caused a firestorm in 1998 by suggesting a possible link. Existence of the measles virus in the gastrointestinal tracts of so many of these children diagnosed with regressive autism certainly supports Dr. Wakefield's controversial assertion that this kind of inflammation in the GI tract can cause autism in children, who described this bowel disease as autism enterocolitis.

Indeed, Dr. Wakefield's findings were highly inconvenient for the pharmaceutical industry, and they responded in kind with allegations of fabricating study data. "The Department of Health and some of the media wanted to dismiss our research as insignificant. The excuse was that no one else had the same findings as us. What they didn't say is that no one else had looked."

The industry's track record with vaccines is notoriously dishonest. For example, these vaccines are rarely scientifically tested using proper placebos such as saline solution. Instead they use other vaccines as their so-called *placebo* in an effort to hide the harmful effects of the vaccines being tested. The ingredients in these vaccines are nothing short of terrifying, including other viruses not listed on the label, DNA from diseased animals, mercury, aluminum and formaldehyde. What's worse, by being directly injected into the body, vaccines bypass the digestive systems that would filter some of the poisons and lessen their toxic impact.

The mainstream media is too conflicted by the heavy funding it receives from Big Pharma to report honestly on these issues, and even governments have an interest in keeping this information hushed in order to avoid the trillions of dollars in damages that would need to be paid to vaccine victims as a result of policies that underwrite their risks. The mere existence of the U.S. Vaccine Injury Compensation Trust Fund, which has paid out tens of millions in reparations to vaccine victims, is basically an admission on the part of the government that vaccines are indeed dangerous – whatever the industry might say. Bottom line: vaccines are a dangerous scheme whose only real intent is accumulation of profits for drug companies. Don't trust them in the least.

For more detailed information about what vaccines can do to the human body and the health of the population, see my book, *Vaccine-nation: Poisoning the Population, One Shot at Time.*

To remove harmful chemicals and toxic metals from the body, I recommend using the zeolite product, Natural Cellular Defense from Waiora, MMS and marine phytoplankton.

The most pressing question we need to ask ourselves is why do the most highly vaccinated countries in the world also have the highest rates of cancer? Those who deny that there exists a cause-effect relationship between known carcinogenic-containing vaccines and cancer must have a vested financial interest in keeping the population from discovering what makes them sick.

Wearing a Bra Impairs Lymph Drainage

There are other factors that affect proper lymph drainage and circulation. Regularly wearing a bra impairs the proper flow of lymph and may greatly increase the chance of developing breast cancer. Several other studies confirm this link. In 1991, C. Hsieh and D. Trichopoulos studied breast size and left/right handedness as risk factors for breast cancer. They noted in their findings that premenopausal women who do not wear a bra had less than half the risk of breast cancer than did their bra-wearing peers [*European Journal of Cancer*, 1991; 27(2):131-5].

Another study published in *Chronobiology International* in 2000 found that wearing a bra decreased melatonin production and increased the core body temperature. Melatonin is a powerful antioxidant and hormone that promotes good sleep, fights aging, boosts the immune system and slows the growth of certain types of cancer, including breast cancer.

The most comprehensive studies on this subject were performed by the husband and wife team of applied medical anthropologists, Sydney Ross Singer and Soma Grismaijer, authors of "Dressed to Kill: The Link Between Breast Cancer and Bras". They found that the Maoris, the indigenous people of New Zealand who integrated into Western culture and began to wear bras, had the same rates of breast cancer as their Western peers. On the other hand, the non-Westernized aboriginals of Australia, interestingly, had practically no breast cancer. The same was true for Westernized Japanese, Fijians and women from other cultures who converted to the practice of bra wearing; when they did so, their rates of breast cancer soared.

In the early 1990s, Singer and Grismaijer studied the bra-wearing habits of 4,500 women in five cities across the U.S. They found that 3 out of 4 women who wore their bras 24 hours per day developed breast cancer. Among those who wore their bras more than 12 hours per day but not to bed, 1 out of 7 developed breast cancer. This is a slightly higher cancer rate than the standard female population of 1 in 8. By comparison, merely 1 out of 152 women who wore their bras less than 12 hours per day had breast cancer, and only 1 out of 168 women who rarely or never wore bras developed cancer of the breast. In other words, women who wore a bra 24 hours per day were 125 times more likely to develop breast cancer than women who rarely or never wore a bra. Interestingly, women who chose to go braless had the same breast cancer rates as men did!

Early Puberty and Breast Cancer

Girls in the United States and other *modern* countries are reaching puberty at very early ages, which has been shown to increase their risk of breast cancer. Just decades ago, biological signs of female puberty – menstruation, breast development and growth of pubic and underarm hair – typically occurred around 13 years of age or older. And in the early 20th century it was more like age 16 or 17. Today, girls as young as eight are increasingly showing these signs. Apparently, African-American girls are particularly vulnerable to early puberty. Girls as young as five or six now go through precocious puberty (also known as early sexual development). Early puberty exposes girls to more estrogen – a major risk for hormone-related breast cancers. According to data published by biologist Sandra Steingraber, girls who have their first menstrual period before age 12 have a 50 percent higher risk of developing breast cancer than those who begin menstruating at age 16. "For every year we could delay a girl's first menstrual period," she says, "we could prevent thousands of breast cancers."

Potential causes for this trend include rising childhood obesity rates and inactivity, cow's milk- and soy-infant formulas, bovine growth hormone commonly found in cow's milk, hormones and antibiotics in beef, and non-fermented soy products, such as soy milk and tofu, which mimic estrogens. Soy's estrogenic effects exceed those produced by the birth control pill by 4 to 5 times. (*Also see the section* Soy – A Carcinogen for Humans *below.*) Other causes may include bisphenol A and phthalates (found in many plastics, such as baby containers, water bottles and the inner lining of soda cans), other man-made chemicals that affect hormonal balance (such as those found in cosmetics, toothpastes, shampoos and hair dyes), stress at home and at school, and excessive TV viewing and media use.

Introducing infants to solid food prematurely can also increase their chances of becoming obese, a key risk factor for developing cancer down the road. In a study published in *Pediatrics,* researchers conclude that formula-fed babies who started solid foods before four months are 600 percent more likely to be obese by age three than children who began solid foods later.

This study also found a striking nutritional difference between human breast milk and conventional infant formula, the latter of which is often loaded with refined sugar and genetically modified ingredients, and which also increases the child's likelihood of obesity by up to 20 percent. Choosing to breastfeed is not only better nutrition, but also natural antibodies found in a mother's breast milk can help infants fight infection in this vulnerable period of their lives.

New Fluorescent Light Bulbs Cause Cancer

If you have replaced your old incandescent light bulbs with compact fluorescent lamps (CFLs) in an effort to save money and live eco-friendly, be aware that a German study found that these light bulbs contain poisonous carcinogens that can cause cancer. These include phenol, a mildly acidic toxin obtained from coal tar, naphthalene, a volatile white crystalline compound also produced by the distillation of coal tar, and styrene, an unsaturated liquid hydrocarbon. These toxins can produce electrical smog that can negatively affect human health.

The researchers therefore suggested using the bulbs as little as possible, in good ventilation, and especially to keep them away from the head. Like other artificial light sources, they can also disrupt the body's melatonin production, known to be another factor in the development of cancer, as well as cause migraines. Further, if these bulbs are broken or cracked, they can release toxic dust that contains mercury.

Poisoned By Sugar

It should come as no surprise that diabetes is a key contributor to the development of cancer. In fact, the journal *Diabetes Care* reported in

May 2011 that the disease can nearly double a person's risk of developing certain kinds of cancers.

Other research suggests that an average American child consumes upwards of four pounds of sugar *every week*. This shocking news is largely a result of the U.S.'s love affair with junk foods, processed meals and sugary soft drinks. And this lifestyle epidemic is creating new cases of diabetes at an alarming rate.

It goes without saying, then, that prevention of diabetes is important in preventing cancer. Interestingly enough, the *miracle drug* mentioned earlier in this book – vitamin D – is one way to do just that. Researchers working at Tufts Medical Center in Boston discovered that 2,000 IU per day of vitamin D given for 12 weeks significantly improved pancreatic function for overweight adults with pre-diabetes. For every 5 ng/ml increase in vitamin D levels, the risk of developing diabetes dropped by 8 percent.

Furthermore, if you have cancer, it is important that you stop eating refined, processed sugar immediately. Refined sugars contain none of the nutrients necessary for the assimilation of the sugar that is ingested. Consuming these sugars drains the body's stores of nutrients and energy (if any are still present), leaving less (or none) for other tasks. Cancer never kills a person; the wasting of organ tissue does. Cancer and wasting go hand in hand. Eating sugar feeds cancer cells while it starves healthy cells.

Natural sweeteners like stevia and Xylitol do not rob the body of its nutrient and energy resources. Stevia has zero calories, so it cannot serve as food for cancer cells. Xylitol contains calories (about 40% less than sugar), but its slow release into the blood gives it a much lower glycemic index. If taken in moderation, Xylitol is unlikely to pose a problem. However, refined carbohydrates, such as pasta, white bread, pastries and cakes, are quickly broken down into glucose and act just as refined sugar does. (Note: complex carbohydrates, as found in whole grains and washed white Basmati rice, are fine, but avoid most other types of polished white rice due to their depleted nutritional value.)

Obviously, sugar-rich foods and beverages, such as chocolate, ice cream and soda, should be avoided. Lymph-congesting dairy products like milk, yogurt and cheese also have no place in the diet of someone seeking to recover from cancer, although unsalted butter is safe. Again, cancer cells are normal body cells that have become anaerobic – they have been forced to stop functioning on oxygen, and gain sustenance from sugars such as lactose and glucose. Therefore, avoiding foods that contain them is just common sense.

Soy – A Carcinogen For Humans?

The food industry, which operates in a similar way to the pharmaceutical industry, has successfully convinced the population that soy is a health food. Soy has even been praised as the miracle food that will save the world from starvation. Soy supporters claim it can provide an ideal source of protein, lower cholesterol, protect against cancer and heart disease, alleviate menopause symptoms and prevent osteoporosis. However, when you look beyond the propaganda, the facts about soy paint a very different picture. In spite of soy's impressive nutritional content, soy products are biologically useless to the body, for reasons explained below. Today, soy is used in thousands of different food products, which has led to a massive escalation of disease in both developed and underdeveloped countries.

Soy contains a number of compounds that interfere with vitamin and mineral absorption. For example, the phytic acid found in soy leads to deficiencies of calcium, magnesium, copper, molybdenum, iron, manganese and especially zinc in the GI tract, as well as vitamins E, K, D and B12. It has also been estimated that a mere 100 grams of soy protein provides the estrogen equivalent of one birth control pill. It also contains haemaglutinin, a clot-promoting substance that can create a higher risk of clogged arteries and stroke.

Given the fact that soybeans are grown on farms that use toxic, cancer-producing pesticides and herbicides – and many are from genetically engineered plants[73] – increasing evidence suggests soy is a major health hazard. What's more, typical soy processing involves acid-washing the beans in aluminum tanks, thereby leaching high levels of toxic aluminum into the product. With a few exceptions, such as miso, tempeh and other carefully fermented soy products, soy is not suitable for human consumption. Eating soy, soy milk and regular tofu increases risks of serious health conditions. In addition, soy is a common food

---

[73] In the U.S., 80% of all soy beans come from genetically engineered soy plants.

allergen. Numerous studies have found that soy products are responsible for:

- Increasing the risk of breast cancer in women, brain damage in both men and women, and abnormalities in infants
- Contributing to thyroid disorders, especially in women
- Promoting kidney stones (because of excessively high levels of oxalates that combine with calcium in the kidneys)
- Weakening the immune system
- Causing severe, potentially fatal food allergies
- Accelerating brain weight loss in aging users

Soy products contain:

- Phytoestrogens (isoflavones) genistein and daidzein, which mimic and sometimes block the hormone estrogen
- Phytic acids, which reduce the absorption of many vitamins and minerals, including calcium, magnesium, iron and zinc, thereby causing mineral deficiencies
- *Antinutrients* or enzyme inhibitors that inhibit enzymes needed for protein digestion and amino acid uptake
- Haemagglutin, which causes red blood cells to clump together and inhibits oxygen uptake and growth
- Trypsin inhibitors that can cause pancreatic enlargement and, eventually, cancer

Phytoestrogens are potent anti-thyroid agents, which are present in vast quantities in soy. Infants exclusively fed on a soy-based formula have 13,000 to 22,000 times more estrogen compounds in their blood than babies fed a milk-based formula. This would be the estrogenic equivalent of at least five birth control pills per day. For this reason, premature development of girls (early puberty) has been linked to the use of soy formula, as has the underdevelopment of males. Infant soy formula and soy milk have been linked to autoimmune-thyroid disease, and also to death.

In 2007, two parents were convicted of murder and given life sentences in prison for starving their 6-week old baby to death by feeding it with soy milk and apple juice. Soy experts are again calling for clear and proper warning labels on all soy milk products, following this and several other babies' hospitalizations or deaths under similar circumstances.

Only soy products, such as miso, tempeh and natto, provide soy nutrients that can easily be absorbed and utilized by the body. To make soy products nutritious and healthy, they must be carefully fermented, according to the traditional preparation methods used in Japan. Typically, soy must be fermented for at least two summers, ideally for 5–6 years, before it becomes beneficial for the body.

A study of 700 elderly Indonesians showed that properly fermented soy, such as tempeh, miso, natto and soybean sprouts (not genetically modified), helped improve memory, particularly in participants over 68 years of age. The study also affirms that high tofu consumption (at least once a day) was associated with diminished memory, particularly among those over age 68. The study was published in *Dementia and Geriatric Cognitive Disorders*, June 27, 2008; 26(1):50-57. If you want to avoid dementia, avoid all processed soy milks, tofu, soy burgers, soy ice cream, soy cheese and all other soy-containing junk foods.

In spite of the documented scientific evidence that shows non-fermented soy to be carcinogenic and also cause DNA and chromosome damage, the multi-billion dollar soy industry has managed to turn this generally worthless food into one of the most widely used *nutritious foods* of all times. In a written statement, a spokesman for Protein Technologies, Inc. said that they had "... teams of lawyers to crush dissenters, could buy scientists to give evidence, owned television channels and newspapers, could divert medical schools and could even influence governments ..."

Lipid specialist and nutritionist, Mary Enig, Ph.D., explains one of the main reasons behind the soy revolution. She says, "The reason there's so much soy in America is because they (the soy industry) started to plant soy to extract the oil from it and soy oil became a very large industry. Once they had as much oil as they did in the food supply, they had a lot of soy protein residue left over, and since they can't feed it to animals, except in small amounts, they had to find another market." In other words, the human population became an effective garbage dumpster for the food industry, while making the medical industry increasingly profitable as a result of treating the many soy-caused illnesses. This is not unlike the pouring of the poison fluoride – a hazardous waste product from aluminum plants – into the municipal water system to *save* children from developing bad teeth. To dispose of fluoride in any other way would be extremely costly.

Animals that naturally ferment their foods in their stomach before absorbing them can break down the enzyme inhibitors that soy contains and, in turn, make use of the proteins. Not all foods that grow on this planet are beneficial for human beings. In fact, animals inhabited the planet long before humans did; therefore, most foods were actually designed to feed and sustain the animal kingdom. The recent addition of large amounts of non-fermented soy in the human food chain has already had disastrous consequences on the health of millions of people and will continue to do so unless the masses educate themselves about the deceptive practices of the food industry and government agencies that are supposed to protect us from harm.

Why French Fries Can Cause Cancer

French fries and other fried, baked or roasted carbohydrate-rich foods contain the chemical acrylamide, which has been implicated to be a human carcinogen. Women who eat approximately one portion of chips a day may drastically double their risk of ovarian and endometrial cancer (cancer of the uterus lining), according to a study published in the journal *Cancer Epidemiology, Biomarkers & Prevention*.

Acrylamide was accidentally discovered in foods in April 2002 by scientists in Sweden when they found large amounts of the chemical in potato chips, French fries and bread that had been heated at temperatures above 120 degrees centigrade (250 degrees Fahrenheit). Prior to that, acrylamide was believed solely to be an industrial chemical. The production of acrylamide in the heating process was shown to be clearly temperature-dependent. Over-cooking and microwaving foods may also produce large amounts of acrylamide. Boiled and unheated foods don't contain acrylamide.

In this study, researchers examined data gathered by the Netherlands Cohort study on diet and cancer occurrence among 62,573 women. The women who ingested the most acrylamide, 40.2 micrograms per day, had a 29 percent higher risk of endometrial cancer and a 78 percent higher risk of ovarian cancer. Surprisingly, women who had never smoked had a 99 percent higher risk of endometrial cancer and a 122 percent higher risk of ovarian cancer among those with the highest acrylamide intake.

The March 15, 2005 issue of the *Journal of the American Medical Association (JAMA)* contained an article entitled "Acrylamide Intake and Breast Cancer Risk in Swedish Women," written by Lorelei A. Mucci, ScD, MPH. The study cohort consisted of 43,404 Swedish women in the Women's Lifestyle and Health Cohort. The women's greatest single source of acrylamide was from coffee (54% of intake), fried potatoes (12% of intake) and crisp bread (9% of intake).

Electric Light and Cancer

As explained before, a strong link exists between low levels of the hormone melatonin and cancer. Melatonin protects genetic material from mutation, according to Russell Reiter, professor of cellular and structural biology at the University of Texas. "Night light suppresses the body's production of melatonin and thus can increase the risk of cancer-related mutations," he told a gathering in London. Scott Davis, chairman of the department of epidemiology at the University of Washington, stated that "while the link between light at night and cancer may seem like a stretch on the surface, there is an underlying biological basis for it." Both Davis and Reiter have been studying how night lighting affects the production of female hormones which, in turn, can affect the risk of breast cancer. "We have found a relationship between light at night and night-shift work to breast cancer risk," Davis said. "The studies indicate that night work disrupts the activity of melatonin, which leads to excessive production of hormones in women."

Melatonin secretion controls the normal sleeping/waking cycle in the body and impacts blood pressure, body temperature and insulin sensitivity. A single light emission during sleep is enough to disturb all-important circadian rhythms and negatively affect melatonin production. The body needs 7 to 9 hours of uninterrupted sleep without light distraction in order to regenerate itself and maintain optimal health. Staying true to this simple principle can tremendously improve your general state of health and *joie de vivre*, not to mention greatly reduce your risk of cancer.

Melatonin, which is produced at around 9:30 p.m. and reaches peak level secretions at around 1 a.m., also controls a powerful gene that ensures cells don't live beyond their normal lifespan. If they live longer than they should, they become cancerous. The message here is to get at least eight hours of sleep every day, starting before 10 p.m. Shut off or block out any artificial lighting around you in order to maximize the benefits of a good night's sleep.

In addition, as mentioned before, get regular exposure to sunlight without using sunglasses and sunscreen lotions. These are two of the most effective measures for the treatment and prevention of cancer. Germicidal ultraviolet (UV-C) light kills the cells of germs by damaging their DNA. The light initiates a reaction between two molecules of thymine, one of the bases that make up DNA. UV light at this wavelength (shortwave UV or UV-C) causes adjacent thymine molecules on DNA to dimerize. The resulting thymine dimer is very stable. If enough of these defects accumulate on a microorganism's DNA, its replication is inhibited, thereby rendering it harmless.

The longer the exposure to UVC light, the more thymine dimers are formed in the DNA. If cellular processes are disrupted because of DNA damage, the cell cannot carry out its normal functions. If the damage is extensive and widespread, the cell will die.

Both the germicidal UV-C and the tanning plus vitamin D generating UV-B are involved in this process. Interestingly, the implication of conventional wisdom is that the populations in hot climates where sun exposure is highest would have the highest rates of melanoma, but they don't. In fact, as previously noted, skin cancers occur mostly in people living in the least sun-exposed parts of the world, in those who suffer from chronic vitamin D deficiency, who use sunscreens to *protect* their skin, and who live mostly indoors.

There are also certain foods (such as strong acids like trans fats from eating fried foods, meat, melted cheese, chips, sodas, alcohol, etc.) and chemicals that when ingested or put on the skin in the form of carcinogen-packed sunscreens, react with the UV rays, which can lead to an inflammatory response or cell mutation.

The assumption that cell mutation alone can lead to cancer is now being disputed by research. It is one necessary factor, but cell environmental changes must be in place before the mutation can progress to abnormal cell division and tumor growth. Again, it is misleading and false to claim that the sun can cause cancer. In my view, cell mutation is a biological adjustment response for cells to survive exposure to very toxic, harmful substances and to deal with the bio-chemical effects of emotional and physical stress.

The sun only helps to make this response possible, but cannot cause it without other co-factors in place. Deficient vitamin D and emotional stress, both of which suppress the immune system, are co-factors, and so are lack of sleep, eating junk foods, medical drugs and liver bile duct congestion. The cancer, if it occurs, is a healing mechanism, not the *cause*, of a disease. If it is suppressed or attacked and the root causes remain intact, the healing stops and symptoms vanish or diminish, which is misconstrued as remission, only to recur with a vengeance. If the co-factors are removed and the cancer is supported through its various healing stages, it will disappear on its own and won't recur.

Air Pollution and Stress in Cities

As reported by NaturalNews.com in May 2008, a Canadian study has shown that women with breasts composed of 25 percent or more dense tissue have five times the breast cancer risk of women with fattier breasts. The study also found that women with dense breasts were 18 times more likely to have a breast tumor detected within one year of a negative mammogram.

Research conducted by the Princess Grace Hospital in London (U.K.) in 2007 and presented to the Radiological Society of North America showed that women who live and work in cities have a significantly higher risk of developing breast cancer than women who live in the countryside. To determine the reasons for this occurrence, researchers examined the breast tissue of 972 British women between the ages of 45 and 54. They found that the breasts of women who were living and working in cities were more than twice as likely to have 25 percent or more dense tissue.

Researchers hypothesized that city dwellers may have increased breast density because of hormone-disrupting toxins contained in air pollution. They also cited stress as a possible factor.

I might add that the forceful mammogram procedure could also contribute to breast cancers in women with denser breast tissue, by injuring it. Softer, fattier breast tissue can tolerate the potentially injurious mammography screening much better.

Microwave Ovens

Do you ever wonder what microwaves do to water, food and your body? Russian researchers have found decreased nutritional value, cancer-making compounds and brain-damaging radiolytics in virtually all microwave-prepared foods. Eating microwave-prepared meals can also cause loss of memory and concentration, emotional instability and a decline in intelligence, according to the research. In studying the nutritional value of foods cooked with microwaves, the Russian scientists found significant dimming of their *vital energy field*. This was noted in up to 90 percent of all microwave-prepared foods.

In addition, the B complex, C and E vitamins linked with stress-reduction and the prevention of cancer and heart disease, as well as the essential trace minerals needed for optimum brain and body functioning, were rendered useless by microwaves, even at short cooking durations. Microwave-cooked food is reduced to the nutritional equivalent of cardboard. One study demonstrated this by comparing plants watered with microwaved water to plants watered regularly; in the study, the plants that received microwaved water died within seven days.

If you do not want to develop nutrient deficiencies, you may be better off removing this appliance from your kitchen. In addition, all microwave ovens have unavoidable leakages. Hence, the radiation accumulates in the kitchen furniture, becoming a source of radiation in itself.

Microwave usage in the preparation of food leads to lymphatic disorders and an inability to protect the body against certain cancers. The research found increased rates of cancer cell formation in the blood

232

of people eating microwave-cooked meals. The Russians also reported increased rates of stomach and intestinal cancers, more digestive and excretive disorders, and a higher percentage of cell tumors, including sarcoma.

The Germans were the first to use microwave technology in the 1930s. At the beginning of World War II, German scientists developed a radar system based on technically-generated microwaves. During the extremely cold wintertime, soldiers gathered around the radar screens to get warm, but they developed blood cancers. Subsequently, the German army abandoned the use of radar. However, after German scientists learned that microwaves heated human tissue, they thought these waves could also heat food, and so they invented the microwave oven with the intention of providing German soldiers with warm meals during the battles against the Soviet Union. However, the soldiers who ate foods heated in microwave ovens also developed cancers of the blood, just like the radar technicians. As a result of this discovery, the use of microwave ovens was banned in the entire Third Reich.

Are microwaves any safer today than they were 80 years ago? Certainly not; they use the same technology. Microwaves rip apart the molecular bonds that make food the nourishing substance that it is. They hurl high-frequency microwaves that boil the moisture within food and its packaging by whipsawing water molecules dizzyingly back-and-forth at more than a billion reversals per second. This frantic friction fractures food molecules, rearranging their chemical composition into weird new configurations unrecognizable as food by the human body. By destroying the molecular structures of food, the body cannot help but turn the food into waste – not harmless waste, but *nuclear waste*.

Other side effects of microwave exposure include:

- High blood pressure
- Adrenal exhaustion
- Heart disease
- Migraines
- Dizziness
- Memory loss
- Disconnected thoughts
- Anxiety
- Increased crankiness
- Depression
- Sleep disturbance
- Stomach pain
- Appendicitis
- Cataracts

- Attention disorders
- Brain damage
- Hair loss
- Reproductive disorders

Eating microwave-damaged foods can lead to a considerable stress response in the body and, in so doing, alter the blood chemistry. For example, eating organic vegetables zapped by microwaves will send your cholesterol soaring. According to Swiss scientist Dr. Hans U. Hertel, "Blood cholesterol levels are less influenced by cholesterol content of the food than by stress factors." While the Russian government banned microwave ovens in 1976 for a very good reason, these appliances play a prominent role in the daily cooking routines in 90 percent of American homes.

Reporting for the *Forensic Research Document of Agricultural and Resource Economics* (AREC), William P. Kopp states: "The effects of microwaved food by-products are long-term, permanent within the human body. Minerals, vitamins, and nutrients of all microwaved food is reduced or altered so that the human body gets little or no benefit, or the human body absorbs altered compounds that cannot be broken down."

Microwaves turn healthy food into deadly poison. Seeing the unprecedented cancer epidemic in the U.S. and other countries that largely rely on microwaves for cooking foods, it would be wise if we stopped using microwave ovens altogether.

Dehydration

Cancer growth usually occurs in areas of severe dehydration. Many people suffer from dehydration without being aware of it. Dehydration is a condition in which body cells do not receive enough water for basic metabolic processes. The cells can run dry for a number of reasons:

- Lack of water intake (anything less than six glasses of pure water per day)
- Regular consumption of beverages that have diuretic effects, e.g., coffee, caffeinated tea, carbonated beverages such as soda pop, and alcohol, including beer and wine

- Regular consumption of stimulating foods or substances, such as meat, hot spices, chocolate, sugar, tobacco, narcotic drugs, soda pop, artificial sweeteners and the like
- Stress
- Taking any of a number of pharmacological drugs
- Excessive exercise
- Overeating and excessive weight gain
- Watching television daily for several hours

Dehydration is obviously associated with thirst, dry skin, dark-colored or foul-smelling urine, and fatigue. However, there are also many commonly overlooked symptoms of chronic dehydration, such as heartburn, constipation, urinary tract infections, premature aging, high cholesterol and weight gain.

Dehydration thickens the blood, thereby forcing cells to give up water. The cellular water is used to restore blood thinness. To avoid self-destruction, however, the cells begin to hold onto water. They do this by increasing the thickness of their membranes. The clay-like substance, cholesterol, starts to envelop the cells; and this prevents loss of cellular water. Although this emergency measure may preserve water and save the cell's life for the time being, it also reduces the cell's ability to absorb new water as well as much-needed nutrients. Subsequently, some of the unabsorbed water and nutrients accumulate in the connective tissues surrounding the cells, causing swelling of the body and water retention in the legs, kidneys, face, eyes, arms and other parts. This leads to considerable weight gain. At the same time, the blood plasma and lymph fluids become thickened and congested. Dehydration also affects the natural fluidity of bile, thereby promoting the formation of gallstones. All of these factors combined are sufficient to trigger the survival mechanism of cell mutation.

Tea, coffee, carbonated beverages and chocolate share the same nerve toxin and stimulant, caffeine. Caffeine, which is readily released into the blood, triggers a powerful immune response that helps to counteract and eliminate this irritant. The toxic irritant stimulates the adrenal glands, and, to some extent, the body's many cells, to release the stress hormones, adrenaline and cortisol, into the bloodstream. The resulting sudden surge in energy is commonly referred to as the fight-or-flight response.

If consumption of stimulants continues on a regular basis, however, this natural defense response of the body becomes overused and ineffective. The almost constant secretion of stress hormones, which are highly toxic compounds in and of themselves, eventually alters the blood chemistry and causes damage to the immune, endocrine and nervous systems. The primitive brain doesn't distinguish petty stress from serious fight-or-flight situations, and responds to both by secreting the hormone cortisol, which stops protein synthesis as it prepares the body to react to the stressor. When this happens chronically, future defense responses are weakened, and the body becomes more prone to infections and other ailments, including cell mutation.

The boost in energy experienced after drinking a cup of coffee is not a direct result of the caffeine itself; rather, it is the immune system's attempt to get rid of it that provides this effect. However, an overexcited and suppressed immune system eventually fails to provide the *energizing* adrenaline and cortisol boosts needed to free the body from the acidic nerve toxin, caffeine. At this stage, people say that they are *used* to a stimulant, such as coffee. They tend to increase their intake of it to feel the *benefits*. The often-heard expression, "I am dying for a cup of coffee," reflects the true peril of their situation.

Since the body's cells constantly have to give up some of their own water for the removal of the nerve toxin caffeine, regular consumption of coffee, tea or sodas causes them to become dehydrated. For every cup of tea or coffee a person ingests, the body has to mobilize about 2–3 cups of water just to remove the caffeine, a luxury it cannot afford. This also applies to soft drinks, pharmaceutical drugs, or any other substance or activity that brings about the release of stress hormones, including watching TV for many hours. As a rule, all stimulants have a strong dehydrating effect on the bile, blood and digestive juices. To heal a cancerous growth, stimulants are counterproductive, and it is best to avoid them.

To prevent dehydration, be sure to drink about 6–8 glasses of water, filtered and not chilled, every day. Also avoid drinking regular tap water or bottled water. Much of regular tap water and bottled water in the United States contains arsenic, chlorine, aluminum, fluoride, prescription and OTC drugs, disinfection byproducts (DBPs), and Bisphenol A, a harmful chemical commonly known as BPA.

How Can I Protect Myself?

When we think of all the different ways our bodies are exposed to toxicity on a daily basis, it's easy to become frustrated. There are, however, a number of ways you can help to protect yourself and your family.

- Make sure to drink plenty of water! Most people simply don't consume enough water to help their body cleanse itself
- Cleanse your liver, colon, kidneys and gallbladder at least once a year
- Store food in glass instead of plastic containers
- Only use naturally-based cleaning products in your home. Vinegar and orange oil are excellent natural cleaners. Health food stores and even some chain retailers also stock natural cleaning products
- Eat a sensible diet of organic produce and free-range, organic foods as often as possible to reduce your exposure to pesticides, GMOs, fertilizers and growth hormones
- Avoid conventional or farm-raised fish, which are often contaminated with PCBs and mercury
- Cut out processed foods and artificial food additives, including artificial sweeteners and MSG
- Toss out your Teflon and opt for safer cookware materials such as ceramic and glass
- Test your tap water and install filters if necessary (including your shower or bath)
- Avoid synthetic fragrances, artificial air fresheners, dryer sheets, fabric softeners, etc.
- Switch to natural shampoo, toothpaste, antiperspirants and cosmetics, using organic products if possible
- Use *green*, non-toxic alternatives to regular paint and vinyl in your home whenever possible
- Eliminate or minimize drugs, both prescription and over-the-counter, as well as vaccines
- Avoid chemical pesticides and insect repellents that contain diethyl(meta)toluamide (DEET)

If you have cancer, especially avoid the following:

Chlorinated water: One of the most powerful cancer-producing chemicals around. Avoid drinking unfiltered tap water, swimming in chlorinated pools or showering without a chlorine-removing filter. (You absorb more chlorine through the skin than you could possibly ingest from drinking tap water.)

Fluoride in municipal drinking water: It is just as carcinogenic as chlorine. Fluoride actually increases your body's uptake of aluminum, implicated in causing Alzheimer's disease. Use a water filter that takes out fluoride.

Electromagnetic radiation: Electromagnetic radiation interferes with the body's own electromagnetic field and undermines basic intercellular communication. Remove all electrical appliances or equipment from the bedroom, including electric blankets and electric alarm clocks. By placing a larger Ionized Stone (See *Other Books and Products by Andreas Moritz* at the end of the book) in, above or below the fuse box in your house, many of the harmful effects of electromagnetic radiation are nullified.

Wireless devices: This is explained in Chapter Four.

Pesticides and other chemical toxins: As found in non-organic foods, conventional household cleaning products, commercial beauty products, hair dyes (see information below), shampoos, skin lotions and other personal care products, these overtax and suppress the immune system when all its energy and resources are needed to heal the cancer. Especially avoid cosmetics with aluminum bases, mineral powders that contain bismuth, and aluminum-laden antiperspirants which are known to increase the risk of developing Alzheimer's disease by as much as 300 percent!

Hair dye: The fact that hairdressers have the highest rate of breast cancer of any profession prompted researchers to study the link between hair dye and cancer. A number of different studies found that women who use hair dye at least once a month are twice as likely to develop bladder cancer as those who do not. The risk triples when women use hair dye regularly for 15 or more years. These risks are the same regardless whether the women use permanent, semi-permanent or rinse applications. The chemicals contained in commercial hair dye products penetrate the scalp and enter the blood stream. The kidneys filter them out and pass them into the urinary bladder where they damage the cells of the bladder, leading to repeated bladder infections and cell mutation.

To minimize the harm from hair dyes, make certain to drink enough water each day, and cleanse your kidneys and the liver on a regular basis. (See directions in *The Amazing Liver and Gallbladder Flush*.) Additionally, choose foiling and highlights, natural plant-based Henna dyes or plant-based dyes, such as from Aveda and Herbatint.

Arsenic, asbestos and **nickel:** These can cause lung and other cancers. You wouldn't think that arsenic is something you would ingest somehow, unless someone intended to poison you. Well, if you regularly eat commercially-grown chicken (not organically-grown free-range), you actually take a lot of arsenic into your body. The poultry industry loves arsenic because it acts as a massive growth stimulant. Dr. Ellen Silbergeld, a researcher from the Johns Hopkins School of Public Health, commented about the industry's practice of using arsenic compounds in its feed: "It's an issue everybody is trying to pretend doesn't exist." Yet, inorganic arsenic exposure is a known risk factor for diabetes mellitus. It is also considered one of the prominent environmental causes of cancer mortality in the world. If you have prostate cancer, for example, or don't want to develop it, avoid eating chicken raised on industrial farms.

As shocking as this is, according to a report issued on June 9, 2011 by CBS News and the Associated Press, the FDA has finally admitted that chicken meat sold in the USA contains arsenic, a powerful toxin and carcinogen that is fatal in high doses. Cancer-causing arsenic has been added intentionally to chicken since the 1940s. Whereas the FDA has previously insisted that arsenic only shows up in chicken litter, not in chicken meat, it has now completely reversed its position.

Of course, every sane person knows that if you give arsenic to another person or to an animal, it won't just come right out of them along with the feces; it will actually poison them. That's why arsenic has been used in the past to poison people. I don't believe for a minute that FDA scientists actually assumed arsenic would somehow, for some magical reason, bypass the digestive system of the chicken; they knew all along why it is being fed to them – that is, to kill parasites and make them grow fat faster. To make them grow faster, the arsenic must obviously be absorbed into the blood and carried to liver. The FDA seemed surprised, though, that their research found there was arsenic in chicken liver.

With regard to the FDA's claim that the amount of arsenic found in commercially-grown chicken is still safe for human consumption, why then is the arsenic-containing chicken feed Roxarsone suddenly being pulled off the shelves? Roxarsone is produced by a subsidiary of Pfizer, *Alpharma LLC*, the same company that makes vaccines and other toxic drugs. Now that they have actually been found out to be systemically and slowly rendering the population sick with a known carcinogen, keeping this product on the market any longer could lead to huge class action law suits against them for causing cancers among poultry consumers.

As always, pharmaceutical companies only profit when the population is sick. Making and keeping it sick is an old trick of their trade. Pfizer still sells the arsenic ingredient in about a dozen other countries. It remains to be seen whether it will continue to do so.

While the FDA continues to claim that arsenic-fed chicken is safe for human consumption, the agency continues to conduct armed raids against manufacturers of foods and food supplements, like elderberry juice, cherry juice and walnuts, whose websites and food labels cite scientific evidence that these products were shown to have specific positive health benefits. The FDA claims it is illegal to state, for example, that honey can clear up skin infections, even though there are dozens of clinical studies to suggest honey does so more effectively than antibiotics.

Now if you think that eating hamburgers and beefsteak are arsenic-free, think again. It is common farming practice to use arsenic-laced chicken litter for cattle feed. Why waste all that precious arsenic? The motto is, "Use it twice, it's a lot cheaper."

Benzene: Benzene is among the 20 most widely used chemicals in the United States. It can cause leukemia and other cancers. Cigarette smoke and secondary smoking are major sources of exposure to benzene.

Formaldehyde: This can cause nasal and nasopharyngeal cancer. Formaldehyde is commonly used in the production of more complex chemicals, such as polymers and resins. Resins are used in adhesives, such as those found in plywood and carpeting. Formaldehyde is also used in sanitary paper products, such as facial tissue, table or dinner napkins, and roll towels. Most insulation material, molded products and paints contain formaldehyde derivatives, too.

Environmental/food toxins: Many babies are born toxic due to the toxic load of their mothers. Blood samples from newborns contained an average of **287 toxins, including mercury, fire retardants, pesticides and Teflon chemicals**, according to a 2004 study by the Environmental Working Group (EWG).

Teflon: This chemical in cooking pots is also carcinogenic. Food should never be prepared in Teflon cookware. Use glass, cast iron, carbon steel, titanium and enamel cookware.

PVC shower curtains: These emit a strong smell and can cause serious damage to your liver as well as to the nervous, reproductive and respiratory systems. The smell comes from deadly chemicals, including toluene, ethylbenzene, phenol, methyl isobutyl ketone, xylene, acetophenone and cumene, all named dangerous air pollutants by the EPA. Polyvinyl chloride (PVC) shower curtains are sold at Kmart, Bed Bath & Beyond, Wal-Mart, Sears and Target. "One of the curtains tested released measurable quantities of as many as 108 volatile organic compounds into the air, some of which persisted for nearly a month," according to a *New York Sun* article. To be safe, replace your PVC curtains with cloth curtains or glass doors.

Artificial sweeteners, such as aspartame and Splenda: Once in the body, they break down into powerful carcinogenic compounds.[74] The link between diet soda and increased risk of cancer is especially well-documented. It has also been associated with health problems ranging from headaches and memory loss, to seizures, asthma, sleep disorders, abdominal cramps and diabetes, to name just a few. Nevertheless, these artificial sweeteners remain on the market due to strong political and financial pressures, and show up under a variety of brand names: NutraSweet, Equal, AminoSweet, Natra Taste, Spoonful, Canderel and Neotame, among others.

Alcohol consumption: This causes liver bile duct congestion, suppresses the immune system and reduces magnesium in the body – all risks for developing cancer.[75] In 2002, the *British Journal of Cancer*

---

[74] For details about the effects of artificial sweeteners, see *Timeless Secrets of Health & Rejuvenation.*

[75] A Swedish study showed that women with the highest magnesium intake had a 40 percent lower risk of developing cancer than those with the lowest intake of the mineral. And researchers from the School of Public Health at the University of Minnesota found that diets rich in magnesium reduced the occurrence of colon cancer.

reported that 4 percent of all breast cancers in the United Kingdom – about 44,000 cases a year – are due to alcohol consumption. And, according to findings presented in San Diego at the 2008 annual meeting of the American Association for Cancer Research, alcohol, consumed even in small amounts, may significantly increase the risk of breast cancer – particularly estrogen-receptor/progesterone-receptor positive breast cancer.

The study followed more than 184,000 postmenopausal women for an average of seven years. Those women who had less than one drink per day had a 7 percent increased risk of breast cancer compared to those who did not drink at all. Women who drank 1–2 drinks a day had a 32 percent increased risk, and those consumed 3 or more glasses of alcohol a day had up to a 51 percent increased risk. The risk was seen mostly in those 70 percent of tumors classified as estrogen receptor- and progesterone receptor-positive. The study showed no difference in risks whether women consumed beer, wine or hard liquor.

Growth hormones in cow's milk: Samuel Epstein, M.D., a scientist at the University of Illinois School of Public Health, points out that rBGH milk is "supercharged with high levels of a natural growth factor (IGF-1), excess levels of which have been incriminated as major causes of breast, colon and prostate cancers."

Synthetic vitamins: Manufactured vitamins (non-methylated, inexpensive junk vitamins) can rob your body of energy and actually cause the vitamin deficiencies you want to avoid by taking these vitamins. Natural vitamins, as found in fruits and vegetables, on the other hand, *donate* energy to your cells.

Synthetic vitamin pills contain as much as 90 percent pure filler. The absorption rate of these vitamins is often less than 5 percent. Taking many vitamin supplements can also greatly burden the digestive system, liver and kidneys. Besides, it is virtually impossible to produce vitamin products that have the right balance between the various vitamins they contain. Each person's vitamin requirement is uniquely different and changes all the time; therefore, no vitamin product can ever match and meet that requirement. Leaving it up to the body to decide how many vitamins to extract from food is the only really safe way to ingest them.

It is always best to get your vitamins from the foods you eat. Vitamins are naturally toxic, acidic and reactive. Fruits and vegetables contain natural, neutralizing agents to keep the vitamins from causing harm to the body. Even a high quality methylated vitamin (one that uses the coenzyme of the vitamin) is stripped of these agents and can trigger an imbalanced response by the body, such as irritation and removing existing vitamins, thereby causing a vitamin deficiency.[76]

Grilling meat, poultry or fish: In April 2008, the American Institute of Cancer Research urged everyone to rethink the pastime of barbecuing meat. After analyzing the results of 7,000 studies, the Institute concluded that grilling any meat – whether red, white or fish – creates potent cancer-producing chemicals. Apparently, the high heat of grilling reacts with proteins in red meat, poultry and fish, producing heterocyclic amines, which are linked to cancer. Another form of cancer-causing agents, polycyclic aromatic hydrocarbons, are created when juices from meats drip and hit the heat source. They then rise in smoke and can stick to the meat.

The Institute took particular aim at processed meats, such as hot dogs, sausages, bacon, ham, pastrami, salami and any meat that has been salted, smoked or cured. The chemicals used to preserve meat increase the production of cancer-causing compounds, regardless of how the meat is cooked. The Institute's report said it "could find no amount of processed meat that is safe to eat."

High intake of fructose and sucrose: Consumption of these sugars may increase the risk of developing pancreatic cancer, according to a study conducted by researchers from the University of Hawaii and the University of Southern California. Fructose naturally occurs in fruits, while sucrose is usually extracted from sugarcane or sugar beets. Researchers analyzed dietary data on 162,150 people who had participated in the Hawaii–Los Angeles Multiethnic Cohort Study, looking for evidence that a diet with a high glycemic load increases the risk of pancreatic cancer. Participants who consumed the most fructose had a significantly higher pancreatic cancer risk than those who consumed the least. Participants who drank more fruit juice also had a higher risk of pancreatic cancer. Meanwhile, among obese and overweight patients, high sucrose intake was correlated with a higher risk of pancreatic cancer. Fructose, in particular, can also have a highly

---

[76] For detailed information, read the section, Hidden Perils of Vitamin Pills in Chapter Fourteen of my book, *Timeless Secrets of Health & Rejuvenation*.

negative effect on the neurological system and actually shut down parts of the brain.

Smoking cigarettes: This increases the incidence of any type of cancer by undermining the blood's ability to carry oxygen to the cells of the body, and inflaming them. In addition, smoking and inhaling second-hand smoke causes cadmium poisoning, a major risk for developing cancer. Having said that, the hysteria of most anti-smoking campaigns is unnecessarily extreme. While it is not exactly beneficial, smoking is not the unavoidable cause of lung cancer as we have been led to believe. Indeed, many countries with high percentages of smokers, such as Iceland, Japan, Israel and Greece, also have some of the world's longest life expectancies.

Sunscreens: Cancer of all types increased dramatically when sunscreens and sunglasses were introduced to the masses. (See Chapter Two for details.)

Night shift work: The World Health Organization's International Agency for Research on Cancer (IARC) has added working the night shift to a list of possible carcinogens, based on an analysis of the existing research on the topic. The IARC reviewed studies on night workers, primarily nurses and airline crews, and found that night workers were more likely to develop cancer than day workers. "There was enough of a pattern in people who do shift work to recognize that there's an increase in cancer," said IARC carcinogen classifications unit head Vincent Cogliano. Apparently, years of overnight work among women is particularly linked to higher breast cancer, with a similar effect on prostate cancer in men.

Blood transfusions: If you opt for cancer surgery and receive a blood transfusion, please be aware that this may significantly increase your risk of heart attack and death. Research shows that blood transfusions increase the risk of complications and reduce survival rates. Almost immediately after it is donated, blood begins to lose its ability to transport oxygen to the cells of the patient's body. The longer the blood has been stored, the higher the risk of heart attack, heart failure, stroke and death.

Nitric oxide in red blood cells is critical to the delivery of oxygen to the body's tissues. If blood is stored for more than two weeks, its nitric oxide concentration drops to a level that may endanger the life of the patient. It is accepted practice to store blood for transfusion for up to six weeks. The above risk could be reduced by enriching the blood with nitric oxide, but very few hospitals do so.

In a study reported in the March 20, 2008 *New England Journal of Medicine*, researchers found that patients who were given older units of blood had higher rates of in-hospital mortality. In one year, mortality was significantly less in the patients given newer blood. In another study, at the University of Bristol, researchers found that patients receiving a red blood cell transfusion were three times more likely to experience complications from lack of oxygen to key organs, such as heart attack or stroke. And an earlier study at Duke University in 2004 found that patients who receive a blood transfusion to treat blood loss or anemia were twice as likely to die during their first 30 days of hospitalization. They were also more than three times as likely to suffer a heart attack within 30 days, when compared to those who did not receive a transfusion.

Please note: There are alternative options to blood transfusion that carry a much lower risk, such as auto-transfusion and hemodilution. (See details in *Timeless Secrets of Health & Rejuvenation.*)

Ionizing radiation: Exposure can increase the risk of certain cancers. **X-rays** used to treat disorders such as acne or adenoid enlargement can increase the risk of certain types of leukemias and lymphomas. Your doctor will not tell you this, but x-rays accumulate in the body, and each x-ray taken increases the risk, regardless of whether it has been given for your teeth, gallbladder, spine, lungs or bones.

In 2006, over 62 million CT or CAT scans were performed in the United States, which has greatly increased the personal radiation dose experienced by the average U.S. resident. The radiation dose from a CT scan is 50 to 100 times larger than from a conventional x-ray. Ionizing radiation can produce free radicals and break important chemical bonds in the body, causing tremendous damage to molecules that regulate cell processes (such as DNA, RNA and proteins). Though the body can easily repair this damage when incurred at low levels, the high levels of radiation emitted by these medical technologies can create irreversible damage to important tissues. A surge in the use of CT scans in the last 25 years has led to millions of patients per year being unnecessarily exposed to dangerous radiation that increases their risk of cancer, according to a paper published in the *New England Journal of Medicine*.

There are no *harmless* MRIs or mammograms. Other studies reveal that children exposed to x-rays are more likely to develop breast cancer as adults. Microwave ovens that heat and radiate your food are just as damaging and can cause cancer of the blood, as well as tumors in the brain and other parts of the body.

Facts about mammography:

- Each x-ray you are exposed to increases your risk of abnormal cell growth. One standard mammography test results in approximately 1 rad (radiation absorbed dose) exposure, about 1,000 times greater than that from a chest x-ray.
- The National Cancer Institute (NCI) reports that among women under 35, mammography could cause 75 cases of breast cancer for every 15 it identifies.
- A Canadian study found a 52 percent increase in breast cancer mortality in young women who have received annual mammograms.
- Dr. Charles B. Simone, a former clinical associate in immunology and pharmacology at the National Cancer Institute, said, "Mammograms increase the risk for developing breast cancer and raise the risk of spreading or metastasizing an existing growth."
- After reviewing 117 studies conducted between 1966 and 2005, an expert panel from the American College of Physicians (ACP) found that the data on mammography screening for women in their 40s are so unclear that the effectiveness of reducing breast cancer death could be either 15 percent or "… nearly zero."
- Researchers at the Nordic Cochrane Centre in Denmark found that for every 2,000 women who received mammograms over a 10-year period, only one would have her life prolonged, but 10 would endure unnecessary and potentially harmful treatments. The study examined the benefits and negative effects of seven breast cancer screening programs on 500,000 women in the United States, Canada, Scotland and Sweden.
- The Breast Cancer Detection Demonstration Project, a large epidemiological study first done in the 1970s, found that a combination of mammography and clinical breast exam failed to

detect at least 20 percent of cancers. This statistic has remained fairly constant to the present day. Mammography isn't foolproof.

- One of the top cancer experts in the world, Dr. Samuel Epstein of the Cancer Prevention Coalition claims, "Screening mammography poses significant and cumulative risks of breast cancer for premenopausal women. ....The premenopausal breast is highly sensitive to radiation, each 1 rad exposure increasing breast cancer risk by about 1 percent, with a cumulative 10 percent increased risk for each breast over a decade's screening."

- The strong compression of breasts during the mammography procedure may help disperse existing cancer cells. Medical schools teach doctors to always handle a woman's breasts with great care for this reason.

- Research has identified a gene, called oncogene AC, that is extremely sensitive to even small doses of radiation. A significant percentage of women in the United States have this gene, which could increase their risk of mammography-induced cancer. An estimated 10,000 AC carriers will die of breast cancer each year *due to* mammography.

- Since mammogram screening was introduced, the incidence of a form of breast cancer called ductal carcinoma in situ (DCIS) has increased by 328 percent.

- Each year, thousands of women unnecessarily undergo mastectomies, radiation and chemotherapy after receiving false positives on a mammogram.

- A meta-analysis of 117 studies published in *Annals of Internal Medicine* (2007) reported that false-positive results on mammograms range from 20 percent to 56 percent in women 40 to 49 years of age.

- In July 1995, *The Lancet* wrote about mammograms, saying: "The benefit is marginal, the harm caused is substantial, and the costs incurred are enormous ..."

- Mammograms are known to shorten life spans much more often than they improve them; for every woman who benefits, 10 others' lives will be cut short. Nevertheless, the FDA approved new mammogram technology at twice the radiation dose.

- Magnetic resonance mammography (MRM), which is being peddled to young women deemed at higher risk for breast cancer, has a frighteningly high false-positive rate of around 25 percent. This inevitably leads to a higher rate of completely unnecessary mastectomy surgeries.
- As published in October 2007 by *The Cochrane Library and PubMed*, breast self-exams don't benefit mortality rates from breast cancer either. Two large population-based studies (388,535 women) from Russia and Shanghai that compared breast self-examination found that death rates from breast cancer were the same among women who rigorously self-examined as those who did not. Almost twice as many biopsies (3,406) with benign results were performed in the screening groups compared to the control groups (1,856).

In addition to the high risk of a false-positive diagnosis that may result in unnecessary surgery, disfigurement, and extremely harmful fear and stress, the MRI procedure itself is very dangerous. Indeed, the risk of anaphylaxis from the dye injected as part of an MRI procedure is even higher than that from vaccinations. What's worse, these tests provide basically no medical benefit to women.

Dr. Epstein, who is also a professor emeritus of Environmental and Occupational Medicine at the University of Illinois School of Public Health, has been warning about the risks of mammography since at least 1992. Commenting on the official mammography guidelines, Epstein says: "They were conscious, chosen, politically expedient acts by a small group of people for the sake of their own power, prestige and financial gain, resulting in suffering and death for millions of women. They fit the classification of **crimes against humanity**."

Experts no longer recommend following a strict examination routine, but rather for women to get to know what is normal, and feel their breasts regularly for signs of any changes. They should look out for a new lump or hard knot found in the breast or armpit, or unusual changes in the size, color, shape or symmetry of the breast and nipple, such as swelling or thickening of the breast.

Is there a good alternative screening method?

Yes, there is a side effect-free and inexpensive screening technology that is far more effective than mammography: High-resolution Digital

248

Infrared Thermal Imaging (DITI). DITI measures the radiation of infrared heat from your body and translates this information into anatomical images. If there is an abnormal growth of some sort in your breast, it will stand out clearly on the thermographic image as a *hot spot*. This type of thermography is simple and non-invasive.

Although accepted by Duke University, this diagnostic tool is not a mainstream technology. "…The establishment ignores safe and effective alternatives to mammography, particularly trans illumination with infrared scanning," Dr. Epstein points out.

Thanks to the discoveries of the North Carolina Institute of Technology (NCIT), a privately funded research center, thermal imaging, done using the protocol established by NCIT, may find developing breast cancer 10 years earlier than mammography.

It is important to note, though, that I personally don't endorse any screening method to diagnose cancer, for reasons already explained in this book – it creates unnecessary and damaging paranoia that can spur disease, while an undiscovered cancer can clear up on its own. Just having the fear and expectation that you may have breast cancer, when you really do not, focuses your mind on the disease, and this is often enough to actually trigger the very illness in your body that you are so afraid of.

Just think about what fear can get you: shallow breathing, sweaty palms, upset stomach, irritability, headache, inability to speak, inability to think clearly, disorientation, confusion, depression, uncontrollable shaking, panic attacks, inability to move, anger, and feeling weak and worthless. If ongoing, any of these distressing experiences are enough for your body to release the stress hormone cortisol, which again prevents the uptake of food proteins and breaks down existing cell proteins to the point of wasting. In other words, the fearful response to a cancer diagnosis can be the very mechanism that makes it terminal.

In addition, the pressure that doctors and loved ones may put on you to get the *proper treatment* can be so overwhelming that you feel you have no other choice but to go ahead with it. Feeling trapped or cornered while feeling physically ill is certainly not conducive to healing. It is far more beneficial to attend to the underlying causes of congestion and emotional conflict, as outlined in this book, than to treat the symptoms of cancer. The same principle holds true for every so-called *disease*.

Disease is but a perception of fear, but it can just as well turn into a perception of healing, improvement and a new direction in life.

Chapter Six

What You Need
To Know To Heal Yourself

Cancer – Who Cures It?

Those who have gone into complete remission of cancer and remained free from it are the most likely candidates to reveal the mechanisms that cause and cure cancer.

Anne was 43 when she was diagnosed with an incurable form of lymphoma and given only a short time to live. Her doctors strongly recommended that she have radiation and chemotherapy treatments, the two most commonly used methods of combating cancer cells. Anne was aware that the treatments could not only substantially increase the risk of secondary cancer, but also have potentially severe side effects. She refused the treatment, arguing that if the cancer was incurable anyway, why treat it and unnecessarily suffer the horrendous side effects.

Having accepted that she had an incurable disease, which meant that she had come to terms with death, Anne felt free to look for alternative ways to make the *transition* easier. Rather than passively accepting her fate, she decided to focus on feeling well and began taking an active role in improving her well-being. She tried everything from acupuncture, cleansing of her organs, and herbal medicine, to meditation and visualization, which were all definite signals of caring attention sent to her body's cells. Anne's cancer went into remission a few months later. Within a year, all apparent signs of cancer had disappeared, much to the astonishment of her oncologist. Now, over two decades later, she is not only without a trace of cancer, but also feels that she has never been healthier and more vital.

When she was just 38 years old, Linda was diagnosed with a malignant melanoma (the most aggressive form of skin cancer). After several unsuccessful operations, she was informed that her cancer had progressed to the point where it was *terminal* and that she had only about one year to live. Linda also refused treatment with chemotherapy and radiation and, instead, focused on the more positive approaches to healing, including yoga, prayer, a vegetarian diet, cleansing her organs, meditation and daily visualizations. Today, 22 years after having outlived her *death sentence*, she is as healthy as can be with no trace of even a skin irritation.

Both Anne and Linda have changed their entire attitude toward life – from being passive victims of an uncontrollable, *invasive* disease, to being active participants in the creation of a healthy body and mind. Taking self-responsibility was their first step to remove the focus from cancer and direct it toward consciously creating healthfulness.

To call remissions such as these *miracle cures* is certainly not appropriate. Today there is ample documentation of remarkable recoveries from every type of cancer and nearly every other disorder, from diabetes to warts, and even to AIDS. The fact that a spontaneous remission of cancer can occur, even in the final stages of the illness, shows that the immune system not only has the potential to quickly and effectively clear the body of existing tumors, but also to prevent new ones from forming, provided their causes are addressed. A shift in attitude from having to attack and kill cancer cells, to leaving them in peace and eliminating the energy-depleting influences in one's life, may be a strong enough stimulant for the immune system to do away with the symptom (the cancerous tumor). Without its root causes, cancer is as harmless as a simple cold.

People like Anne and Linda do not have to be the exception; they can be the rule. So-called *spontaneous* remissions rarely occur spontaneously, or for no apparent reason. The body regards the causes of cancer as emotional and physical obstructions that can be overcome through a healing crisis, and cleansing the body as well as the mind and spirit. Active participation in the healing process and taking self-responsibility (an expression of love for oneself) are absolute necessities in the treatment of every major disorder, including cancer. If you are afflicted with cancer, it in no way means that you are helpless.

When George, the Cypriot businessman, came to me with kidney cancer, he was in the weakest condition of his entire life. Despite his hopeless diagnosis, George was still breathing. As long as one breathes, there is a chance of recovery. George not only recovered, but started to live his life afresh, with more awareness, love and joy.

Cancer has the tremendous potential of creating deeper meaning and purpose in a person's life, while bringing up and releasing longstanding fears of survival and death. It can transform a pessimistic outlook on life into an optimistic one that allows the person facing cancer to perceive the positive reason behind it and everything else that happens to him in life. This inner transformation no longer allows for perceiving oneself as a helpless victim at the mercy of oncologists or surgeons. Healing cancer or a similar life-threatening condition is perhaps one of the most powerful and meaningful accomplishments a person can achieve in life.

Removing the Need For Cancer

Because cancer is a natural consequence of an unhealthy lifestyle, the most sensible way of making sure you never become a cancer statistic is simply to ensure that you are doing everything you can to nourish your body and help it to run as cleanly and efficiently as possible. A healthy, organic diet that provides plenty of nutrients and fiber without unnatural additives and sugars is the key, as is optimizing your vitamin D levels and exercising regularly. Minimize your exposure to environmental toxicity as much as possible. Go outdoors. Stretch. Dance. Smile at the sun. Take a walk. Get enough sleep. Live with balance. The body is designed to sustain itself; it will only resort to such extreme measures as cancer if you give it no other choice. Really, it's just common sense.

Having examined a considerable number of cancer patients in my European practice during the 1990s, I discovered that all of them, regardless of the type of cancer, had accumulated large quantities of gallstones in the liver and gallbladder. By removing *all* stones from the liver and gallbladder through a series of liver cleanses, and cleansing the colon and kidneys before and after each liver flush,[77] a person creates the

---

[77] See directions for these cleanses in *The Amazing Liver and Gallbladder Flush*.

physical preconditions for almost every type of cancer to go into spontaneous remission. This also applies to cancers that are commonly considered terminal.

If the health-seeker continues to maintain a healthy diet and lifestyle, the cure is likely to be permanent. Evidence abounds that plenty of fruits and vegetables have cancer-curing and cancer-preventive properties. Research carried out at Britain's Institute of Food Research has revealed that brassica vegetables such as cabbage, kale, broccoli and Brussels sprouts contain anti-carcinogenic compounds, which prompt or stimulate cancer cells to commit suicide. These vegetables have strong purifying effects on the tissues and blood. Eating them regularly greatly reduces overall toxicity and eliminates the body's need for cancer cells. Another study published in the *Journal of the American Dietetic Association* suggests that eating apples, cauliflower and broccoli is particularly potent in preventing colon cancer, the third most common cancer.

In addition to these foods, numerous herbs and plants have powerful cleansing and anticancer properties. Out of 2,500,000 plants tested, roughly 3,000 have proven anticancer properties. The mechanisms by which they achieve their effects vary. Some arrest the fermentation process upon which the cancer cells depend for survival (cancer cells use lactic acid to generate cellular energy), others have direct toxic effects on tumor cells, still others inhibit the division of cancer cells while permitting healthy cells to reproduce normally, and finally, some affect the pH (acid/alkaline milieu) in such a way as to reduce or prevent the risks of cancer cells growing in other parts of the body. Usually, though, most of these plants have all of the effects mentioned above. A few of these are listed here:

- Agaricus Blasai Mushroom
- Aloe vera
- Astragalus
- Basil
- Black cohosh* (for breast

- Ginseng[79]
- Goji juice
- Grape seed extract
- Graviola (See section below)
- Green tea[80]

---

[79] Ginseng can increase cell oxygenation by 25 percent, which is very beneficial for any type of cancer.
[80] Recent studies have shown a significant preventive effect against colorectal and oral cancer in women who drank green tea regularly; and a 48 percent reduction in risk of developing advanced prostate cancer in men who drank five or more cups a day (over 14 years).

cancer)
- Black walnut hull
- Burdock root
- Cat's claw
- Cardamom
- Chaparral
- Citrus Medica**
- Coconut oil
- *Cogumelo do Sol* (Mushrooms of the Sun)
- Cumin, black (nigella sativa)[78]
- Dandelion***
- Dill
- Ellagic acid
- Essiac herbs
- Fennel
- Ginger****
- Herbal cancer treatment Carctol (Ayurvedic herbs)
- Lingzhi mushroom[81]
- Licorice root (powder)[82]
- Marjoram
- Oregano (also oregano oil)
- Parsley and Celery*****
- Pau d'Arco
- Red clover
- Rosemary
- Sage
- Schizandra berry
- Shiitake or Maitake mushrooms
- Tumeric
- Vinegar and Carbon Dioxide
- Walnuts[83]
- Andreas Moritz Kidney Cleanse Tea (www.presentmoment.com)
- Andreas Moritz Liver Cleanse Tea (www.presentmoment.com)

*More on black cohosh:

A French study published in the journal *Phytomedicine* showed that extract of black cohosh may prevent and halt the growth of breast cancer cells. The study was funded by the National Institutes of Health and the Susan G. Komen Breast Cancer Foundation. Black cohosh has already

---

[78] Researchers at Thomas Jefferson University in Philadelphia have discovered that an extract of nigella sativa seed oil, known as thymoquinone, can remedy one of the most virulent and difficult to treat cancers: pancreatic cancer. The extract does this by blocking pancreatic cell growth, and actually enhancing the built-in cellular function that causes programmed cell death, or apoptosis.

[81] Japan's National Cancer Center subjected this mushroom to pharmacological testing; they found that it was actually a potent immune system builder and cancer fighter. Scientists at Japan's University School of Medicine tested the mushrooms on mice. They discovered that it retarded tumor growth by 8 percent after 20 days. Cancerous guinea pigs experienced recovery rates of over 99 percent. Lingzhi can be found in many Asian markets as well as Western health stores. Extracts of 'lingzhi', which may also be called 'reishi', are also available.

[82] Licorice root powder is a powerful curative herb for both cancer and diabetes. It is more effective than chemotherapy drugs in destroying cancer cells, yet without injuring or destroying healthy cells.

[83] Walnuts May Lower Breast Cancer Risk:
http://www.webmd.com/breast-cancer/news/20090421/walnuts-fight-breast-cancer

earned a reputation for helping with gynecological problems, kidney problems, sore throat and somewhat easing the symptoms of menopause. It isn't advised to completely eliminate the symptoms of menopause since they have proven to reduce the risk of breast cancer by at least 50 percent. (**Contraindications:** Do not use black cohosh if you also use either of the two chemotherapy drugs, doxorubicin and docetaxel, or if you are pregnant.)

**More on Citrus Medica fruit juice:
This Ayurvedic herbal treatment is used in treating all kinds of liver diseases, including liver cirrhosis, jaundice, damaged liver function, viral hepatitis B and C, primary and secondary liver malignancies.

***More on dandelion
This common weed, known as a good liver tonic, is a cancer-fighter too. Research conducted by a Windsor University biochemist on leukemia blood samples and dandelion root extract[84] showed that leukemia cells were forced into apoptosis, or cell suicide, whereas non-cancerous cells were left unaffected. In other words, the dandelion root extract targeted only the *bad* cancer cells, unlike chemotherapy drugs that kill even the *good* cells.

****More on ginger:
Ginger naturally inhibits COX-2, an enzyme responsible for inflammation and pain [*Food and Chemical Toxicology* 40: 1091-97, 2002]. Ginger's active ingredient, gingerol, inhibits the spread of cancer cells and makes it impossible to distinguish cancer cells from normal healthy cells [*Cancer Research* 61: 850-53, 2001]. Ginger root extract (gingerol) blocks inflammation and thins the blood much like aspirin does, except without the harmful side effects that result from the use of aspirin [*Pharmazie* 60: 83-96, 2005]. Ginger juice produces better recovery from symptoms of nausea than ondansetron, a drug commonly prescribed during chemotherapy [*Journal Ethnopharmacology* 62: 49-55, 1998]. It has been shown to inhibit the growth of tumors in the colon in animal studies [*Clinica Chimica Acta* 358: 60-67, 2005]. Gingerol inhibits the growth of

---

[84] http://www.naturalnews.com/035754_dandelion_cancer_prevention.html

Helicobacter pylori in the digestive tract, which is a bacterium linked to stomach cancer [*Anticancer Research* 23: 3699-702, 2003].

*****More on parsley and celery
Celery and parsley contain apigenin, a flavonoid, which is also found in many other natural foods. In animal studies, it slowed cancer growth and shrank cancerous tumors, even deadly, fast-growing breast tumors. Injections of the substance could be a safe alternative to toxic chemotherapy, as it showed no signs of side effects, even at high doses. The researchers are having trouble finding funding to continue research in humans as pharmaceutical companies have no interest in providing funds for this potential natural cancer cure.[85]

Curcumin – Nature's 'Wonder Drug'

In India, where turmeric is commonplace in the diet, the prevalence of four of the U.S.'s most common cancers (breast, colon, prostate and lung) is 10 times lower. This is largely because of a compound contained in turmeric known as curcumin, whose anticancer benefits are, by now, well documented. A mere 9–12 grams of curcumin extract daily can be enough to provide potent anticancer benefits. According to studies, curcumin also helps to reduce cholesterol levels; suppress diabetes, Alzheimer's disease, MS, tumor formation, rheumatoid arthritis, HIV; and enhance wound healing and bile secretion, among other things. As an added bonus, it's delicious. How's that for smart health?

Menopausal Symptoms Actually Prevent Breast Cancer

If you are among those women who have suffered through menopausal symptoms or are going through them right now, breathe a

---

[85] http://articles.mercola.com/sites/articles/archive/2012/06/04/apigenin-on-breast-cancer-treatment.aspx?e_cid=20120604_DNL_art_2

sigh of relief. Unbeknownst to many doctors and their patients who consider menopause a disease, the uncomfortable symptoms associated with menopause may actually prevent you from developing menopausal breast cancer.

If you ask your doctor to give you hormones to suppress these symptoms, he is unlikely to tell you that by reducing them you will actually increase your risk of breast cancer.

A 2011 study, published in *Cancer Epidemiology, Biomarkers & Prevention* [20(2); 1-10; ©2011 AACR], clearly emphasizes the potentially enormous health benefits of menopause-related hot flashes, night sweats, insomnia, depression, vaginal dryness, irregular or heavy menstrual bleeding and anxiety.

Prior studies have already shown that women with menopausal symptoms have lower estrogen levels because they go through menopause, compared with women who do not experience them. However, this new study by a team of researchers from the University of Washington and the Fred Hutchinson Cancer Research Center, Washington, was the first one to evaluate the association between menopausal symptoms and breast cancer risk.

The results of this research that was funded by the National Cancer Institute showed that women who ever experienced menopausal symptoms had significantly lower risks of invasive ductal carcinoma, invasive lobular carcinoma and invasive ductal-lobular carcinoma compared with women who did not. The risk reduction shown was a whopping 40–60 percent.

These reductions in risk were independent of timing of hormone therapy use, age at menopause and body mass index, which are known risk factors for breast cancer.

The research paper further points out that increasing intensity of hot flashes among women who ever experienced hot flashes was also associated with decreasing risks of all three breast cancer subtypes.

"In particular we found that women who experienced more intense hot flashes – the kind that woke them up at night – had a particularly low risk of breast cancer," senior author Christopher I. Li, M.D., Ph.D., a breast cancer epidemiologist in the Hutchinson Center's Public Health Sciences Division, said in a statement to the media.

The researchers came to the conclusion: "This is the first study to report that women who ever experienced menopausal symptoms have a substantially reduced risk of breast cancer, and that severity of hot flashes is also inversely associated with risk." "If confirmed," suggested the researchers, "these findings could enhance our understanding of breast cancer etiology and factors potentially relevant to prevention."

"While menopausal symptoms can certainly have a negative impact on quality of life, our study suggests that there may be a silver lining if the reduction in breast cancer risk is confirmed in future studies," Dr. Li said.

We can learn a great lesson from this important piece of research. Instead of immediately misconstruing that those symptoms of discomfort must be a sign there is something wrong with the body, we can trust that the body does not make mistakes, even if we don't understand the reasons why it comes up with such unusual symptoms like hot flashes and night sweats.

In other words, count yourself blessed, not cursed, if you experience these symptoms. Focus instead on taking care of your body by eating healthfully, going to sleep early, exercising regularly, remaining hydrated and getting enough vitamin D from regular sun exposure.

Sunlight – Nature's Cancer Treatment

According to a study published in the prominent *Cancer Journal* (March 2002; 94:1867-75), insufficient exposure to ultraviolet radiation may be an important risk factor for cancer in Western Europe and North America. The findings, covering mortality rates from cancer in North America, directly contradict official advice about sunlight. The research showed that deaths from a range of cancers of the reproductive and digestive systems were approximately twice as high in New England as in the Southwest, despite a diet that varies little between regions.

An examination of 506 regions found a close inverse correlation between cancer mortality and levels of UV-B light. The likeliest mechanism proposed by scientists for a protective effect of sunlight is vitamin D, which is synthesized by the body when exposed to ultraviolet B rays. According to the study's author, Dr. William Grant, the northern parts of the United States may be so dark during the winter months that vitamin D synthesis shuts down completely.

While the study focused mainly on white-skinned Americans, the researchers found that the same geographical trend affects dark-skinned Americans whose overall cancer rates are significantly higher. As mentioned earlier, or as explained in my book, *Heal Yourself with Sunlight*, dark-skinned individuals require more sunlight to synthesize vitamin D.

The same study showed that at least 13 malignancies are affected by a lack of sunlight, mostly reproductive and digestive cancers. The strongest inverse correlation is with breast, colon and ovarian cancer, followed by tumors of the bladder, uterus, esophagus, rectum and stomach.

To obtain the disease-curbing benefits of sunlight, you need to be outside at least three times a week for a minimum of 15–20 minutes (each time). **Avoid using sunscreens and sunglasses; otherwise you will not gain the benefits from sunlight exposure.**

To learn about the healing powers of the sun in much more detail and, specifically, how UV-light actually prevents and cures skin cancer, along with why most skin cancers are caused by sun protection creams and lotions, see Chapter Eight of my book, *Timeless Secrets of Health & Rejuvenation*.

While vitamin D supplementation may be necessary for those living in cold climates or during the darker months, it is not necessarily the best choice. In fact, for decades now it has been well-established by reliable research that Hypervitaminosis D through supplementation can have toxic effects, and even be fatal.

In no way do I trust the Recommended Dietary Allowance (RDA) for vitamins, but I have personally seen many cases where vitamin D deficiency has led to at least some of the mentioned side effects. In addition, in my book, *Heal Yourself with Sunlight,* I discuss the research which shows that, when taken as a supplement, vitamin D can suppress the immune system. Although I am aware that supplementation can quickly remove certain disease symptoms, they also replace these with others that are equally serious, if not more so.

By suppressing the immune system, similar to vaccination, the body may no longer mount an appropriate response that would naturally involve inflammation, pain, weakness, swelling, etc. This, however, should not be misconstrued as *improvement of a condition*, but as worsening it. Sunshine or vitamin D lamp-induced vitamin D would never do this.

There is a huge movement behind pushing synthetic vitamin D supplements into the population; and substantial financial interests are involved in conducting studies to *prove* its value, not unlike the manipulated drug trials. I am one of the greatest fans of vitamin D (which is actually a steroid hormone), and I have written extensively about it for 15 years, so I don't need to be convinced about its importance. I just recommend to be discerning when it comes to ingesting steroid hormones, even as precursor drugs like D2. Steroids were once considered miracle drugs with their amazing effects, but now we know they cause far more damage than good. I just hope we won't fall into yet another trap.

Getting Enough Sleep

Ask any workaholic or college student how much they sleep, and chances are they'll tell you how few hours of sleep they can *run on* as a source of pride. But this fundamental part of a natural, healthy lifestyle is far too ignored, and the consequences of treating good sleep as an unaffordable luxury are extremely dangerous. Sleep deprivation has been linked to higher risk of heart disease, diabetes, obesity and, of course, cancer.

Researchers in one study found, for example, that those who got less than six hours of sleep per night were 50 percent more likely to develop colon polyps, precancerous growths that can turn malignant if left untreated. This makes chronic sleep deprivation a major risk factor in the development of cancer.

It follows, then, that simply ensuring a good night's sleep can help prevent and even treat cancer. Research shows that the immune system needs 8–9 hours of sleep in *total* darkness to recharge completely. A weak immune system cannot keep the body clean inside, and the resulting congestion threatens cellular life.

The recurring alteration of day and night regulates our natural sleep/wake cycles and essential biochemical processes. The onset of daylight triggers the release of powerful hormones (glucocorticoids), of which the main ones are cortisol and corticosterone. Their secretion has a marked circadian variation. These hormones regulate some of the most important functions in the body, including metabolism, blood sugar level and immune responses. Peak levels occur between 4 a.m. and 8 a.m. and gradually decrease as the day continues. The lowest level occurs between midnight and 3 a.m.

By altering your natural daily sleep/wake schedule, the peak of cortisol's cycle changes as well. For example, if you continually go to sleep after midnight, instead of before 10 p.m., and/or you arise in the morning after 8 a.m. or 9 a.m., instead of with or before sunrise between 6 a.m. to 7 a.m., you will enforce a hormonal time shift (continual jet lag) that can lead to chaotic conditions in the body. Waste materials that tend to accumulate in the rectum and urinary bladder during the night are normally eliminated between 6 a.m. and 8 a.m. With a changed waking/sleeping cycle, the body has no other choice but to hold on to that waste matter and possibly reabsorb part of it. When you disrupt your natural sleep/wake cycles, the body's biological rhythms desynchronize with the larger circadian rhythms that are controlled by the daily periods of darkness and light. This can lead to numerous types of disorders, including chronic liver disease, respiratory ailments, heart trouble and cancer.

One of the pineal gland's most powerful hormones is the neurotransmitter melatonin. The secretion of melatonin starts between 9:30 p.m. and 10:30 p.m. (depending on age), inducing sleepiness. It reaches peak levels between 1 a.m. and 2 a.m. and drops to its lowest levels at midday. The pineal gland controls reproduction, sleep and motor activity, blood pressure, the immune system, the pituitary and thyroid glands, cellular growth, body temperature and many other vital functions. All of these depend on a balanced melatonin cycle. By going to sleep late (past 10 p.m.) or working the night shift, you throw this and many other hormonal cycles out of balance.

The ongoing Nurses' Study has shown that nurses working the night shift have a more than 50 percent higher risk of developing cancer, but have among the lowest levels of melatonin in the blood. Higher levels of melatonin are linked with a lower risk of cancer. Blind women, for example, whose melatonin levels are naturally high (melatonin responds to darkness), have a 36 percent lower risk of breast cancer compared to sighted women. Taking a melatonin supplement has no cancer-preventive benefits, but may increase the risk because it inhibits the body's own melatonin secretion.

If you have cancer or don't want to develop it, this is about the most important advice you can get: Get a full night's rest every night (with the occasional exception), beginning at no later than 10 p.m.!

The conveniences provided by the onset of electrical lighting came with the great risk of ruining the health of millions of people. The human body and all the other organisms on the planet evolved to adjust themselves to predictable patterns of light and darkness, in a physiological cycle known as the circadian rhythm. The irregular lifestyle of modern living bypasses or ignores the body's vital need to be in sync with the daily, monthly and yearly changes of the environment. A part of the brain called the Suprachiasmatic Nucleus (SCN) controls your biological clock by closely monitoring the light and dark signals of your environment. Therefore, light and darkness have the most powerful influence on our hormonal system and, in turn, on the health and vitality of every cell in the body.

When your eyes stop seeing light as it is getting dark outside, your pineal gland will begin to produce melatonin, but stops secretion altogether when you switch on a light, watch television or use a light-up device such as a smart phone. As a result, the sleep-inducing effect of melatonin becomes inhibited, and you may not feel sleepy at all for several more hours. In fact, the stimulation from light at this time of the night may actually prevent you from falling asleep and cause you to develop a permanent sleeping disorder. Sleep deprivation is a common condition that afflicts 47 million American adults. And as more recent research indicates, it is so serious that it greatly raises their risk of cancer.

Among many other functions, melatonin triggers a nocturnal reduction in your body's estrogen levels, which significantly lowers its ability to ward off or heal *estrogen-related cancers.* By exposing yourself to nighttime light, your melatonin levels drop while your estrogen levels rise.[86] Medical scientists could not believe it at first when they learned that natural hormones such as estrogen and insulin could actually be carcinogens, but it is now official. In December 2002, the National Institute of Environmental Health Sciences (NIEHS) added estrogen to its list of known cancer-causing agents. Strong epidemiological evidence associates the hormone to breast, endometrial and uterine cancers.

---

[86] Both men and women produce estrogen hormones.

The liver regulates numerous hormones, including estrogens and progesterone. A woman with unbalanced hormone levels[87] may experience a low sex drive (low libido), cardiovascular disease, menopausal symptoms, menstrual discomforts, PMS, breast cysts, breast cancer, fibroids, endometriosis, emotional problems, female anxiety, nervous disorders, skin problems, hair loss and bone disorders. But it's certainly not the liver's fault when hormonal imbalance occurs. If you deprive yourself of sleep, especially the two hours before midnight, you also prevent the liver from doing its vital jobs – 500 of them.

There is no part of the body that doesn't suffer when liver functions are affected by not going to sleep on time, including the liver itself. For example, the liver removes insulin from the bloodstream. But when you interfere with its nocturnal activities (by not sleeping on time), insulin causes fat to be deposited in the liver; this prevents the liver from removing insulin from the bloodstream. Elevated insulin levels lead to heart attacks, abdominal obesity, diabetes and cancer.

Apart from making melatonin, the brain also synthesizes serotonin, which is a very important neurotransmitter (hormone) related to our state of physical and emotional well-being. It affects day and night rhythms, sexual behavior, memory, appetite, impulsiveness, fear and even suicidal tendencies. Unlike melatonin, serotonin increases with the light of day; physical exercise and sugar also stimulate it. If you get up late in the morning, the resulting lack of exposure to sufficient amounts of daylight reduces your serotonin levels throughout the day. Moreover, since melatonin is a breakdown product of serotonin, this lowers your levels of melatonin during the night. Any deviation from the circadian rhythms causes abnormal secretions of these important brain hormones. This, in turn, leads to disturbed biological rhythms, which can upset the harmonious functioning of the entire organism, including digestion, metabolism and endocrine balance. Suddenly, you may feel *out of sync* and become susceptible to a wide variety of disorders, ranging from a simple headache, bloating and indigestion to depression and a fully grown tumor.

Note: Over 90 percent of serotonin is produced in the digestive system, with peak levels at noontime when the sun at its highest position.

---

[87] The underlying imbalance consists of a relative excess of estrogen and an absolute deficiency in progesterone.

Lack of exposure to natural light or sleeping during daytime can lead to severe gastrointestinal problems, thereby affecting the health of every cell in the body.

The production of growth hormones, which stimulates growth in children and helps to maintain healthy muscle and connective tissue in adults, depends on proper sleeping cycles. Sleep triggers growth hormone production. Peak secretion occurs around 11 p.m., provided you go to sleep before 10 p.m. This short period coincides with dreamless sleep, often referred to as *beauty sleep*. It is during this period of the sleep cycle that the body cleanses itself and does its main repair and rejuvenation work.

If you are sleep-deprived, growth hormone production drops dramatically. To cure cancer, the body must be able to produce sufficient growth hormones. Getting enough sleep at the right time of the night is one of the best cancer-preventing and cancer-curing approaches. Moreover, it will cost you nothing and benefit you in many other ways. (For a detailed description of the body's biological rhythms and an ideal daily routine, see *Timeless Secrets of Health & Rejuvenation*.)

Maintaining Regular Meal Times

The body is controlled by numerous circadian rhythms, which regulate its most important functions in accordance with pre-programmed time intervals. Sleep, secretion of hormones and digestive juices, elimination of waste and many other bodily processes all follow a specific daily routine. If these cyclic activities become disrupted more often than they are adhered to, the body becomes imbalanced and cannot fulfill its essential tasks. All physical activities in the body are naturally aligned with and depend on the schedule dictated by the circadian rhythms.

Having regular meal times makes it easy for the body to prepare for the production and secretion of the right amounts of digestive juices for each meal. Irregular eating habits, on the other hand, confuse the body. Furthermore, its digestive power becomes depleted by having to adjust to a different schedule each time you eat. Skipping meals here and there, eating at different times, or eating between meals especially disrupts the cycles of bile production by the liver cells. The result is the formation of gallstones.

By maintaining a regular eating routine, the body's 60–100 trillion cells are able to receive their daily ratio of nutrients according to schedule, which helps cell metabolism to be smooth and effective. Many metabolic disorders, such as diabetes or obesity, result from irregular eating habits and can be greatly improved by matching eating times with the natural circadian rhythms.

It is best to take the largest meal of the day around midday and only light meals at breakfast (no later than 8 a.m.) and dinner (no later than 7 p.m.). Eating the main meal of the day in the evening, when the digestion of food is naturally weak, leads to an overload of the gastrointestinal tract with undigested, fermenting and putrefying food. The bacteria engaged in decomposing the undigested food produce poisons that not only affect intestinal health, but also are the main cause for developing lymphatic congestion. This spawns unhealthy weight gain and disturbs basic metabolism. Cancer is a metabolic disorder that can originate in regularly eating the main meal at night and eating between meals or before going to sleep.

Overeating, especially junk foods, usually leads to intestinal congestion, the proliferation of destructive bacteria and yeast, as well as cravings for *energizing* foods (which really means energy-depleting) foods and beverages, such as sugar, sweets, white flour products, potato chips, chocolate, coffee, tea and soft drinks. Constant cravings for any of these foods or beverages indicate cellular starvation. Such starvation at the cellular level may force the weakest cells in the body to undergo genetic mutation.

Even though it is complete common sense, a study published in the *British Medical Journal* spent a fortune to investigate and report on the cancer-producing effects of a couch-potato lifestyle and smoking. The results of the study, which involved 80,000 women aged 50–79, showed that these factors boost cancers of the breast, colon and many others. Why do we need expensive studies to prove that the modern way of life makes us sick?

The *Journal of Clinical Oncology* published a study of over 9,000 cancer survivors, evaluating their lifestyles following treatment. They found that even the survivors of this most feared disease often made little to no change in their lifestyle following remission. Less than one-fifth were consuming the recommended amount of fruits and vegetables, and only 1 in 20 had followed all the main aspects of a healthy lifestyle.

It is imperative that we change our attitudes about cancer and its causes if we want to rid ourselves and our society of the real issue – a toxic, imbalanced, indulgent lifestyle that forces the body's own tissues to resort to sustaining cancer in a desperate attempt to sustain itself. If we are unwilling to take responsibility for our health, we will suffer the consequences. The choice is ours.

Eating a Vegan-Vegetarian Diet

It is a well-known fact that many plant foods have potent cancer-fighting benefits. For example, a huge study done on 300,000 men and women from eight countries in Europe found that those who ate the most fruit and vegetable servings also had the lowest rates of heart disease, which as we know shares many of the same causes as cancer. The variety of colors they come in are not only appealing, but also indicates their nutrient, phytochemical and antioxidant content. Many of these compounds are especially beneficial when it comes to cancer prevention and cure. Some of the most potent fruit and vegetable cures for cancer are discussed later in this chapter.

It goes without saying, then, that the higher your intake and variety of fruits and vegetables, the more likely you are to be protected by all of their benefits, thereby enjoying a healthier, happier lifestyle.

Vegetarians have believed all along that living on a purely vegetarian diet can improve health and the quality of life. More recently, medical research has found that a properly balanced vegetarian diet may in fact be the healthiest diet. This was demonstrated by the over 11,000 volunteers who participated in the *Oxford Vegetarian Study* which for a period of 15 years analyzed the effects of a vegetarian diet on longevity, heart disease, cancer and various other diseases.

The results of the study stunned the vegetarian community as much as the meat-producing industry: "Meat eaters are twice as likely to die from heart disease, have a 60 percent greater risk of dying from cancer and a 30 percent higher risk of death from other causes." Another study

267

directly linked red meats and processed meats to a much higher risk of prostate cancer – with ground beef being the greatest culprit. In addition, the incidence of obesity, which is a major risk factor in many diseases, including cancer, gallbladder disease, hypertension and adult onset diabetes, was found to be much lower in those following a vegetarian diet.

In a study of 50,000 vegetarians, the National Institutes of Health (NIH) found that vegetarians live longer and have an impressively lower incidence of heart disease. They also have significantly lower rates of cancer than meat-eating Americans.

What we eat has a critical impact on our health. According to the American Cancer Society, up to 35 percent of the nearly 900,000 new cases of cancer each year in the United States could be prevented by following proper dietary recommendations. Researcher Rollo Russell writes in his *Notes on the Causation of Cancer:* "I have found of twenty-five nations eating flesh largely, nineteen had a high cancer rate and only one had a low rate, and that of thirty-five nations eating little or no flesh, none of these had a high rate."

Furthermore, T. Colin Campbell, Ph.D. and Thomas M. Campbell, authors of *The China Study*, succinctly sum up the results of their groundbreaking research in the field of nutrition science: "The people who eat the most animal protein have the most heart disease, cancer and diabetes." Not surprisingly, they recommend a whole foods and plant-based diet. Their research indicates that "the lower the percentage of animal-based foods that are consumed, the greater the health benefits – even when that percentage declines from a mere 10% to 0% of calories. So it's not unreasonable to assume that the optimum percentage of animal-based products is zero, at least for anyone with a predisposition for a degenerative disease."

Could cancer lose its grip on modern societies if they turned to a balanced vegetarian diet? The answer is "yes" according to two major reports, one by the World Cancer Research Fund and the other by the Committee on the Medical Aspects of Food and Nutrition Policy in the U.K. The reports conclude that a diet rich in plant foods and the maintenance of a healthy body weight could prevent four million cases of cancer worldwide. Both reports stress the need for increasing one's intake of plant fiber, fruits and vegetables, and reducing red and processed meat consumption to less than 80–90 grams per day.

Eating a balanced vegetarian diet is one of the most effective ways to prevent cancer. If you feel you cannot solely live on foods that are of vegetable origin, then at least try to substitute chicken, rabbit or turkey for red meat, for a period of time. Eventually, you may feel confident enough to eat a fully vegetarian diet. All forms of animal protein decrease the solubility of bile, which is a major risk factor for developing gallstones, as well as lymph and blood vessel wall congestion. These are the main causes of cell mutation, which lead to cancer.

For complete guidelines on how to eat a healthy, life-sustaining diet according to your body type's unique requirements, see *Timeless Secrets of Health & Rejuvenation.*

Exercise and Cancer

Is exercise beneficial to cancer patients or is it harmful? Notable research clears up any controversy and points to the benefits of exercise as a means of fighting cancer, according to a 2007 online report issued by Johns Hopkins University. It can increase chances of recovery by 30 percent.

For cancer patients undergoing chemotherapy, exercise is one of the best ways to combat treatment-related fatigue. "It's not recommended that you begin an intense, new exercise regimen while undergoing chemotherapy, but if you exercised before your cancer diagnosis, try and maintain some level of activity," says Deborah Armstrong, M.D., Associate Professor of Oncology, Gynecology and Obstetrics at Johns Hopkins. "If you haven't been exercising, try low-level exercise, such as walking or swimming."

The benefits of exercise are not limited to helping treatment-related fatigue. In fact, they actively contribute to curing cancer and preventing its recurrence. Several groundbreaking studies attest to this fact. This hardly comes as a surprise, since cancer cells are typically oxygen-deprived, and exercise is a direct way to deliver extra oxygen to cells throughout the body and to improve the immune response. Researchers also believe that exercise can regulate the production of certain hormones that, unregulated, may spur tumor growth.

Exercise should not be strenuous, however. Exercising for half an hour each day or several hours a week may be all that is needed to significantly increase cell oxygenation. (See Chapter Six of my book, *Timeless Secrets of Health & Rejuvenation*, for proper guidance on healthy exercising programs suitable for specific body types, and breathing exercises that greatly enhance oxygenation of cells.)

In one study, published in the *Journal of the American Medical Association,* researchers followed 2,987 women with breast cancer. Women who, for example, walked more than one hour a week after their cancer diagnosis were less likely to die of their breast cancer. In another study of 573 women, those who followed a moderate exercise program for more than six hours a week after a colon cancer diagnosis were 61 percent less likely to die of cancer-specific causes than women who exercised less than one hour per week. In all cases, exercise was found to be a protective factor regardless of the patient's age, stage of cancer, or weight. A third study, published in the *Journal of Clinical Oncology,* confirmed the above findings after examining the effects of exercise on 832 men and women with stage 3 colon cancer.

Restoring Chi, The Life Force

Samuel Hahnemann, founder of homeopathy, once said, **"It is the life force which cures diseases because a dead man needs no more medicines."** In other words, when the life force, Chi, is depleted, not even the best of medicines can restore a sick man's health or bring a dead man back to life. The life force is the only power in the body that is capable of healing it from an illness.

Ener-Chi Art is a unique method of healing art based on energized oil paintings that I created to help restore a balanced flow of Chi or vital energy through the organs and systems in the body. With any cancer, Chi flow is severely disrupted throughout the body. When applied in the context of physical cleansing and healing, I consider this unique approach a very important and effective tool in facilitating a more successful outcome of any treatment or healing method.

When the cells of the body experience a balanced flow of Chi, they are better able to remove toxic wastes, absorb more of the oxygen, water and the nutrients they need, do the necessary repair work, and increase their overall performance and vitality. Although I consider the combination of liver/colon/kidney cleanses to be one of the most effective tools to help the body return to balanced functioning, years of congestion and deterioration may hinder the body from fully restoring its Chi. My 10 years of research with this method, which took me almost two years to develop, has shown that Ener-Chi Art may very well accomplish this balanced Chi flow.

Its rate of effectiveness so far has been 100 percent for every person who has been exposed to the artwork. Due to their unique healing effects, all the Ener-Chi Art paintings were once exhibited for over a month at the prestigious *Abbott Northwestern Hospital* in Minneapolis, Minnesota for all the patients to view. Three of my original paintings – for the immune system, the lymphatic system and blood circulation/small intestine – hung in the cancer ward, affording all cancer patients the opportunity to experience their healing properties.

Ener-Chi Art is perhaps one of the most profound and instantly effective healing programs to balance the life force, Chi, in the following organs, parts and systems of the body:

- Back
- Blood
- Brain and nervous system
- Ears
- Eyes
- Endocrine system
- Heart
- Immune system
- Joints
- Kidneys and bladder
- Large intestine
- Liver
- Lymphatic system
- Muscular system
- Neck and shoulders
- Nose and sinuses
- Respiratory system
- Small intestine and circulatory system
- Skeletal system
- Skin
- Spleen
- Stomach
- Tongue

I have also created one painting for general health, and two additional pictures, *Beyond the Horizon* and *Portrait of Power*, which can be used with any problem, emotional difficulty, physical ailment, and mental or spiritual block. *Portrait of Power* provides a Portrait of All

Possibilities, supporting enhanced engagement in life and greater vitality; *Beyond the Horizon* is for transmuting emotional and physical trauma. Still other paintings were created to balance our relationship with the water and air elements, the rocks and mountains, the animal kingdom, the plant kingdom, and the world of nature spirits. Fully energized prints for each of these paintings are available through my website.[88] **The desired benefits occur while viewing the Ener-Chi Art paintings for about 30 seconds.**[89]

Sacred Santémony –
For Emotional Healing and More

Sacred Santémony is a unique healing system that uses sounds from specific words to balance deep emotional/spiritual imbalances. The powerful words in Sacred Santémony are produced from whole-brain use (involving both hemispheres of the brain) of the letters of the *ancient languages* – languages that are comprised of the basic sound frequencies that underlie and bring forth all physical manifestation. The letters of the ancient language vibrate at a much higher level than our modern languages, and when combined to form whole words, they generate feelings of peace and harmony (Santémony) to calm the storms of unrest, violence and turmoil – both internal and external.

I began this system of healing in April 2002 when I spontaneously began to chant sounds in ancient languages, including Native American, Tibetan, Sanskrit and others. Within two weeks, I was able to bring forth sounds that would instantly remove emotional blocks and resistance or aversion to certain situations, people, foods, chemicals, thought forms, beliefs, etc. The following are a few examples of conditions Sacred Santémony has improved:

---

[88] For more information on Ener-Chi Art and to order the pictures, see my website http://www.ener-chi.com or the section, *Other Books and Products by Andreas Moritz* at the end of this book.
[89] Editor's note: Ener-Chi Art pictures have all been compiled in a special edition book, *Art of Self-Healing*, which took over three years to bring to fruition in order to fully meet Andreas' exceptionally high quality photo-reproduction requirements. To order the book, see http://www.ener-chi.com/books/art-of-self-healing/.

- Reducing or removing fear related to the past or future, death, disease, the human body, foods, harmful chemicals, parents and other people in one's life, lack of abundance, impoverishment, phobias and environmental threats
- Clearing or reducing the pain from a recent or current hurt, disappointment, or anger resulting from past emotional trauma or negative experiences in life
- Cleansing of the *Akashic Records* (a recording of all experiences the soul has gathered throughout all life streams) from persistent fearful elements, including the idea and concept that we are separate from and not one with Spirit, God or our Higher Self
- Setting the preconditions for the individual to resolve his/her karmic issues, not through pain and suffering, but through creativity and joy
- Improving or clearing up allergies and intolerances to foods, gluten, chemical substances, pesticides, herbicides, air pollutants, radiation, medicinal drugs, pharmaceutical by-products, etc.
- Alleviating the psycho-emotional root causes of chronic illness, including cancer, heart disease, MS, diabetes, arthritis, brain disorders, depression, and the like
- Resolving other difficulties or barriers in life by converting them into the useful blessings that they really are

Note: The benefits of Sacred Santémony become amplified when combined with the viewing of Ener-Chi Art pictures. While there is no CD of the Sacred Santémony, since I was unable to source and create the high quality reproduction values that I sought over the years, there is a radio interview which includes the Sacred Santémony sound healing chant. This is the only recording that is available (via YouTube link):

Michelle Skaletski-Boyd Interviews Andreas Moritz
Soul Felt Series interview with Michelle Skaletski-Boyd
Time: 1:33:01
http://www.youtube.com/user/enerchiTV/videos?query=Soul+F elt+Series+interview+with+Michelle+Skaletski-Boyd+

The Sacred Santémony chant is toward the end of the interview, at around 1 hour 25 minutes.

Fruit and Vegetable Therapies

By now, fruit is well-known for containing antioxidant compounds that can boost health and wellness with regular consumption. A few of these common favorites contain compounds that are especially helpful in healing cancer, including lemon and raspberry.

Lemon, a powerful antimicrobial and stress reliever, has long been one of alternative medicine's best kept secrets, and pharmaceutical companies are catching on. One of the world's largest drug manufacturers discovered that it destroys the malignant cells in 12 cancers, including colon, breast, prostate, lung and pancreatic. Lemon compounds proved 10,000 times more effective in destroying malignant cells than the chemo drug Adriamycin, and did so without harming healthy tissue. The industry's response to these findings, of course, is to create a synthetic version of lemon compounds that can be sold at exorbitant profits. Feel free to skip the middleman on this one.

Raspberry is another commonplace fruit that has proven to be a powerful remedy for cancer. In tests at Clemson University in South Carolina, researchers discovered that raspberry extracts successfully destroyed around 90 percent of stomach, colon and breast cancer cells. In addition to powerful antioxidants, they contain ellagic acid that can help treat a wide variety of different cancers, including skin, breast, esophageal, oral, bladder and lung cancer – even leukemia.

Another potent cancer therapy is found within the pits of **peaches, nectarines, plums** and **apricots**. Break open these large seeds and you will find an almond-shaped kernel inside. This kernel contains high concentrations of a naturally occurring chemical known most commonly as laetrile, amygdalin or vitamin B17. Research has shown that laetrile induces programmed cell death in cancer cells while leaving healthy ones intact – without the harmful side effects of chemotherapy. In keeping with their affinity for demonizing effective but relatively unprofitable cures for cancer, the FDA banned laetrile in 1971. Yet research has proven that laetrile is safe, and certainly much safer than toxic chemotherapy.

Likewise, certain vegetables contain particularly potent compounds that can help fight cancer: **asparagus, broccoli** and **cabbage**. Taking four tablespoons twice daily of pureed asparagus has been shown to cure symptoms of a number of cancers, including Hodgkin's disease, bladder cancer and lung cancer, even when traditional treatments were failing.

Broccoli is also well-known for its anticancer effects. It contains an enzyme known as myrosinase that activates broccoli's cancer-preventive and anti-inflammatory compound sulforaphane. It is necessary to cook the broccoli to unlock these components. However, overcooking broccoli can destroy this enzyme and prevent the body from utilizing these benefits. Researchers recommend gently steaming broccoli in order to maximize its effectiveness. They also suggested combining it with other sulforaphane-rich foods like mustard, radishes, arugula, wasabi and broccoli sprouts to maximize absorption.

Both **red and white cabbage** are also potent cruciferous vegetable cures for cancer. They contain a variety of powerful compounds known as anthocyanins that are known to prevent and treat cancer in humans. They also contain isothiocyanates, which help to hinder carcinogens inside the body and speed up their removal. This is in addition to the fact that they are already rich in beneficial antioxidants.

Graviola – More Effective Than Chemo

If you suffer from cancer and feel you need to have a specific treatment that is both natural and at least as effective as chemotherapy or radiation, you may wish to consider the use of the herbal remedy graviola. Graviola is a plant indigenous to most of the warmest tropical areas in South and North America, including the Amazon.

Scientists have been studying graviola's properties since the 1940s and discovered it has numerous active compounds and chemicals. Graviola has presented a large variety of benefits for many different ailments, one of which is cancer. Graviola contains a set of chemicals called *annonaceous acetogenins*. It makes these compounds in its leaves, stem, bark and fruit seeds. In a total of eight clinical studies, several independent research groups have confirmed that these chemicals have significant anti-tumor properties and selective toxicity against various types of cancer cells without harming healthy cells. Purdue University, in West Lafayette, Indiana, has conducted a great deal of research on these chemicals known asacetogenins, much of which has been funded by The National Cancer Institute (NCI) and/or the National Institutes of Health (NIH). Thus far, Purdue University and/or its staff have filed at least nine U.S. and/or international patents for their work on the anti-tumor and insecticidal properties and uses of these acetogenins.

One of America's billion-dollar drug companies attempted to produce an anticancer drug from graviola after it discovered that this compound was 10,000 times more toxic to colon cancer cells than a common chemo drug. It found graviola to be lethal to 12 different kinds of malignant cells, especially those that cause lung, prostate and breast cancers, and to be safe enough to protect healthy cells instead of killing them. With graviola, the patient experiences no nausea or hair loss, and no major weight loss or weakness. Rather than compromising the immune system, graviola actually strengthens it.

For seven years, this drug company tried to develop a synthetic patented prescription version of graviola's anticancer chemicals (it being against the law to patent natural compounds), but all attempts failed and the project was terminated. Instead of making their findings public, the researchers boxed up their results and put their research away for good. Eventually, though, the story leaked out and graviola is increasingly receiving the recognition it deserves among health professionals and researchers alike.

Many terminal cases of cancer have been reversed through the use of graviola, even in people 85 years or older. When cancerous tumors break up, the body may be flooded with poisons, causing the patient to feel quite weak. To minimize the intensity of the healing crisis, it is important to cleanse the colon every day, perhaps through such approaches as enemas, colemas or colosan. The kidneys should be supported by drinking the kidney cleanse tea. (For this kidney cleanse tea recipe, see *Timeless Secrets of Health & Rejuvenation* or *The Amazing Liver and Gallbladder Flush.*) If possible, the liver should be cleansed as well.

Please note: Graviola has cardio-depressant, vasodilator and hypotensive (lowers blood pressure) actions. The dosage should be increased gradually. Overly large dosages can cause nausea and vomiting. Use this treatment only when under the supervision of a health practitioner who understands its value, the above actions and its possible interaction with other drugs.

Master Mineral Solution (MMS)

All cancers have three things in common:

1. The immune system is weak and depleted.
2. The body is overwhelmed with toxins and waste matter.
3. There is a massive presence of pathogens (infecting agents) inside and around cancer cells. These may include parasites, viruses, bacteria, yeast and fungi.

One mineral substance − sodium chlorite − may have the most balanced and immediate effects on all these disease-causing factors. Apart from the topics already discussed, other important requirements for healing cancer and most illnesses, both serious and minor, include the following:

- Neutralize the toxins and poisons that weaken the immune system and feed or attract the pathogens.
- Strengthen the immune system to remove all pathogens and keep them at bay.
- While detoxifying, kill off all harmful parasites, viruses, bacteria, fungi, molds and yeast, and eliminate them from the body.

To be successful, all of these need to occur at the same time.

The product Master Mineral Solution (MMS) is a stabilized oxygen solution of 28 percent sodium chlorite (*not* sodium chloride, which is common salt) in distilled water. When a small amount of lemon juice, lime juice or citric acid solution is added to a few drops of MMS, chlorine dioxide is formed. Once ingested, the chlorine dioxide instantly oxidizes harmful substances such as parasites, bacteria, viruses, yeast, fungi and molds within a matter of hours, while boosting the immune system at least tenfold. By doing so, MMS has removed, for example, any strands of the malaria and HIV viruses from the blood within less than 48 hours in nearly every person tested. MMS has also been used successfully for many other serious illnesses, including Hepatitis A, B & C, typhoid, most cancers, herpes, pneumonia, food poisoning, tuberculosis, asthma and influenza.

The following is a quote from a book by Jim Humble, the discoverer of MMS and the *author* of the book, *Breakthrough . . . The Miracle Mineral Solution of the 21st Century:*

"While first developed to address Malaria in Africa, it has now been shown to address any disease condition that is directly or indirectly related to pathogens. There is documentation of over 75,000 cases of Malaria being overcome in Africa. Often in as little as 4 hours, all symptoms are gone, and the patient is tested clear of Malaria. It is now known that MMS can be used to overcome the symptoms of AIDS, Hepatitis A, B & C, Typhoid, most cancers, herpes, pneumonia, food poisoning, tuberculosis, asthma, colds, flu and a host of other conditions. Even conditions not directly related to pathogens seem to be helped due to the huge boost to the body's immune system, for example, macular degeneration, allergies, lupus, inflammatory bowel disorders, diabetes, snake bites, abscessed teeth and fibromyalgia. Please note that MMS doesn't cure anything, but rather it allows our body to heal itself. Notice how I carefully step around the words 'cure' and 'heal', even though that is what is really happening."

Humble says, "Separate tests conducted by the Malawi government produced 99% cure results for malaria. Over 60% of AIDS victims treated with MMS in Uganda were well in 3 days, with 98% well within one month. More than 90% of the malaria victims were well in 4 to 8 hours. Dozens of other diseases were successfully treated and can be controlled with this new mineral supplement."

The inventor believes that this information is too important to the world for any one person or group to control. The free ebook download gives complete details of this discovery. Please help to ensure that it gets to the world free. Many medical breakthroughs have been suppressed, and this invention must not be added to that list. The name of the ebook is *The Miracle Mineral Solution of the 21st Century.*[90] You can download Part One of the book free of charge at www.miraclemineral.org, or ask a friend to download and print it for you if you don't have a computer. Jim Humble's book tells the story of the discovery and how to make and use it. I recommend that every person read this book. Jim has no personal, vested interest in making MMS available to the world. Rather, he wants to use his discovery to end disease and poverty.

Ojibwa Herb Tea – 8-Herb Essiac

One Remedy for Many Ailments

Ojibwa Indian herb tea is a 280 year old Native American Indian root and herb tea remedy that was made in the 1700s by the Ojibwa Indian medicine society. Ojibwa people used it to survive a smallpox genocide started by the early European settlers.

Native Americans have since used the tea formula to cure all types of cancers, type 1 and type 2 diabetes, liver infections and other liver/gallbladder conditions, tumors, arthritis, gout, asthma and other respiratory ailments, obesity, high blood pressure, elevated cholesterol, fibromyalgia and chronic fatigue syndrome, ulcers, irritable bowel syndrome (IBS), kidney and bladder disorders, sinus congestion, influenza (flu) and chest colds, measles, mumps, chicken pox, smallpox, herpes, diarrhea, constipation, lymphedema (fluid retention), heart disease, allergies, skin diseases, auto immune diseases such as lupus and AIDS, Lyme disease, addiction to substances such as alcohol, drugs and tobacco, clinical depression and much more.

8-herb Essiac contains the following ingredients:

Blessed Thistle is used for digestive problems such as gas, constipation and an upset stomach. This herb is also used to treat liver and gallbladder diseases.

---

[90] Editor's note: The new title is *The Master Mineral Solution of the 3rd Millennium (2011)*, an update to Jim Humble's first book, *The Miracle Mineral Solution of the 21st Century.*

Burdock Root is a mild diuretic. It increases the production of both urine and sweat, potentially making it useful for treating swelling and fever. Burdock root might play a role in preventing liver damage caused by alcohol, chemicals or medications. The exact reason for this protective effect is not known, but it is thought to involve opposition to a chemical process called oxidation, which occurs in the body as a natural function of metabolism. Although oxidation is a natural process, it does not mean that it is *not* harmful to the body! One result of oxidation is the release of oxygen free radicals, which are chemicals that may suppress immune function. Antioxidants such as burdock root may protect body cells from damage caused by oxidation.

Kelp is a sea vegetable that is a concentrated source of minerals, including iodine, potassium, magnesium, calcium and iron. Kelp as a source of iodine assists in making the thyroid hormones, which are necessary for maintaining normal metabolism in all cells of the body. This increases energy levels and makes it easier to maintain a healthy body weight. Kelp is the most nutrient-dense of all the Native Ojibwa tea ingredients – and it is found in the 4-herb formulas of the tea.

Red Clover is a source of many valuable nutrients, including calcium, chromium, magnesium, niacin, phosphorus, potassium, thiamine and vitamin C. Red clover is also one of the richest sources of isoflavones (water-soluble chemicals that act like estrogens and are found in many plants). The isoflavones found in red clover have been studied for their effectiveness in treating some forms of cancer. It is thought that the isoflavones prevent the proliferation of cancer cells and may even destroy them.

Sheep Sorrel is a rich source of oxalic acid, sodium, potassium, iron, manganese, phosphorous, beta carotene and vitamin C. This Native Ojibwa tea ingredient is a mild diuretic, mild antiseptic and mild laxative.

Slippery Elm Bark has been used as a poultice for cuts and bruises. It is also useful for aching joints due to gout or other conditions. Besides being a Native American tea ingredient, this herb is often used to alleviate sore throats. Slippery elm bark is found in many lozenges that claim to soothe throat irritation. Since a sore throat and a cough are often linked, slippery elm bark has also been used in cough remedies. Furthermore, it regulates the elimination phase of the digestive process, easing both constipation and diarrhea.

Turkish Rhubarb Root is a detoxifying herb that is world-famous for its healing properties. Rhubarb root purges the body of bile, parasites and putrefying food in the stomach by stimulating the gall duct to expel toxic waste matter. It alleviates chronic liver problems by cleansing the liver. Rhubarb root improves digestion and helps regulate the appetite. It has also helped to heal ulcers, alleviate disorders of the spleen and colon, relieve constipation and heal hemorrhoids and bleeding in the upper digestive tract.

Watercress is high in vitamin C, and is used as a general tonic. Its bitter taste is thought to regulate appetite and improve digestion. It can be used to alleviate nervous conditions, constipation and liver disorders. Watercress is a popular remedy for cough and bronchitis. It contains a remarkable substance called rhein, which appears to inhibit the growth of pathogenic bacteria in the intestines. It is believed that rhein is also effective against Candida Albicans (yeast infection), fever and inflammation, and pain.

Note: As with other sources of food and remedies that contain soluble fiber, such as slippery elm bark, Ojibwa tea can interfere with the absorption of other medicines within the gut if they are taken at the same time. Because of this, take prescription medications at an alternate time to consuming this tea.

Where to find it: One company sells this tea formula under the name Essiac tea at http://www.premium-essiac-tea-4less.com. **For those who wish to purchase these herbs separately, the exact ratio of the herbs is available at** http://www.biznet1.com/p2699.htm. **This site also sells the Ojibwa tea in larger quantities.**

The Bicarbonate Maple Syrup Treatment

As I have explained earlier, cancer cells can only operate in an acidic and oxygen-deprived environment. Since they are anaerobic by nature, they cannot use oxygen to metabolize glucose (sugar) and produce energy; instead, they have to ferment it. Compared with aerobic cells, which use oxygen and glucose to produce energy, cancer cells require about 15 times the amount of glucose as healthy cells to generate the same amount of metabolic energy. The cancer cells' excessive hunger for glucose robs other healthy cells of this vital nutrient, thereby causing them to become weak, die or also mutate into cancer cells. The starvation or weakening of healthy cells caused by the cancer cells' incessant draining of nutrients from the tissue fluids greatly diminishes the affected organ's glucose and energy reserves. This is the main reason behind the failure of organs associated with cancer.

Although sugar intake strongly stimulates cancer cell growth, the combination of baking soda (sodium bicarbonate) and maple syrup has the exact opposite effect; it makes it actually very difficult for cancer cells to function and survive.

To prepare this simple, inexpensive but powerful remedy, combine 5 parts of 100% pure maple syrup (ideally B-grade), with 1 part of pure baking soda (with no added aluminum!).[91] Place the mixture in a saucepan and heat it on a medium flame for five minutes. Stir briskly. The mixture will greatly spread out and become foamy. Store in a cool place and take one teaspoon twice daily. For very serious conditions, take one teaspoon three times a day. Take uninterruptedly for at least 7–8 days, which is often sufficient to collapse tumors of the size 1–2 inches. You may experience a strong die-off, consisting of dead cancer cells, bacteria and toxins, usually expelled via the intestinal tract. Don't be concerned if diarrhea occurs. This is the body's way of relieving itself of the acid burden that's behind the cancer. Other seemingly unrelated health conditions may improve, too.

The maple syrup is capable of transporting bicarbonate into all parts of the body, including the brain and nervous system, bones, teeth, joints, eyes and solid tumors. It may also help with other conditions of acidosis. Sodium bicarbonate therapy is harmless and so quick-acting because it is extremely diffusible.

The greatest advocate of sodium bicarbonate as a cancer therapy is the prominent oncologist Dr. Tullio Simoncini in Rome, Italy. The basic concept of his therapy consists of administering a solution of sodium bicarbonate directly into tumors. He believes that cancer is a fungus which can be destroyed by direct exposure to sodium bicarbonate.

Dr. Simoncini is certainly correct about fungus playing a major role in nearly all cancers. There are over 1.5 million different species of fungus. One of them is Candida Albicans which grows in the intestinal tract to

---

[91] Bob's Red Mill or other brands state 'aluminum-free' on their labels.

help ferment undigested sugars or starches. This intestinal yeast can spread to other parts of the body and set up colonies wherever the need for decomposing organic waste arises.

Certain fungi, in particular *white rot* fungi, can degrade insecticides, herbicides, pentachlorophenol, creosote, coal tars and heavy fuels, and turn them into carbon dioxide, water and basic elements. Fungi occur in every environment on Earth and play very important roles in most ecosystems, including the internal ecosystem of the body. Along with bacteria, fungi are the major decomposers in most terrestrial and some aquatic ecosystems. As decomposers, they play an indispensable role in nutrient cycling, especially as saprotrophs and symbionts, degrading organic matter to inorganic molecules. They become essential when the body accumulates organic waste matter, heavy metals and chemical compounds.[92] They will also turn up when cells decay or die, and may not be readily removed via the body's lymphatic system. Congested lymphatic ducts almost always cause fungal proliferations in the cells and tissues of organs. The fungi that grow in the tissues of organs always show up as a white mass. That's why cancerous tumors are always white (although on scanning images they show up as dark masses or shadows).

While doing their precious job, fungi produce compounds with biological activity. Several of these compounds are toxic and are therefore called mycotoxins, referring to their fungal origin and toxic activity. Particularly infamous are the aflatoxins, which are insidious liver toxins and highly carcinogenic metabolites. In other words, the fungal toxins can damage cells and cause them to mutate into cancer cells. In essence, fungi grow inside and outside polluted tissue to feed on the harmful toxins and chemicals. But they also produce poisons which can further damage cells and cause them to mutate. Thus, while the fungal activity helps remove the causes of the original cancer (toxins), the poisons that the fungi produce contribute to the cancer's proliferation.

---

[92] When compared with healthy tissue, cancer tissue contains a much higher concentration of toxic chemicals, pesticides and heavy metals. In 1973, a study conducted by the Department of Occupational Health at Hebrew University-Hadassah Medical School in Jerusalem found a significantly higher concentration of such toxic compounds as DDT and PCBs in cancerous breast tissue of women, compared with the normal breast and adjacent adipose tissue in the same women.

Bicarbonate of soda can bind to and remove toxins, chemicals and organic acidic waste matter, and quickly raises the pH of cancer cells and their environment. The extracellular pH of solid tumors is significantly more acidic compared to normal tissues. By altering the pH of a tumor, it becomes exposed to more oxygen, which can cause its destruction.

To get as close as possible to the tumor tissue, Dr. Simoncini places a small catheter directly into the artery that nourishes the tumor, and administers high doses of sodium bicarbonate to the deepest recesses of the tumor. He claims that most tumors treated in this way will break up within several days, similar to the maple syrup bicarbonate treatment.

Organic Sulfur Crystals

Another therapy that has proven successful in treating cancer is the consumption of organic sulfur crystals. The idea was discovered by a researcher who was diagnosed with terminal testicular cancer. Unwilling to give up, he started taking one tablespoon of these crystals twice a day. The results were startling. Because sulfur crystals produce oxygen, they were essentially able to aerate the body, creating an aerobic environment in the body and destroying anaerobic cancer cells.

A 2006 study done at the University of Southampton in the U.K. also demonstrated that, in addition to their cancer-fighting benefits, organic sulfur crystals produce all essential amino acids, including highly beneficial omega-3 fatty acids and B vitamins. Diabetes patients who tried them reported at least a 20 percent reduction in their insulin requirements – some were able to eliminate their need for insulin entirely. They also proved effective in treating high blood pressure and depression.

Over 70,000 people have participated in the ongoing 12-year study testing organic sulfur crystals, and except for the initial discomfort of the body's detoxification process, there have been no complaints of side effects. (For more information on Organic Sulfur Crystals, see http://www.ener-chi.com/wellness-products/organic-sulfur-crystals/.)

Thermotherapy

In the 19th century, a doctor noticed that patients who got high fevers from other infections (such as scarlet fever) often were cured of their cancer. This simple observation that cancer cells cannot tolerate heat has developed into a form of cancer treatment known as hyperthermia or thermotherapy, which destroys cancer cells without harming healthy tissue.

During the treatment, the patient's body temperature is slowly raised to about 105 degrees Fahrenheit, approximating a high fever. This temperature is maintained for two hours while doctors carefully monitor the patient's vitals and ensure hydration. This kills cancer cells by the millions, and any left are so weak that simple vitamin therapy, such as vitamin C, can finish them off. This type of therapy is effective, safe and painless – unlike chemo and radiation, which as we know have a slew of deadly side effects.

Ashwagandha – An Ayurvedic Cure

Researchers at Emory University have found that a plant compound commonly used by Ayurveda practitioners can prevent breast cancer cell metastasis. This compound is known as Withaferin A and derives from the roots of *withania somnifera*, also known as *ashwagandha*, Indian ginseng or winter cherry. The plant is a short shrub in the nightshade family which produces small green flowers and orange-red fruit. It has been used in India for medicinal purposes for thousands of years. Researchers in the study were successful in using it to prevent the spread of breast cancer.

Marine Phytoplankton – Nature's Ultimate Superfood

Marine phytoplankton is considered to be one of the most powerful foods on Earth because it is loaded with high-energy super anti-oxidants, vitamins, minerals and proteins in microscopic form. It is a tiny little plant (about the size of a red blood cell) that naturally grows in the ocean and is the beginning of the food chain, whereas all other living creatures in the ocean feed on other living things that feed on this little plant. It is responsible for over 70 percent of the planet's oxygen and, because of its unique nutritional properties and microscopic size, is believed to penetrate the cellular level of the body, thereby enabling fast nutritional support to all the body's organs and systems.

By strengthening the cells directly, phytoplankton's nutrients can help restore health and vitality in the entire body. Ultimately, cancer and other disorders occur when nutrients are missing on the cellular level. Since phytoplankton contains nearly all nutrients that exist on the planet, and delivery of these nutrients does not depend on the efficiency of the digestive system, this superfood may quickly provide whatever the body may be missing.

Other Useful Cancer Therapies

Dozens of other natural cancer therapies have helped millions of people regain their health, without aggressive medical intervention. Although this book's purpose is to reveal the true causes of cancer and how to address them, I also wish to acknowledge the great potential benefits that these natural cancer remedies have. I have already described some of them in more detail, but this in no way diminishes the value of others. These include:

- Ayurveda's Pancha Karma treatment and herbal remedies
- Ayurvedic massage and meditation
- Massage
- Art therapy
- Music therapy
- Dance therapy
- Yoga
- Physical exercise, ideally in natural light
- The Coley Vaccine
- The Camphor Therapy of Gaston Naessens
- Burton's Immuno-augmentative therapy
- Livingston therapy
- Issels' Whole Body therapy
- Metabolic therapy by Hans Nieper, M.D.
- Live Cell therapy
- Chelation therapy
- Hyperthermia

- Regular exposure to sunlight, without using sunscreens
- Hypnosis
- Biofeedback
- Hydrazine Sulfate
- Antineoplaston therapy by Dr. Bursynski
- Acupuncture
- Bioelectric therapy
- Bioresonance therapy
- Royal Rife Machine therapy
- Gerson therapy
- Hoxsey therapy
- Hemp oil
- Therapies using Iscador (Mistletoe), Pau d'Arco, Chaparral, Aloe Vera, Graviola
- DMSO therapy
- The Cesium Chloride Protocol
- Oleander Treatment (oleander plant)
- Intravenous Hydrogen Peroxide
- IP6
- Dr. Simoncini's Baking Soda treatment
- Homeopathy
- Edgar Cayce's Castor Oil Packs
- Dr. Budwig Diet
- Dr. Clark's Parasite/Cancer treatments
- Moerman's Anticancer Diet
- Red Clover Tea[93]
- Zeolite
- and more….

It's important to point out that alternative cancer therapies would appear a lot more successful than they are if patients didn't use them as a last resort, after all other approaches have failed. Unfortunately, almost every person diagnosed with cancer picks the mainstream medical approach. Most cancer patients believe that the doctor-prescribed orthodox treatments offer them a 40 percent chance of *beating that thing*. However, the true likelihood of surviving the cancer and, more importantly, the cancer treatment, is actually less than 3 percent.[94] And there is no guarantee for the 3 percent who survive that

---

[93] Although red clover's anticancer effects are anecdotal, they are being confirmed as a traditional cancer remedy. Women with breast cancer were able to stop cancer growth by drinking red clover tea in place of water. Take one cup of clover herb and place it in one gallon of boiling water; allow it to seep for 20 minutes, strain and refrigerate. Drink 6–8 glasses (8 oz.) per day, at room temperature or warm.

[94] This is the average 5-year survival rate for all medically treated cancers. It may be higher or lower, given the type of cancer. It excludes the millions of non-fatal skin cancers which the orthodox medical system conveniently includes in their statistical calculations to boost their success rate.

they will not suffer from a new bout of cancer or a different, equally debilitating illness in the future.

The side effects resulting from orthodox cancer therapy are so severe that those surviving cancer patients then choosing alternative cancer treatments are often disappointed that the new, natural treatments just *didn't work*. The problem is that over 95 percent of cancer patients seeking help from natural cancer therapies have already been given up by orthodox medicine. In other words, the medical treatment has destroyed their body to a point that healing is very difficult to achieve. Their immune system is severely compromised, liver functions have been impaired, and the digestive system is too weak to make proper use of the food they eat. Unless a potent alternative therapy includes restoring these important parts and functions, the chances of it bringing about a complete cure are indeed slim. The true cure rate using natural approaches could exceed 90 percent if the body's key healing systems weren't severely damaged or destroyed by previously administered medical treatments. The less damage these treatments have caused, the stronger is the likelihood of recovery.

While I bring the above-listed alternative, natural approaches to your attention, I also wish to recommend that you don't lose sight of the true nature, origins and progressive stages of cancer and general illness, as described in this and my other books, *The Amazing Liver and Gallbladder Flush* and *Timeless Secrets of Health & Rejuvenation*.

It is easy to become so overwhelmed by the physical appearance and reality of a cancerous tumor that you may impatiently focus on finding a *cure* and forsake attending to the ultimate, less obvious causes of cancer. The cancerous tumor already is the body's attempt at curing the real cancer – toxicity. The intention to combat cancer, even with such relatively natural methods as listed above, is similar to trying to enforce peace by waging a war. But we all know that this strategy rarely works. If you choose one or more of these methods, make certain you don't use them with the intention to kill something, especially a tumor. Any of these approaches may or may not be useful in supporting the body to heal, but you must never forget that, ultimately, the healing is done in the body and by the body, and is especially determined by what is going on in your heart and mind.

The intention behind your decision is more powerful than what you choose as your therapeutic tool. If fear motivates your decision-making, you may be better off taking no action at all until you can face, embrace and transform that fear into trust and confidence. Fear has a paralyzing effect and undermines the body's ability to heal. It is well-known that the body cannot heal well when it is under stress. Stress hormones suppress digestive functions, eliminative functions, the immune system and blood circulation to vital organs. Perceiving a cancer as a threat to your life makes it stressful. Perceiving it as a healing attempt by the body, or a solution to an underlying unresolved conflict, gives it meaning and purpose, and, therefore, it will not invoke a stress response.

Eventually, there will come a time when you no longer perceive the lump in your chest or the tumor in your colon or brain as a problem, but as an essential part of the solution to a deeper unresolved issue in your life – an issue that may have been buried so deep inside you that you weren't even aware of it. Cancer can bring to the surface what was concealed for a long time and allow you to make peace with it, accept it and even embrace it. A lump in the breast or a tumor in the brain is merely a manifestation of resistance – resistance against yourself, against others, or against situations and circumstances. When it no longer matters to you whether a lump is getting bigger or smaller, you will practically stop feeding it with your energies.

Healing occurs when there is no more need to fix what you believe is broken. The need to fix it still reflects an incomplete perception or acceptance of yourself, based on the fear of not being good enough, strong enough, or deserving enough. The lump or tumor helps you to be in touch with that insecurity and vulnerability, and transform these into courage and confidence. It challenges you to live happily and enjoy your life even with the cancer. When you have risen to meet this challenge, which is achieved through simple acceptance of its deeper meaning and purpose, the need for the cancer will be gone along with the insecurity.

To repeat, the lump or tumor is not the problem. What is important is how you react to it. If you could live with it comfortably and without much concern or wanting to kill it off, you are close to experiencing a spontaneous remission. The size of a tumor is quite irrelevant. In fact, it can increase in size when it is healing, due to increased lymphocyte activity. And then it may vanish quickly. I once saw a bladder tumor displayed live on an ultrasound screen. It was the size of a grapefruit, and it completely disintegrated and disappeared within 15 seconds. This was during a sound-energy healing session by a group of Chinese Qigong masters.

Know that the body is always on your side, and never against you, however bad the situation may appear to be. In fact, nothing in your life is ever against you; even pain is a way of breaking your resistance to what is actually good for you, but you cannot yet see it that way. You can learn from everything that happens to you, including cancer.

In any case, it is far more important to identify and address whatever prevents the body from healing or, rather, to supply whatever helps it to feel whole and vital, than to fix the symptomatic appearance of a cancer.

Summary and Concluding Remarks

Healing the Ultimate Cause

My intention in writing this book was to offer an alternative view of what cancer is, one that reflects the intelligence and purpose of nature's laws. Important and commonsense reasons govern the constructive forces of natural law; the same is true of natural law's destructive forces. If it were otherwise, growth would not occur, and the universe as we know it would have vanished long ago. Everything has meaning, regardless of how meaningless it may appear to be.

An apple, for example, can only grow (constructive force of natural law) after the blossom that precedes it has been destroyed (destructive force of natural law). **He who finds purpose and meaning in the occurrence of a cancer will also find the way to cure it.** That is the promise of this book. It is a matter of tracing a cancer back to its origins – the various layers of preceding causes and effects.

The ultimate cause of cancer is *fear* – fear of not being good enough, fear of loss, fear of being hurt, fear of hurting others, fear of loving, fear of not loving enough, fear of disappointment, fear of success, fear of failure, fear of dying, fear of food, fear of being disappointed, and fear of life and existence. Each of these fears is but an offspring of fear of the unknown.

The fear of the unknown is not a tangible thing that you can just get rid of by deciding to. More often than not, you manifest what you are afraid of. Negative expectations are self-fulfilling prophecies. When these prophecies or expectations become fulfilled, it may give you the idea that they would have occurred anyway, as if you had no choice. Yet, you always have a choice. You are never a victim of anything or anyone, even it feels that way, which is the point. You can only be a victim when you feel like one. Although we often create what we fear through subconscious programming, we can just as easily change the program and create what we love.

291

To heal cancer, you must first know deep within yourself that your body does not have the ability to do you any harm. Therefore, you need not be afraid of it. Through the eyes of acceptance, you will be capable of seeing any negative situation in life, such as the occurrence of a cancerous tumor, in a positive light.[95] This inner transformation of perspective immediately dispels the fear of the unknown. Once you accept an injury or an illness as something that can benefit you, e.g., strengthen you in an area of your life where you have felt weak, incompetent or anxious before, you will start connecting with it. This connection with the *problem* then allows your energy and emotion to flow into it and release the emotional barriers to spontaneous healing.

As mentioned before, healing cannot occur when the life force is absent. Life force is unavailable when you are *absent*, when you separate yourself from the body and its predicament or illness. You do this when you perceive or imagine it to be turning against you, or even trying to kill you. Whenever you are afraid of the body, you will try either to protect yourself from it or fight against it. In either case, this strong feeling of being alienated from the body sucks the life force out of every cell. Your cells go into protection or fighting mode, commonly known as the fight-or-flight response; hence, their life force energy is wasted, which prevents them from growing, healing and regenerating themselves.

Tumors of any kind are direct manifestations of fear. Fear is synonymous with separation and defensiveness. Cancer cells do not like what they have become, but your resistance to them keeps them in that state. They heal spontaneously when your resistance disappears and you are able to replace this attitude with one of acceptance and, yes, love. When you consciously accept and embrace what or whom you resist in your life (what or whom you resist is merely a mirror image of yourself),[96] you will not only lose the fear, but also your body's cells can return to their natural, balanced growth mode.

---

[95] To develop this ability, see *Lifting the Veil of Duality – Your Guide to Living Without Judgment.*
[96] For details, see *Lifting the Veil of Duality – Your Guide to Living Without Judgment.*

Balanced growth always results in homeostasis or health. Cleansing, pampering and nourishing the body are acts of accepting responsibility for what is happening to you, and they return to you true ownership of your body. Taking your power back where it belongs and letting go of external crutches like suppressive drugs, aggressive treatments, surgery, etc., is essential for healing yourself – healing your body, mind and emotions.

The power of thoughts, feelings and emotions is many times stronger than any physical influence can be. Yes, you may have a tumor in your breast or in your brain, but you are still more powerful and influential than the tumor is. In fact, your own energy of fear or resistance has created it and sustains it.

In the same way you feed the tumor, your energy of love and acceptance can crumble its foundation and undo it. Do not fall into the trap of believing the body is causing you problems that you cannot heal. The theory that cancer is a life-threatening disease that has a separate power or agenda other than your own is just an acquired belief. And yet beliefs shape reality. The body does not have the power to cause you any ailments; on the contrary, it is ever vigilant to resolve them in the best possible way it can.

You are the creator of your circumstances. It is for you to decide every morning when you wake up whether to spend the day recounting the difficulties you have with the parts of your body that no longer work properly, or to be thankful for the ones that do. The same applies to every other problem in your life. It is within your power to choose between watering the roots of a withering plant or lamenting over its falling leaves.

You can do much in terms of self-healing that you may never have thought of before. Show your body that you are not afraid of it. Place both hands over your *dis-eased* organ or gland. Thank the cancer cells for the precious work they have done for you. Give thanks to all the cells that have managed to keep you alive, despite the toxins and congestion that have impeded their work. Infuse them with the life force that is inside you by appreciating them and accepting them back into your awareness and presence.

The DNA of your cells can hear you just as well as you can hear someone speaking to you. The body primarily runs by vibration. Expressing gratitude to the cells of your body, and for the challenges and blessings life presents you with, acts as one of the most powerful vibrations you can produce. The energy of "thank you" actually reconnects you with whatever you have separated yourself from. This makes gratitude the major secret and prerequisite for healing to occur.

With a renewed, more loving and compassionate attitude toward your cancer cells – remember, they are still your body's cells – you can truly start healing the physical and non-physical causes of cancer. You, yourself, will become living proof that **cancer is not a disease.**

WISHING you PERFECT HEALTH, ABUNDANCE AND HAPPINESS !

Andreas Moritz

References, Links and Resources

References

Anderson, J. W., J. E. Blake, et al. (1998). "Effects of soy protein on renal function and proteinuria in patients with type 2 diabetes." Am J Clin Nutr 68(6 Suppl): 1347S-1353S.

Anderson, J. W., B. M. Johnstone, et al. (1995). "Meta-analysis of the effects of soy protein intake on serum lipids." N Engl J Med 333(5): 276-82.

Arjmandi, B. H., R. Birnbaum, et al. (1998). "Bone-sparing effect of soy protein in ovarian hormone-deficient rats is related to its isoflavone content." Am J Clin Nutr 68(6 Suppl): 1364S-1368S.

Baird, D. D., D. M. Umbach, et al. (1995). "Dietary intervention study to assess estrogenicity of dietary soy among postmenopausal women." J Clin Endocrinol Metab 80(5): 1685-90.

Bloedon, L. T., A. R. Jeffcoat, et al. (2002). "Safety and pharmacokinetics of purified soy isoflavones: single-dose administration to postmenopausal women." Am J Clin Nutr 76(5): 1126-37.

Brown, N. M. and K. D. Setchell (2001). "Animal models impacted by phytoestrogens in commercial chow: implications for pathways influenced by hormones." Lab Invest 81(5): 735-47.

Cassidy, A., S. Bingham, et al. (1995). "Biological effects of isoflavones in young women: importance of the chemical composition of soyabean products." Br J Nutr 74(4): 587-601.

Chiang, C. E., S. A. Chen, et al. (1996). "Genistein directly inhibits L-type calcium currents but potentiates cAMP-dependent chloride currents in cardiomyocytes." Biochem Biophys Res Commun 223(3): 598-603.

Cook, J. D., T. A. Morck, et al. (1981). "The inhibitory effect of soy products on nonheme iron absorption in man." Am J Clin Nutr 34(12): 2622-9.

Divi, R. L., H. C. Chang, et al. (1997). "Anti-thyroid isoflavones from soybean: isolation, characterization, and mechanisms of action." Biochem Pharmacol 54(10): 1087-96.

Freni-Titulaer, L. W., J. F. Cordero, et al. (1986)."Premature thelarche in Puerto Rico.A search for environmental factors." Am J Dis Child 140(12): 1263-7.

Gumbmann, M. R., W. L. Spangler, et al. (1986). "Safety of trypsin inhibitors in the diet: effects on the rat pancreas of long-term feeding of soy flour and soy protein isolate." Adv Exp Med Biol 199: 33-79.

Kennedy, A. R. (1998). "The Bowman-Birk inhibitor from soybeans as an anticarcinogenic agent." Am J Clin Nutr 68(6 Suppl): 1406S-1412S.

Khalil, D. A., E. A. Lucas, et al. (2002). "Soy protein supplementation increases serum insulin-like growth factor-I in young and old men but does not affect markers of bone metabolism." J Nutr 132(9): 2605-8.

Maake, C., H. Yamamoto, et al. (1997). "The growth hormone dependent serine protease inhibitor, Spi 2.1 inhibits the des (1-3) insulin-like growth factor-I generating protease." Endocrinology 138(12): 5630-6.

Morton, M. S., O. Arisaka, et al. (2002). "Phytoestrogen concentrations in serum from Japanese men and women over forty years of age." J Nutr 132(10): 3168-71.

Pagliacci, M. C., M. Smacchia, et al. (1994). "Growth-inhibitory effects of the natural phyto-oestrogen genistein in MCF-7 human breast cancer cells." Eur J Cancer 30A(11): 1675-82.

Paillart, C., E. Carlier, et al. (1997). "Direct block of voltage-sensitive sodium channels by genistein, a tyrosine kinase inhibitor." J Pharmacol Exp Ther 280(2): 521-6.

Picherit, C., C. Bennetau-Pelissero, et al. (2001). "Soybean isoflavones dose-dependently reduce bone turnover but do not reverse established osteopenia in adult ovariectomized rats." J Nutr 131(3): 723-8.

Santen, R. J., J. V. Pinkerton, et al. (2002). "Treatment of urogenital atrophy with low-dose estradiol: preliminary results." Menopause 9(3): 179-87.

Scheiber, M. D., J. H. Liu, et al. (2001). "Dietary inclusion of whole soy foods results in significant reductions in clinical risk factors for osteoporosis and cardiovascular disease in normal postmenopausal women." Menopause 8(5): 384-92.

Seiberg, M., J. C. Liu, et al. (2001). "Soymilk reduces hair growth and hair follicle dimensions." Exp Dermatol 10(6): 405-13.

Setchell, K. D. (1998). "Phytoestrogens: the biochemistry, physiology, and implications for human health of soy isoflavones." Am J Clin Nutr 68(6 Suppl): 1333S-1346S.

Setchell, K. D. (2001). "Soy isoflavones--benefits and risks from nature's selective estrogen receptor modulators (SERMs)." J Am Coll Nutr 20(5 Suppl): 354S-362S; discussion 381S-383S.

Setchell, K. D., S. J. Gosselin, et al. (1987). "Dietary estrogens--a probable cause of infertility and liver disease in captive cheetahs." Gastroenterology 93(2): 225-33.

Shulman, K. I. and S. E. Walker (1999)."Refining the MAOI diet: tyramine content of pizzas and soy products." J Clin Psychiatry 60(3): 191-3.

Su, S. J., T. M. Yeh, et al. (2000). "The potential of soybean foods as a chemoprevention approach for human urinary tract cancer." Clin Cancer Res 6(1): 230-6.

Wangen, K. E., A. M. Duncan, et al. (2000). "Effects of soy isoflavones on markers of bone turnover in premenopausal and postmenopausal women." J Clin Endocrinol Metab 85(9): 3043-8.

Links and Resources

Introduction

CNN Health June 6, 2012

http://articles.mercola.com/sites/articles/archive/2012/06/13/keep-young-girls-away-from-xrays-as-new-study-shows-them-to-increase-breast-cancer-risk.aspx?e_cid=20120609_DNL_artTest_A1

http://www.naturalnews.com/036137_CT_scans_brain_cancer_children.html#ixzz2wtJw17Hc

Chapter One

http://www.naturalnews.com/032700_National_Cancer_Institute_Dr_Samuel_Epstein.html#ixzz1PHz
GApM3

http://articles.mercola.com/sites/articles/archive/2011/10/15/mayo-clinic-finds-massive-fraud-in-cancer-research.aspx

http://articles.mercola.com/sites/articles/archive/2011/10/21/seeing-red-over-pink-the-dark-side-of-breast-cancer-awareness-month.aspx

http://earcommunity.com/microtiaatresia/more/cat-scan-information/cat-scan-articles/?ak_action=reject_mobile

http://jama.ama-assn.org/

http://www.naturalnews.com/032577_genetic_testing_disease.html#ixzz1O4BMMKaF

http://www.medicalnewstoday.com/articles/243962.php

http://www.naturalnews.com/031230_cough_medicines_infants.html#ixzz1DHezD1A5

http://www.naturalnews.com/031596_cough_medicines_FDA.html#ixzz1G3hDgobv

http://www.naturalnews.com/032067_chemotherapy_murder.html

http://www.naturalnews.com/031354_vitamin_D_pregnancy.html#ixzz1E8SETh00

http://www.naturalnews.com/031250_vitamin_D_multiple_sclerosis.html#ixzz1DPw9bc4L

http://www.naturalnews.com/030598_vitamin_D_Institute_of_Medicine.html

http://www.naturalnews.com/031577_vitamin_D_scientific_research.html#ixzz1Fa7yUzHD

http://www.naturalnews.com/031

23_drugs_death_risk.html#ixzz1DEAHPYL4

http://www.naturalnews.com/031485_experimental_drugs_cancer.html#ixzz1EuwyVDcb

http://archive.wired.com/medtech/health/news/2004/03/62296?currentPage=all

http://www.dca.med.ualberta.ca/Home/Updates/2007-03-15_Update.cfm

http://pediatrics.aappublications.org/content/107/6/1241.abstract

http://www.ncbi.nlm.nih.gov/pubmed/16490323

http://www.ncbi.nlm.nih.gov/pmc/articles/PMC1742910/pdf/v079p00672.pdf

http://www.netdoktor.de/News/Freie-Radikale-Harmloser-al-1136130.html

Chapter Two

http://articles.mercola.com/sites/articles/archive/2011/03/30/the-war-on-cancer-a-progress-report-for-skeptics.aspx

http://www.naturalnews.com/025633_cancer_olive_oil_brst.html#ixzz1QZx7HuwX

http://www.naturalnews.com/031132_cholesterol_Alzheimers.html

http://articles.mercola.com/sites/articles/archive/2011/02/01/statins-raise-stroke-risk.aspx

http://www.naturalnews.com/032996_sunscreen_cancer_risk.html#ixzz1S7W6LwaZ

http://www.naturalnews.com/031448_colon_cancer_vitamin_D.html#ixzz1EvVdE4DK

http://www.naturalnews.com/031339_milkweed_sap_skin_cancer.html

http://www.naturalnews.com/032764_drugs_nutritional_deficiencies.html#ixzz1Pv3kqNcm

http://www.naturalnews.com/033511_melatonin_cancer.html#ixzz1XILlw6k8

http://www.naturalnews.com/031287_pharmacogenomics_medicine.html#ixzz1Dl7KxFYw

http://www.naturalnews.com/pancreatic_cancer.html

http://www.naturalnews.com/032414_acetaminophen_blood_cancer.html#ixzz1McVj6meS

Chapter Three

http://articles.mercola.com/sites/articles/archive/2011/05/18/how-properly-prescribed-prescription-drugs-ruined-a-famous-rock-super-star.aspx

http://www.naturalnews.com/032327_sugar_health.html#ixzz1Ls0QJZIB

Chapter Four

http://www.naturalnews.com/032018_prostate_cancer_surgery.html

http://www.naturalnews.com/033660_prostate_biopsy.html#ixzz1YlR6YvFm

http://www.naturalnews.com/030877_PSA_screening.html#ixzz19jeL2XKT

http://www.naturalnews.com/032953_nettle_root_prostate_health.html

http://www.naturalnews.com/031026_prostate_cancer_prevention.html#ixzz1BJEjCcTu

http://www.naturalnews.com/032436_coffee_prostate_cancer.html#ixzz1MirN0bpz

http://articles.mercola.com/sites/articles/archive/2012/01/09/x-ray-mammography-screenings-finding-cancers-not-there.aspx

Chapter Five

http://www.naturalnews.com/032732_styrofoam_chemicals.html#ixzz1PeiDYhBI

http://www.naturalnews.com/033821_BPA_chemicals.html

http://www.naturalnews.com/033818_canned_foods_BPA.html

http://www.naturalnews.com/033726_sodium_benzoate_cancer.html#ixzz1ZKlycODI

http://www.naturalnews.com/032793_sedentary_lifestyle_health_risks.html#ixzz1QD8y34jr

http://www.naturalnews.com/031113_vaccines_science.html

http://www.naturalnews.com/031313_swine_flu_vaccine_narcolepsy.html#ixzz1DqqkCDqa

http://www.naturalnews.com/031564_Jonas_Salk_medical_experiments.html

http://articles.mercola.com/sites/articles/archive/2011/06/20/uk-scraps-pneumonia-vaccines-because-they-dont-work.aspx

http://www.forbiddenknowledgetv.com/page/998.html

http://www.naturalnews.com/autism.html

http://www.naturalnews.com/measles.html

http://www.dailymail.co.uk/news/article-388051/Scientists-fear-MMR-link-autism.html#ixzz1Bajg4Fra

http://www.naturalnews.com/031173_vaccines_science.html#ixzz1CjXO6MXL

http://www.naturalnews.com/031274_babies_food_health.html#ixzz1Db6dhF9U

http://www.naturalnews.com/032405_diabetics_cancer.html#ixzz1MiImBhfY

http://diabetes.webmd.com/news/20110628/study-vitamin-d-may-cut-risk-of-diabetes

http://www.naturalnews.com/031087_night_lights_cancer.html#ixzz1BxBa541d

http://www.naturalnews.com/031929_microwaved_water_plants.html

http://www.cancer.org/cancer/cancercauses/othercarcinogens/intheworkplace/benzene

http://ezinearticles.com/?Why-Are-So-Many-People-Being-Diagnosed-With-Cancer?-Is-It-The-Cleaning-Products?&id=1135065

http://www.naturalnews.com/031372_diet_soda_stroke.html#ixzz1EFc11afs

http://articles.mercola.com/sites/articles/archive/2011/10/23/rgbh-in-milk-increases-risk-of-breast-cancer.aspx

http://articles.mercola.com/sites/articles/archive/2011/02/28/new-study-confirms-fructose-affects-your-brain-very-differently-than-glucose.aspx

http://articles.mercola.com/sites/articles/archive/2012/03/03/experts-say-avoid-mammograms.aspx

http://articles.mercola.com/sites/articles/archive/2011/07/12/for-every-woman-who-benefits-from-mammograms-ten-womens-lives-will-be-shortened.aspx

http://www.naturalnews.com/031628_mammograms_radiation.html

http://www.naturalnews.com/030992_MRI_scans_surgery.html#ixzz1AxF2hac5

http://www.sciencedaily.com/releases/2011/10/111004132532.htm

http://www.naturalnews.com/034190_MRIs_breast_cancer.html

Chapter Six

http://www.naturalnews.com/033764_fruits_and_vegetables_colon_cancer.html

http://www.ayurveda-cancer.org/cancerbysystem6.htm

http://www.naturalnews.com/032197_curcumin_cancer.html#ixzz1Kp3s5nv2

http://www.naturalnews.com/031367_colon_cancer_sleep.html#ixzz1EJJywWzz

http://www.naturalnews.com/032561_lifestyle_changes_patients.html#ixzz1Ny9WoySv

http://www.naturalnews.com/032010_plant-based_diet_cancer.html

http://www.naturalnews.com/031284_fruits_vegetables.html#ixzz1Dl8njiSG

http://www.naturalnews.com/033616_stroke_risk_foods.html#ixzz1YNziw9zV

http://www.naturalnews.com/034549_prostate_cancer_processed_meat_diet.html

http://fitness.mercola.com/sites/fitness/archive/2011/09/02/the-new-natural-wonder-drug-for-cancer.aspx

http://www.naturalnews.com/031272_cancer_raspberries_power.html#ixzz1Db8OJG6H

http://www.naturalnews.com/035554_laetrile_cancer_cure_cyanide.htmlCyanide fears

http://www.naturalnews.com/033123_laetrile_vitamin_B17.html#ixzz1T98SaGts

http://www.naturalnews.com/031498_broccoli_cancer.html#ixzz1EysznXUL

http://www.naturalnews.com/032377_cabbage_anti-cancer_food.html

http://www.naturalnews.com/031441_organic_sulfur_crystals.html#ixzz1EmZ3nn00

http://www.naturalnews.com/031169_thermotherapy_chemotherapy.html

http://www.naturalnews.com/032582_Ayurveda_breast_cancer.html#ixzz1O7uXkOme

Other Books and Products by Andreas Moritz

Timeless Secrets of Health & Rejuvenation
Breakthrough Medicine for the 21st Century

This book meets the increasing demand for a clear and comprehensive guide that can help people become self-sufficient regarding their health and well-being. It answers some of the most pressing questions of our time: How does illness arise? Who heals, and who doesn't? Are we destined to be sick? What causes aging? Is it reversible? What are the major causes of disease, and how can we eliminate them? What simple and effective practices can I incorporate into my daily routine that will dramatically improve my health?

Topics include: The placebo effect and the mind/body mystery; the laws of illness and health; the four most common risk factors for disease; digestive disorders and their effects on the rest of the body; the wonders of our biological rhythms and how to restore them if disrupted; how to create a life of balance; why to choose a vegetarian diet; cleansing the liver, gallbladder, kidneys, and colon; removing allergies; giving up smoking, naturally; using sunlight as medicine; the new causes of heart disease, cancer, diabetes, and AIDS; and a scrutinizing look at antibiotics, blood transfusions, ultrasound scans, and immunization programs.

Timeless Secrets of Health & Rejuvenation sheds light on all major issues of healthcare and reveals that most medical treatments, including surgery, blood transfusions, and pharmaceutical drugs, are avoidable when certain key functions in the body are restored through the natural methods described in the book. The reader also learns about the potential dangers of medical diagnosis and treatment, as well as the reasons why vitamin supplements, *health foods*, low-fat products, *wholesome* breakfast cereals, diet foods, and diet programs may have contributed to the current health crisis rather than helped to resolve it. The book includes a complete program of healthcare, which is primarily based on the ancient medical system of Ayurveda and the vast amount of experience Andreas Moritz has gained in the field of health restoration during the past 30 years.

The Amazing Liver and Gallbladder Flush
A Powerful Do-It-Yourself Tool to Optimize Your Health and Well-being

In this updated edition of his bestselling book, *The Amazing Liver Cleanse,* Andreas Moritz addresses the most common but rarely recognized cause of illness – gallstones congesting the liver. Although those who suffer an excruciatingly painful gallbladder attack are clearly aware of the stones congesting this vital organ, few people realize that hundreds if not thousands of gallstones (mainly clumps of hardened bile) have accumulated in their liver, often causing no pain or symptoms for decades. Most adults living in the industrialized world, and especially those suffering a chronic illness, such as heart disease, arthritis, MS, cancer or diabetes, have gallstones blocking the bile ducts of their liver. Furthermore, 20 million Americans suffer from gallbladder attacks every year. In many cases, treatment consists merely of removing the gallbladder, at the cost of $5 billion a year. This purely symptom-oriented approach, however, does not eliminate the cause of the illness and, in many cases, sets the stage for even more serious conditions.

This book provides a thorough understanding of what causes gallstones in both the liver and gallbladder and explains why these stones can be held responsible for the most common diseases so prevalent in the world today. It provides the reader with the knowledge needed to recognize the stones and gives the necessary, do-it-yourself instructions to remove them painlessly in the comfort of one's own home. The book also shares practical guidelines on how to prevent new gallstones from forming. The widespread success of *The Amazing Liver and Gallbladder Flush* stands as a testimony to the strength and effectiveness of the cleanse itself. This powerful yet simple cleanse has led to extraordinary improvements in health and wellness among thousands of people who have already given themselves the precious gift of a strong, clean, revitalized liver.

Lifting the Veil of Duality
Your Guide to Living Without Judgment

"Do you know that there is a place inside you – hidden beneath the appearance of thoughts, feelings, and emotions – that does not know the difference between good and evil, right and wrong, light and dark? From that place you embrace the opposite values of life as One. In this sacred place you are at peace with yourself and at peace with your world." – *Andreas Moritz*

In *Lifting the Veil of Duality*, Andreas Moritz poignantly exposes the illusion of duality. He outlines a simple way to remove every limitation that you have imposed upon yourself during the course of living in the realm of duality. You will be prompted to see yourself and the world through a new lens: the lens of clarity, discernment and non-judgment. You will also discover that mistakes, accidents, coincidences, negativity, deception, injustice, wars, crime and terrorism all have a deeper purpose and meaning in the larger scheme of things. So naturally, much of what you will read may conflict with the beliefs you currently hold. Yet you are not asked to change your beliefs or opinions. Instead, you are asked to have an *open mind*, for only an open mind can enjoy freedom from judgment.

Our personal views and world views are currently challenged by a crisis of identity. Some are being shattered altogether. The collapse of our current world order forces humanity to deal with the most basic issues of existence. You can no longer avoid taking responsibility for the things that happen to you. When you *do* accept responsibility, you also empower and heal yourself.

Lifting the Veil of Duality shows how you create or subdue your ability to fulfill your desires. Furthermore, you will find intriguing explanations about the mystery of time, the truth and illusion of reincarnation, the oftentimes misunderstood value of prayer, what makes relationships work and why so often they don't. Find out why injustice is an illusion that has managed to haunt us throughout the ages. Learn about our original separation from the Source of life and what this means with regard to the current waves of instability and fear that so many of us are experiencing.

Discover how to identify the angels living amongst us and why we all have light-bodies. You will have the opportunity to find the ultimate God within you and discover why a God seen as separate from yourself keeps you from being in your Divine Power and happiness. In addition, you can find out how to heal yourself at a moment's notice. Read all about the *New Medicine* and the destiny of the old medicine, the old economy, the old religion, and the old world.

It's Time to Come Alive
Start Using the Amazing Healing Powers of Your Body, Mind and Spirit Today!

In this book, Andreas Moritz brings to light man's deep inner need for spiritual wisdom in life and helps the reader develop a new sense of reality that is based on love, power, and compassion. He describes our relationship with the natural world in detail and discusses how we can harness its tremendous powers for our personal and humanity's benefit. *It's Time to Come Alive* challenges some of our most commonly held beliefs and offers a way out of the emotional restrictions and physical limitations we have created in our lives.

Topics include: What shapes our destiny, using the power of intention, secrets of defying the aging process, doubting – the cause of failure, opening the heart, material wealth and spiritual wealth, fatigue – the major cause of stress, methods of emotional transformation, techniques of primordial healing, how to increase the health of the five senses, developing spiritual wisdom, the major causes of today's Earth changes, entry into the new world, the 12 gateways to heaven on Earth, and much more.

Simple Steps to Total Health
Andreas Moritz with co-author John Hornecker

By nature, your physical body is designed to be healthy and vital throughout life. Unhealthy eating habits and lifestyle choices, however, lead to numerous health conditions that prevent you from enjoying life to the fullest. In *Simple Steps to Total Health*, the authors bring to light the most common cause of disease, which is the buildup of toxins and residues from improperly digested foods that inhibit various organs and systems from performing their normal functions. This guidebook for total health provides you with simple but highly effective approaches for internal cleansing, hydration, nutrition and living habits.

The book's three parts cover the essentials of total health: Good Internal Hygiene, Healthy Nutrition, and Balanced Lifestyle. Learn about the most common disease-causing foods, dietary habits and influences responsible for the occurrence of chronic illnesses, including those affecting the blood vessels, heart, liver, intestinal organs, lungs, kidneys, joints, bones, nervous system and sense organs.

To be able to live a healthy life, you must align your internal biological rhythms with the larger rhythms of nature. Find out more about this and many other important topics in *Simple Steps to Total Health*. This is a must-have book for anyone who is interested in using a natural, drug-free approach to restore total health.

Heart Disease – No More!
(With excerpts from Timeless Secrets of Health & Rejuvenation)

Less than 100 years ago, heart disease was an extremely rare illness. Today it kills more people in the developed world than all other causes of death combined. Despite the vast financial resources spent on finding a cure for heart disease, the current medical approaches remain mainly symptom-oriented and do not address the underlying causes.

Even worse, overwhelming evidence shows that the treatment of heart disease or its presumed precursors, such as high blood pressure, hardening of the arteries, and high cholesterol, not only prevents a real cure, but also can easily lead to chronic heart failure. The patient's heart may still beat, but not strongly enough for him to feel vital and alive.

Without removing the underlying causes of heart disease and its precursors, the average person has little, if any, protection against it. Heart attacks can strike whether you have undergone a coronary bypass or have had stents placed inside your arteries. According to research, these procedures fail to prevent heart attacks and do nothing to reduce mortality rates.

Heart Disease – No More!, with excerpts from the author's bestselling book, *Timeless Secrets of Health & Rejuvenation*, puts the responsibility for healing where it belongs: on the heart, mind and body of each individual. It provides the reader with practical insights about the development and causes of heart disease. Even better, it explains simple steps you can take to prevent and reverse heart disease for good, regardless of a possible genetic predisposition.

Diabetes – No More!
Discover and Heal Its True Causes
(Excerpted from Timeless Secrets of Health & Rejuvenation)

According to bestselling author Andreas Moritz, diabetes is not a disease; in the vast majority of cases, it is a complex mechanism of protection or survival that the body chooses in order to avoid the possibly fatal consequences of an unhealthy diet and lifestyle.

Despite the body's ceaseless self-preservation efforts (which we call *diseases*), millions of people suffer or die unnecessarily from these consequences. The imbalanced blood sugar level in diabetes is but a symptom of illness, and not the illness itself. By developing diabetes, the body is neither doing something wrong, nor is it trying to commit suicide. The current diabetes epidemic is man-made, or rather, factory-made, and, therefore, can be halted and reversed through simple but effective changes in diet and lifestyle. *Diabetes – No More!* provides you with essential information on the various causes of diabetes and how anyone can avoid them.

To stop the diabetes epidemic, you need to create the right circumstances that allow your body to heal. Just as there is a mechanism to becoming diabetic, there is also a mechanism to reverse it. Find out how!

Ending The AIDS Myth
It's Time To Heal The TRUE Causes!
(Excerpted from Timeless Secrets of Health & Rejuvenation)

Contrary to common belief, no scientific evidence exists to this day to prove that AIDS is a contagious disease. The current AIDS theory falls short in predicting the kind of AIDS disease an infected person may be manifesting, and no accurate system is in place to determine how long it will take for the disease to develop. In addition, the current HIV/AIDS theory contains no reliable information that can help identify those who are at risk for developing AIDS.

On the other hand, published research actually proves that HIV only spreads heterosexually in extremely rare cases and cannot be responsible for an epidemic that involves millions of AIDS victims around the world. Furthermore, it is an established fact that the retrovirus HIV, which is composed of human gene fragments, is incapable of destroying human cells. However, cell destruction is the main characteristic of every AIDS disease.

Even the principal discoverer of HIV, Luc Montagnier, no longer believes that HIV is solely responsible for causing AIDS. In fact, he showed that HIV alone could not cause AIDS. Increasing evidence indicates that AIDS may be a toxicity syndrome or metabolic disorder that is caused by immunity risk factors, including heroin, sex-enhancement drugs, antibiotics, commonly prescribed AIDS drugs, rectal intercourse, starvation, malnutrition, and dehydration.

Dozens of prominent scientists working at the forefront of AIDS research now openly question the virus hypothesis of AIDS. Find out why! *Ending The AIDS Myth* also shows you what really causes the shutdown of the immune system and what you can do to avoid this.

Heal Yourself with Sunlight
Use the Sun's Secret Medicinal Powers to Help Cure Cancer, Heart Disease, Diabetes, Arthritis, Infectious Diseases, and Much More!

This book by Andreas Moritz provides scientific evidence that sunlight is essential for good health, and that a lack of sun exposure can be held responsible for many of today's diseases.

Ironically, most people now believe that the sun is the main culprit for causing skin cancer, certain cataracts leading to blindness, and aging. Only those who take the *risk* of exposing themselves to sunlight find that the sun makes them feel and look better, provided they don't use sunscreens or burn their skin. The UV rays in sunlight actually stimulate the thyroid gland to increase hormone production which, in turn, increases the body's basal metabolic rate. This assists both in weight loss and improved muscle development.

It has been known for several decades that those living mostly in the outdoors, at high altitudes or near the equator, have the lowest incidence of skin cancers. In addition, studies have revealed that exposing patients to controlled amounts of sunlight dramatically lowered elevated blood pressure (up to 40 mm Hg drop), decreased cholesterol in the blood stream, lowered abnormally high blood sugars among diabetics, and increased the number of white blood cells which we need to help resist disease. Patients suffering from gout, rheumatoid arthritis, colitis, arteriosclerosis, anemia, cystitis, eczema, acne, psoriasis, herpes, lupus, sciatica, kidney problems and asthma, as well as burns, have all been shown to receive great benefit from the healing rays of the sun.

There is ample scientific evidence to demonstrate that vitamin D deficiency due to lack of regular sun exposure is responsible for most diseases prevalent in modern societies where most people spend most of their time indoors. In addition, the use of sunscreens often leads to a life-threatening vitamin D deficiency.

This book reveals the true reasons the masses are fed the misinformation that the sun is harmful to our health.

Hear The Whispers, Live Your Dream
A Fanfare of Inspiration

Listening to the whispers of your heart will set you free. The beauty and bliss of your knowingness and love center are what we are here to capture, take in and swim with. You are like a dolphin sailing in a sea of joy. Allow yourself to open to the wondrous fullness of your selfhood, without reservation and without judgment.

Judgment stands in the way, like a boulder trespassing on your journey to the higher reaches of your destiny. Push these boulders aside and feel the joy of your inner truth sprout forth. Do not allow another's thoughts or directions for you to supersede your inner knowingness, for you relinquish being the full, radiant star that you are.

It is with an open heart, a receptive mind, and a reaching for the stars of wisdom that lie within you, that you reap the bountiful goodness of Mother Earth and the universal I AM. For you are a benevolent being of light and there is no course that can truly stop you, except your own thoughts, or allowing another's beliefs to override your own.

May these expressions of love, joy and wisdom inspire you to be the wondrous being that you were born to be!

Feel Great, Lose Weight
Stop Dieting and Start Living

No rigorous workouts. No surgery. In this book, celebrated author Andreas Moritz suggests a gentle – and permanent – route to losing weight. In this groundbreaking book, he says that once we stop blaming our genes and take control of our own life, weight loss is a natural consequence.

"You need to make that critical mental shift. You need to experience the willingness to shed your physical and emotional baggage, not by counting calories but by embracing your mind, body and spirit. Once you start looking at yourself differently, 80 percent of the work is done."

In *Feel Great, Lose Weight*, Andreas Moritz tells us why conventional weight loss programs don't work and how weight loss experts make sure we keep going back. He also tells us why food manufacturers, pharmaceutical companies and health regulators conspire to keep America toxically overweight.

But we can refuse to buy into the Big Fat Lie. Choosing the mind/body approach triggers powerful biochemical changes that set us on a safe and irreversible path to losing weight, without resorting to crash diets, heavy workouts or dangerous surgical procedures.

Vaccine-nation
Poisoning the Population, One Shot at a Time

Andreas Moritz takes on yet another controversial subject, this time to expose the Vaccine Myth. In *Vaccine-nation*, Moritz unravels the mother of all vaccine lies – that vaccines are safe and they prevent disease. Furthermore, he reveals undeniable scientific proof that vaccines are actually implicated in most diseases today.

This book reveals:

- Statistical evidence that vaccines never actually eradicated infectious diseases, including polio
- How childhood vaccines, flu shots and other kinds of inoculations systemically destroy the body's immune system
- The massive increase of allergies, eczema, arthritis, asthma, autism, acid reflux, cancer, diabetes (infant and childhood), kidney disease, miscarriages, many neurological and autoimmune diseases, and Sudden Infant Death Syndrome (SIDS) is largely due to vaccines
- Why vaccinated children have 120 percent more asthma, 317 percent more ADHD, 185 percent more neurologic disorders and 146 percent more autism than those not vaccinated
- The shocking fact that most outbreaks of infectious diseases occur largely among those who are fully vaccinated
- Vaccines lack long-term safety testing and most vaccine side effects are never reported in order to protect vaccine makers from liability suits

National health agencies still refuse to conduct long-term double-blind control studies to prove vaccines are both safe and work better than the placebo effect. The Centers for Disease Control and Prevention (CDCP) say that we shouldn't test such drugs (vaccines) on human beings because that would be *"unethical"*. However, pumping little children with 35 vaccine shots that are loaded with dangerous toxins and proclaiming that this would cause *no* harm can hardly be considered safe and ethical. We are asked to just trust them on this, in the complete absence of proof that vaccines are safe and effective to prevent disease. Avoiding comparison studies is not really a reasonable excuse today, as many parents *have already* opted out of at least some, if not all, vaccines for their children anyway. So there are many children available for such kind of research.

In *Vaccine-nation*, Moritz minces no words while unraveling these and other skeletons in Big Pharma's closet and cautions you not to buy into the hollow claims of vaccine makers. In his characteristic style, Moritz offers a gentle and practical approach to a disease-free life, which rests on the fulcrum of the mind/body connection, cleansing of the body, and naturally healthy living.

Art of Self-Healing
(Special edition, healing modality book containing all Ener-Chi Art pictures)

Andreas Moritz developed a new system of healing and rejuvenation designed to restore the basic life energy (Chi) of an organ or a system in the body within a matter of seconds. Simultaneously, it also helps balance the emotional causes of illness.

Eastern approaches to healing, such as acupuncture and shiatsu, are intended to enhance well-being by stimulating and balancing the flow of Chi to the various organs and systems of the body. In a similar manner, the energetics of Ener-Chi Art are designed to restore a balanced flow of Chi throughout the body.

According to most ancient systems of health and healing, the balanced flow of Chi is the key determinant for a healthy body and mind. When Chi flows through the body unhindered, health and vitality are maintained. By contrast, if the flow of Chi is disrupted or reduced, health and vitality tend to decline.

A person can determine the degree to which the flow of Chi is balanced in the body's organs and systems by using a simple muscle testing procedure. To reveal the effectiveness of Ener-Chi Art, it is important to apply this kinesiology test both before and after viewing each Ener-Chi Art picture.

To allow for easy application of this system, Andreas created a number of healing paintings that have been *activated* through a unique procedure that imbues each work of art with specific color rays (derived from the higher dimensions). To receive the full benefit of an Ener-Chi Art picture, all it requires is to look at it for less than a minute. During this time, the flow of Chi within the organ or system becomes fully restored. When applied to all the organs and systems of the body, Ener-Chi Art sets the precondition for the whole body to heal and rejuvenate itself.

Alzheimer's – No More!
Discover the True Causes and Empowering Steps You Can Take <u>Now</u>

It is not often that we come across bold statements about serious, even terminal diseases – such as the fact that they can be cured and even reversed. But no one speaks with more authority on the power of self-healing than Andreas Moritz.

In this book, Moritz – author of several books on the power of self-healing and supportive natural remedies, and an internationally acclaimed practitioner of Ayurveda and natural medicine – offers hope to patients of Alzheimer's disease and their families, and provides a roadmap for recovery.

In his typically cogent style, Moritz convincingly exposes the lies of Big Pharma and their vested interest in keeping Alzheimer's patients trapped in their terrifying predicament. He argues against medical doctors whose questionable ethics and diagnoses put the 'death fright' into their patients, virtually coaxing them towards an untimely death. Most importantly, he backs up his statements with empirical research.

Moritz goes on to deconstruct Alzheimer's and demonstrate how the disease is nothing but the body's cry for help. He explains how the condition is a result of sustained toxic overload that suffocates and inflames the brain. Considering modern lifestyles and the careless disregard for health that comes as baggage, this book is more relevant than ever today.

After tracing the genesis of the disease, Andreas Moritz goes on to discuss its prevention and the healing that can be achieved even after its onset. He lists potent remedies that can detoxify a 'dying brain' and provides numerous supporting therapeutic measures that can restore a toxic brain to optimal health. Often, the results can be remarkable!

In this book, Moritz also describes the subtle but powerful role of the mind in Alzheimer's and explores a spiritual connection with the disease. At the heart of his message is the basic truth – the first step to getting back on the road to recovery is to believe in the body's innate ability to heal itself.

Timeless Wisdom from Andreas Moritz
Sage Guidance and Wisdom – Lovingly Shared

A respectful, heartfelt compilation of quotes, carefully selected from Andreas' comments and responses to questions posed on his forums or addressed to him one-on-one. His deep spiritual awareness and compassionate spirit, combined with a thorough understanding of the human body, have inspired thousands of people to lead more vital, uplifting and balanced lives.

"Open up your heart like a flower in the sun;
ask a question in your mind; open this book to any page, and
receive your answer with gratitude."

———

All books are available in paperback format
(except *Alzheimer's – No More!* and *Cancer Is Not a Disease – It's a Healing Mechanism*)
and electronic books/eBooks (except *Art of Self-Healing*)
through the Ener-Chi Wellness Center.

Ener-Chi Ionized Stones

Ener-Chi Ionized Stones are stones and crystals that have been energized, activated and imbued with life force through a special process introduced by Andreas Moritz, the creator of Ener-Chi Art.

Stone ionization has not been attempted before because stones and rocks have rarely been considered useful in the field of healing. Yet, stones have the inherent power to hold and release vast amounts of information and energy. Once ionized, they exert a balancing influence on everything with which they come into contact. The ionization of stones may be one of our keys to survival in a world that is experiencing high-level pollution and destruction of its eco-balancing systems.

In the early evolutionary stages of Earth, every particle of matter on the planet contained within it the blueprint of the entire planet, just as every cell of our body contains within its DNA structure the blueprint of our entire body. The blueprint information within every particle of matter is still there – it has simply fallen into a dormant state. The ionization process *reawakens* this original blueprint information and enables the associated energies to be released. In this sense, Ener-Chi Ionized Stones are alive and conscious, and are able to energize, purify and balance any natural substance with which they come into contact.

**To order Books, Ener-Chi Art and Ener-Chi Ionized Stones,
please visit the Ener-Chi website or contact:**

Ener-Chi Wellness Center, LLC
Website: http://www.ener-chi.com
Toll-free: +1 (866) 258-4006 (USA & Canada)
+1 (709) 570-7401 (worldwide)

To view or order wellness products recommended by Andreas, click:
http://www.ener-chi.com/wellness-products/

About Andreas Moritz

Andreas Moritz was a medical intuitive; a practitioner of Ayurveda, iridology, shiatsu, and vibrational medicine; a writer; and an artist. Born in southwest Germany in 1954, Moritz dealt with several severe illnesses from an early age, which compelled him to study diet, nutrition, and various methods of natural healing while still a child.

By age 20, he had completed his training in both iridology (the diagnostic science of eye interpretation) and dietetics. In 1981, he began studying Ayurvedic medicine in India and finished his training as a qualified practitioner of Ayurveda in New Zealand in 1991. Not satisfied with merely treating the symptoms of illness, Moritz dedicated his life's work to understanding and treating the root causes of illness. Because of this holistic approach, he had great success with cases of terminal disease where conventional methods of healing proved futile.

Since 1988, he began practicing the Japanese healing art of shiatsu, which gave him insights into the energy system of the body. In addition, he devoted eight years to researching consciousness and its important role in the field of mind/body medicine.

Andreas Moritz is the author of the following books on health and spirituality:

- *The Amazing Liver and Gallbladder Flush*
- *Timeless Secrets of Health & Rejuvenation*
- *Cancer Is Not a Disease*
- *Lifting the Veil of Duality*
- *It's Time to Come Alive*
- *Heart Disease – No More!*
- *Diabetes – No More!*
- *Simple Steps to Total Health*
- *Ending The AIDS Myth*
- *Heal Yourself with Sunlight*
- *Feel Great, Lose Weight*
- *Vaccine-nation*
- *Hear the Whispers, Live Your Dream*
- *Art of Self-Healing*

- *Timeless Wisdom from Andreas Moritz*
- *Alzheimer's – No More!*

During his extensive travels throughout the world, Andreas consulted with heads of state and members of government in Europe, Asia, and Africa, and lectured widely on the subjects of health, mind/body medicine and spirituality. Moritz had a free forum, 'Ask Andreas Moritz', on the large health website CureZone.com. Although he stopped writing for the forum around 2006, it contains an extensive archive of his answers to thousands of questions on a variety of health topics.

After moving to the United States in 1998, Moritz began developing his new and innovative system of healing called *Ener-Chi Art* that targets the root causes of many chronic illnesses. Ener-Chi Art consists of a series of light ray-encoded oil paintings that can instantly restore vital energy flow (Chi) in the organs and systems of the body. Moritz is also the creator of *Sacred Santémony – Divine Chanting for Every Occasion,* a powerful system of specially generated frequencies of sound that can transform deep-seated fears, allergies, traumas and mental or emotional blocks into useful opportunities for growth and inspiration within a matter of moments.

In October 2012, Andreas transitioned to the Higher Realms. He released the updated and expanded edition of *The Amazing Liver and Gallbladder Flush* just before his passing, and had completed the manuscripts for *Alzheimer's – No More!* as well as the updated edition of this book, *Cancer Is Not a Disease* which, along with *Timeless Secrets of Health & Rejuvenation* and *The Liver and Gallbladder Flush,* remains the groundbreaking nucleus of his work.

Andreas' legacy comprises a tremendous body of work, which he always generously shared with his readers, colleagues and fans. His YouTube videos, free health information and words of wisdom are available at: www.ener-chi.com, www.youtube.com/user/enerchiTV and www.facebook.com/enerchi.wellness.

The Andreas Moritz Light Trust is a non-profit 501(c)(3) foundation created in 2013 in honor of Andreas and his time-honored kindness, generosity of spirit, profound wisdom, far-reaching teachings and life-transforming insights that have helped countless people around the world.

The goal of the Andreas Moritz Light Trust is to provide meaningful, much-needed assistance to children around the world who have no parents – including nutritious food, healthy and safe living conditions, holistic education, compassionate care and enriching spiritual opportunities.

For more information, please visit www.andreasmoritzlighttrust.org.

Index

Lightning Source UK Ltd.
Milton Keynes UK
UKHW021701191219
355683UK00007B/1339/P